Making Sense of Data

MAKING SENSE OF DATA

*A Self-Instruction Manual
on the Interpretation
of Epidemiological Data*

SECOND EDITION

J. H. ABRAMSON
Professor of Social Medicine
The Hebrew University-Hadassah School
of Public Health and Community Medicine
Jerusalem

New York   Oxford
OXFORD UNIVERSITY PRESS
1994

Oxford University Press

Oxford   New York   Toronto
Delhi   Bombay   Calcutta   Madras   Karachi
Kuala Lumpur   Singapore   Hong Kong   Tokyo
Nairobi   Dar es Salaam   Cape Town
Melbourne   Auckland   Madrid

and associated companies in
Berlin   Ibadan

Copyright © 1988, 1994 by Oxford University Press, Inc.

Published by Oxford University Press, Inc.,
200 Madison Avenue, New York, New York 10016

Oxford is a registered trademark of Oxford University Press

Library of Congress Cataloging-in-Publication Data
Abramson, J. H. (Joseph Herbert), 1924–
Making sense of data : a self-instruction manual on
the interpretation of epidemiological data /
J.H. Abramson. —2nd ed.
p.   cm.
Companion v. to: Survey methods in community medicine/
J. H. Abramson. 4th ed. 1990
Includes bibliographical references and index.
ISBN 0-19-508968-5 (cloth). ISBN 0-19-508969-3 (pbk.)
1. Epidemiology—Statistical methods.
2. Epidemiology–Statistical methods—Problems, exercises, etc.
I. Abramson, J. H. (Joseph Herbert), 1924–
Survey methods in community medicine.
II. Title.
[DNLM: 1. Epidemiologic Methods—programmed instruction.
WA 18   A161m 1994]
RA652.4.A27 1994
614.4'072—dc20   DNLM/DCL   for Library of Congress   93-36497

2 4 6 8 9 7 5 3 1
Printed in the United States of America
on acid-free paper

For Jonathan, Dafna,
Roni, Efrat
Boaz, Tamar,
and Dan

Preface

The purpose of this manual is to provide readers with basic epidemiological concepts and skills that will help them to appraise published reports as well as their own findings. Consideration is given to applications in clinical medicine, public health and community medicine, and research. The book should thus be useful to a wide range of students and other readers.

The aim is to produce competence in the ABCs of data interpretation. The manual is not a textbook of statistics, nor does it cover data-processing techniques or advanced epidemiological methods. It is, in a sense, a companion volume to my book *Survey Methods in Community Medicine*, which deals with the planning of studies and the gathering of data.

This edition includes a new section on meta-analysis (the critical review and integration of the findings of separate studies). Its aim is to provide readers with the basic skills required for making sense of the results of a set of studies and for appraising published reports of meta-analyses and deciding whether to use their results. Minor changes have been made in other sections of the book. Errors have been corrected, elucidative comments added, and references updated.

The book can be used for independent study. In the framework of organized courses, experience indicates that many students prefer to work on the exercises together, in small groups; formal or informal discussions with instructors are helpful.

I am grateful to the many students who participated as involuntary guinea pigs in the testing of the exercises, and to a number of colleagues for their criticism. I am especially indebted to Eric Peritz (despite his insistence that my treatment of statistical matters is too simplistic) and to Anneke Ifrah, Yehuda Neumark, Bella Adler, and Jeremy Kark.

J. H. A.

Jerusalem
October 1993

Contents

Making Sense of Data

Introduction

"Why," said the Dodo, "the best way to explain it is to do it."

(*Carroll, 1865*)

THE AIM OF THIS BOOK

The purpose of this book is to help you to interpret and use data concerning health and disease, health care, and their determinants in populations, population groups, or groups of patients. The book aims to equip you with basic concepts and skills that will enable you to appraise your own data or data collected or published by others, and apply the findings in clinical practice, community medicine and public health, or research.

The book has six sections. Section A, which deals with basic concepts and procedures, presents a basic step-by-step procedure for the appraisal of data, starting with the assessment of single tables and diagrams. It introduces fundamental terms and directs attention to the variety of uses to which epidemiological data may be put. Section B deals with rates and other simple measures used in epidemiology; and Section C, with their accuracy, the appraisal of accuracy, and the ways in which inaccurate measures can bias results. The appraisal of associations between variables is given detailed consideration in Section D, and Section E deals with the appraisal of cause–effect relationships and ways of measuring the impact of causal factors. Section F deals with meta-analysis, or the critical review and integration of the findings of separate studies of the same topic.

By the time you reach the end, you should be competent in the use of basic epidemiological tools and capable of exercising critical judgment when assessing results reported by others. When you read a paper, you should be able to identify shortcomings in the study methods or inferences, and make due allowance for them when drawing your conclusions, but without succumbing, it is to be hoped, to the "I am an epi-

4

demiologist" bias (Owen, 1982) that leads to the complete repudiation of any study with a flaw.

This book does *not* aim to make you an epidemiological expert; it is an introductory manual that tries to deal in a simple way with fundamental epidemiological approaches and procedures for use in data interpretation. It does not pretend to be a comprehensive textbook of epidemiology. It does *not* deal with techniques of data processing. And, it is *not* a textbook of survey methods or statistics.

HOW TO USE THIS BOOK

This is a workbook. There is no point in just sitting down and reading it, skipping the exercises. You will reap little benefit unless you systematically do the exercises.

Each of the book's six sections is made up of numbered units. These contain short exercises, comments on the exercises in the previous unit, and other explanatory text. Preferably, work on the sections in sequence (but this is not essential). Within each section, go through the units in order; each exercise leads to the next one. Most of the exercises are easy; few require much calculation (but have a pocket calculator handy). To derive the most benefit from the exercises, *write down* your answer to each one. And don't peek! Only when you have written down your answer should you read the detailed comments in the next unit. When you are sure that you have learned all there is to learn from one unit, go on to the next.

At the end of each section there is a self-test. This is a checklist of "what you should now be able to do." Test yourself on each item; if you have any doubts, refer back to the respective unit before proceeding to the next section.

The book is intended to be reasonably self-contained, and sufficient explanations, notes, and definitions are included to minimize the need to refer to other books. You are encouraged, however, to consult textbooks and other sources for in-depth explanations.

The book may be used for independent study, but if there is an opportunity to work on the exercises in collaboration with others, you may find this an advantage.

SECTION
A

Basic Concepts and Procedures

The White Rabbit put on his spectacles. "Where shall I begin, please your majesty?" he asked.

"Begin at the beginning," the King said gravely, "and go on till you come to the end; then stop."

(Carroll, 1865)

Unit
A1

INTRODUCTION

This initial series of exercises has three main purposes. First, it introduces a basic approach to the appraisal of data. Step by step, what is the procedure we should use when we look at a table or graph? What are the basic questions to be asked, and in what order? What kinds of explanation should be considered, and how should they be tested?

Second, a number of fundamental terms and concepts that are relevant to the interpretation of epidemiological data are introduced. These include incidence rates, associations, confounding, effect modification, absolute and relative differences, epidemiological models, and many others.

Third, attention is directed to the variety of uses that may be made of epidemiological data. Clinicians, practitioners of public health and community medicine, researchers, and others have different interests, so that though their basic approach to data is the same, they may be interested in asking different questions and reaching conclusions of different kinds.

EXERCISE A1

Table A1 provides information on the occurrence of cases of acute gastroenteritis (diarrhea and vomiting) in Epiville, an imaginary town in a developing region.

When a table or graph is examined, the first steps are to determine what facts are shown, and then to summarize the facts (unless, of course, they are so simple they do not need to be summarized).

Question A1–1

State the facts shown in Table A1.

7

Table A1. Number of Cases of Acute
Gastroenteritis Occurring in Epiville
in Selected Years, 1955–1985

Year	No. of Cases
1955	400
1960	600
1965	800
1970	900
1975	1,000
1980	1,100
1985	1,200

Question A1–2

Summarize these facts.

Unit
A2

DETERMINING WHAT THE FACTS ARE

To be sure of what facts are shown by a table, always read the words as well as the figures. If you read the title of the table, the column and row captions, the footnotes (if there are any), and any explanatory material in the accompanying text, this should enable you to understand *what the numbers represent* and *how they were obtained or calculated.*

The detailed facts shown in Table A1 are easily stated: In 1955, there were 400 cases of acute gastroenteritis in Epiville; in 1960, there were 600; in 1965, 800; in 1970, 900; in 1975, 1,000; in 1980, 1,100; and in 1985, 1,200.

Stating the facts in such detail is, of course, seldom necessary. But what is important is that one should always be sufficiently certain of what the numbers represent to be *able* to spell out the facts in detail. This may not be easy if the table is complicated, badly constructed, or poorly labeled, or if the requisite information is not available.

Unfortunately, Table A1 gives no information on the manner in which the data were obtained. The data are admittedly imaginary, but we are not told from what imaginary source (interviews, a survey of medical records, a case notification system, etc.) they are derived. This uncertainty will have to be taken into account when we later go on to consider possible explanations for the findings. In extreme instances, such serious doubts about the accuracy of the data may arise at this point that further consideration of the findings may be deemed superfluous.

Also, we are unfortunately not told whether the "cases" in Table A1 are *individuals* who had gastroenteritis, or are *episodes* (spells) of illness. If the same child had the disease twice in one year, did he or she count as one case or as two? (In answer to an SOS, the honorary official epidemiologist in Epiville tells us that the table actually refers to spells of illness.)

SUMMARIZING THE FACTS

Obviously, there was a rise in the number of cases per year between 1955 and 1985. A full summary of the facts in Table A1 would mention at least three features of this increase:

1. The continuing, or "monotonic" (see Note A2–1), nature of the increase—that is, the occurrence of a rise between each observation and the next.
2. The overall extent of the increase. This may be expressed in absolute or relative terms. The absolute difference is 800 cases per year (1,200 minus 400). The relative difference can be expressed as a simple ratio: 1,200/400 (i.e., 1,200 divided by 400)—a threefold increase. Alternatively, it can be stated as a percentage change: $[(1,200 - 400)/400] \times 100$—a rise of 200%.
3. The variation in the rate of change. The trend is not uniform: the increase is steeper in earlier than in later periods. This variation is apparent whether we look at the absolute or relative changes in the numbers of cases. The absolute differences between successive observations are 200 for each of the first two intervals, and only 100 for each of the subsequent intervals. If you have not already done so, examine the relative changes as well, by calculating the ratio of each observation to the preceding one, and/or the percentage change between each pair of successive observations. (For answers, see Note A2–2.)

When you listed or summarized the facts, you may have included such items as "sanitary conditions got worse," "the population grew in size," or "the number of deaths from gastroenteritis increased." These are *not* empirically observed facts; they are *inferences*. They may or may not be true, and should not be regarded or reported as facts. It is usually important to consider possible explanations for the observations, but only *after* the facts themselves have been determined. (Sometimes, of course, there is no need to go beyond determining the facts. These may be all we want, and there may be no interest in drawing inferences or finding explanations.)

EXERCISE A2

In Table A1, we saw that initially there was a steep increase in the annual number of cases of gastroenteritis in Epiville, and later the rise became less steep. This change in trend was obvious whether we looked at the absolute changes or the relative ones. Sometimes, however, abso-

Table A2–1. Number of Cases
of Gastroenteritis

	Wuntown	*Nuthertown*
1985	500	5,000
1987	25	4,000

lute and relative differences may give us conflicting messages, and we may have to decide which mean more to us.

Question A2–1

Table A2–1 shows the numbers of cases of gastroenteritis in two imaginary towns in 1985 and 1987. Health programs for preventing gastroenteritis were introduced in both towns in 1986. Calculate the absolute and relative changes in each town. In which town is there stronger evidence that the program was effective in reducing the occurrence of gastroenteritis?

Question A2–2

You are a health administrator concerned with the provision of facilities for health care. Table A2–2 shows the numbers of new patients with end-stage renal disease who required renal dialysis (a life-saving but elaborate and expensive form of treatment) in two regions in 1985 and 1987. Calculate the absolute and relative changes. Looking forward to 1988, in which region would you be more concerned about the increase?

Question A2–3

Table A2–3 shows the numbers of infant deaths in the same two regions in 1985 and 1987; the numbers of births did not change. Programs aimed at reducing infant mortality were started in both regions in 1986.

1. In which region is there more convincing evidence that the reduction in mortality was caused by the program?

Table A2–2. Number of Patients
Requiring Dialysis

	Pepi	*Quepi*
1985	30	2,000
1987	90	3,000

Table A2–3. Number of Infant Deaths

	Pepi	Quepi
1985	300	5,000
1987	60	4,000

2. If the program can be continued in only one region, which would you choose? (Assume that the reductions are caused by the programs.)

Question A2–4

Can you suggest a rule of thumb for deciding when to use the relative difference and when to use the absolute difference?

NOTES

A2–1. *Monotonic sequence.* A sequence is monotonically increasing if each value is more than or equal to the previous one, and monotonically decreasing if each value is less than or equal to the previous one. If each value is more than the preceding one, or if each value is less than the preceding one, the sequence is strictly monotonic (increasing or decreasing).

A2–2. The successive ratios were 1.50, 1.33, 1.12, 1.11, 1.10, and 1.09. The percentage changes were 50%, 33%, 12.5%, 11%, 10%, and 9%.

ABSOLUTE AND RELATIVE DIFFERENCES

In some circumstances we may be more interested in absolute differences; and in others, in relative differences.

In answer to *Question A2–1*, Table A2–1 shows a larger relative decrease in gastroenteritis in Wuntown (95%) than in Nuthertown (20%), and a larger absolute decrease in Nuthertown (1,000) than in Wuntown (475). The evidence that the program was effective is stronger in Wuntown, where most of the disease was apparently prevented. In this context, the relative difference is more meaningful.

In answer to *Question A2–2*, Table A2–2 shows a larger absolute increase in patients needing renal dialysis in Quepi (1,000) than in Pepi (60), and a larger relative increase in Pepi (200%) than in Quepi (50%). The administrator would probably be more concerned with the change in Quepi, where the personnel, equipment and other facilities needed to treat a very large additional number of patients must be found. In this context, the absolute difference is more meaningful.

In answer to *Question A2–3*, the evidence that the program was effective is more convincing in Pepi, where the number of infant deaths decreased by 80%, than in Quepi, where the relative decrease was only 20%. But the program apparently prevented 1,000 deaths in Quepi in 1986, and only 240 in Pepi. If we had to choose, we would probably decide to continue the program in Quepi, where more lives are saved.

In answer to *Question A2–4*, a general rule of thumb is that when we are concerned with the magnitude of a public health problem—how many lives, how many facilities, how much cost—it may be appropriate to give emphasis to absolute rather than relative differences. Relative differences, on the other hand, are of more interest when we wish to study processes of causation—for example, to examine the effect of health care or of a supposed risk factor or protective factor, on the occurrence of diseases or deaths. It is not always easy to choose between the use of relative and absolute differences, and sometimes both are important.

EXERCISE A3

Diagrams are often used to summarize and clarify findings. They provide a useful way of showing trends and differences at a glance.

In this exercise you are asked to draw and interpret diagrams.

Question A3–1

Draw a graph showing the data of Table A1. Put the scale for numbers of cases (i.e., the dependent variable—see Note A3–1) along the *Y* (vertical) axis, and put the scale for time (the independent variable) along the *X* (horizontal) axis. It is customary to use the *Y* axis for dependent variables and the *X* axis for independent variables. Use ordinary (arithmetic) scales along both axes.

Question A3–2

Draw another graph showing the data of Table A1. Again use an ordinary scale for time, but this time use a logarithmic scale for numbers of cases. This is easy if you have semilogarithmic graph paper (see Note A3–2). If you have only ordinary graph paper, plot the logarithms of the numbers of cases instead of the actual numbers (see Note A3–3). If you have forgotten what logarithms are, see Note A3–4.

Question A3–3

Which scale—ordinary or logarithmic—is more appropriate for showing absolute differences, and which one gives a better representation of relative differences? If the answer is not obvious to you, examine the absolute and relative changes displayed by the following two sequences, and then plot them against both kinds of scale. In each instance, use 1, 2, 3, 4, 5, 6, and 7 on the horizontal axis.

Sequence A: 1, 3, 5, 7, 9, 11, 13.

Sequence B: 1, 2, 4, 8, 16, 32, 64.

Question A3–4

Draw a diagram to summarize the data provided in Table A3 on the distribution of gastroenteritis during the year.

Question A3–5

The three graphs in Fig. A3–1 show the changes in the annual number of cases of diseases A, B, and C between 1980 and 1985. Which disease showed the biggest change, and which the smallest?

Table A3. Occurrence of Cases
of Acute Gastroenteritis in Epiville
in 1975

Period	No. of Cases
January–March	60
April–June	150
July	280
August–September	300
October–December	210
Total	1,000

Question A3–6

Figure A3–2 shows the change in mortality from ischemic heart disease of males and females in the Philippines between 1964 and 1976. (At last! Real data!) In which sex was there more change? The actual figures (rates per 100,000) were: males, 33.3 (1964), 40.3 (1968), 55.8 (1972), and 78.0 (1976); females: 15.4, 18.4, 25.2, and 34.5, respectively (Note A3–5).

Figure A3–1. Cases of diseases A, B, and C, 1980–1985.

Figure A3–2. Mortality from ischemic heart disease, Philippines, 1964–1976. M = Males; F = females. (Data from Tuomilehto et al., 1984.)

NOTES

A3–1. A *dependent variable* is "a variable the value of which is dependent on the effect of other [independent] variable(s) in the relationship under study. A manifestation or outcome whose variation we seek to explain or account for by the influence of independent variables"—*A Dictionary of Epidemiology* (Last, 1983).

A3–2. Semilogarithmic paper has a logarithmic scale along the Y (vertical) axis, and an ordinary (arithmetic) scale along the other. You need not look up logs; just plot the numbers against the scale. The paper probably has figures from 1 to 10 printed along the Y axis (starting at the bottom), and then another set of figures from 2 to 10; take the second set to represent 20, 30, 40, and so on—up to 100; if there is a third set, it will represent 200, 300, and so on—up to 1,000. If you had smaller values to plot, you could designate the first set of figures as (say) 0.1 to 1 and the second as 2 to 10. A logarithmic scale has no zero.

A3–3. If you have ordinary graph paper, use a table of logs or a pocket calculator to obtain the logarithms of the numbers of cases, and then plot these logs on an ordinary (arithmetic) scale. Instead of 400, plot its log, which is 2.60; instead of 600, plot 2.78, and so on.

A3–4. To refresh your memory about logarithms, *common logs* use 10 as their base, and the log of 100 to this base is 2, because $100 = 10^2$; 100 is the antilog of 2. Similarly, the log of 1,000 is 3, because $1,000 = 10^3$. Logs and antilogs can be got from tables, calculators, or computers; every number above 0 has a log. Adding two logs is equivalent to multiplying the numbers they represent: if the logs are 2 and 3 (representing 100 and 1,000), their sum is 5, and 10^5 is 100,000, and so is $100 \times 1,000$. If the absolute difference between two logs is x, this means that one of the numbers they represent is antilog (x) times as large as the other; the difference between the logs of 100,000 and 100 is 3, and the ratio of 100,000 to 100 is 1,000, which is the antilog of 3. Hence if a series of logs is equally spaced—that is, if x is constant—this means that each of the numbers they represent has the same ratio to the preceding number in the series; that is, the relative differences between the numbers are the same. Use is often made of *natural logs*, which have a mysterious number called e, the value of which is about 2.718281828, as their base; their antilogs may be called *exponentials*.

A3–5. Data from Tuomilehto et al. (1984). The rates are age-standardized rates for the 35–64 age group.

Unit
A4

DIAGRAMS

The graphs requested in *Questions A3–1* and *A3–2* should have a general resemblance to those shown in Fig. A4–1. In graphs (line diagrams) like these, the slope represents the rate of change: the steeper the slope, the more the change. Rates of change can be compared by comparing different segments of a line, or by comparing different graphs (*but only if they are plotted against the same scales*).

In answer to *Question A3–3*, the slope of a graph plotted against an ordinary (arithmetic) scale represents the rate of absolute change, whereas the slope of a graph plotted against a logarithmic scale represents the rate of relative change. Sequence A (1, 3, 5, 7, etc.) displays a constant rate of absolute change (an increase of 2 between each pair of numbers) and a decreasing rate of relative change (the percentage increase between successive numbers decreases from 200% to 18%). When an arithmetic scale is used, the graph is a straight line, showing that the rate of absolute change is constant; but a logarithmic scale provides a curve that rises steeply at first, and then progressively rises less steeply (Fig. A4–2). Sequence B (1, 2, 4, 8, etc.), on the other hand, displays a constant rate of relative change (each number is double the previous one), and a logarithmic scale therefore provides a straight-line graph.

There is an increasing rate of absolute change (the successive changes increase from 1 to 32), and an arithmetic scale shows a progressively steeper rise.

Both of the graphs based on Table A1 (Fig. A4–1) show a slowing in the tempo of change, providing a pictorial summary of our previous observation that the increase in cases of gastroenteritis was steeper in earlier than in later years, whether we looked at absolute or relative changes.

Various kinds of diagram are shown in Fig. A4–3. You may have used one of these in answering *Question A3–4*. The difficulty, however, is that

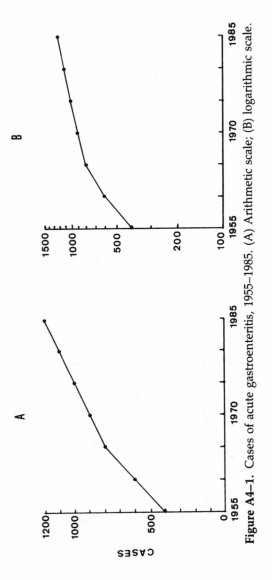

Figure A4–1. Cases of acute gastroenteritis, 1955–1985. (A) Arithmetic scale; (B) logarithmic scale.

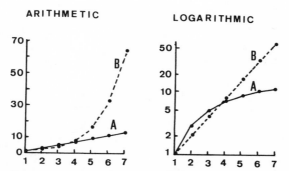

Figure A4–2. Comparison of arithmetic and logarithmic scales. Sequence A: 1, 3, 5, 7, 9, 11, 13. Sequence B: 1, 2, 4, 8, 16, 32, 64.

Table A3 provides data for periods of different lengths. In this instance, therefore, the diagrams in the top row of the figure may be misleading. These are a *bar diagram*, in which the height of the bar portrays the number of cases in each period; a *line graph* (or *curve*), in which each period is represented by a single point; and a *pie chart*, showing the proportion of cases in each period. (To draw a pie chart, calculate the degrees for each segment by multiplying the percentage in the segment by 360/100, i.e., 3.6.) Better solutions are shown in the bottom row of the figure. The best is probably a *histogram*, which comprises adjacent blocks whose widths are proportional to the class interval (the number of months), and whose *areas* are proportional to the number of cases. (This is achieved by plotting, not the number of cases, but the number of cases divided by the class interval—e.g., 20 instead of 60 for the three-month period from January to March.) Note how the bar diagram and histogram give quite different impressions. Use may also be made of a *frequency polygon*, which is a line diagram constructed from a histogram; it is the dotted line in the figure.

Question A3–5 shows how easily graphs can mislead. The three graphs in Fig. A3–1 present identical data—a steady rise from 200 in 1980 to 400 in 1985. The first graph looks flat because the vertical scale is compressed, whereas the third one looks steep because the vertical scale is spread out and because it does not begin at zero. (This is the easiest way to give a deceptive impression of the facts.)

In answer to *Question A3–6*, Fig. A3–2 clearly shows a steeper increase in mortality from ischemic heart disease among men. However, an arithmetic scale was used, and it is only the *absolute* change that is greater. If we plot the same data against a logarithmic curve (Fig. A4–4), we see that the *relative* change—which may be of more interest to us—is about the same in the two sexes.

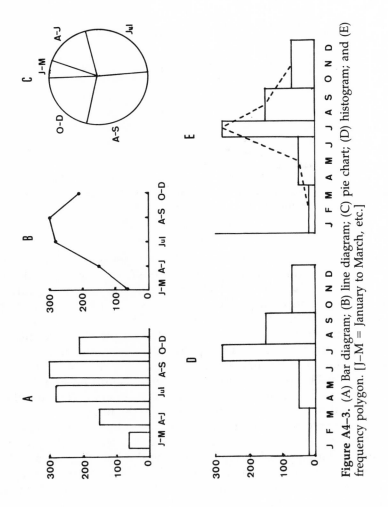

Figure A4–3. (A) Bar diagram; (B) line diagram; (C) pie chart; (D) histogram; and (E) frequency polygon. [J–M = January to March, etc.]

Figure A4–4. Mortality from ischemic heart disease, Philippines, 1964–1976. Logarithmic scale.

EXERCISE A4

Question A4–1

Let us come back to Epiville. Both in words and in pictures, we have summarized the facts about the rise in cases of gastroenteritis between 1955 and 1985 (Table A1). Now let us consider possible explanations. What explanations can you suggest?

Question A4–2

There is an important principle of economy in scientific thinking, often called *Occam's razor*. William of Occam (c.1285–c.1349) was an English philosopher who formulated the maxim, *Entia non sunt multiplicanda praeter necessitatem*—that is, "assumptions to explain a phenomenon must not be multiplied beyond necessity." In 1853, Sir William Hamilton termed this the "law of parsimony" and expressed it as follows: "Neither more, nor more onerous, causes are to be assumed, than are necessary to account for the phenomena." Karl Pearson (1892), in *The Grammar of Science*, calls this canon of economy "the most important in the whole field of logical thought."

Which of the explanations you listed in your answer to Question A4–1 would you test first? What additional information do you need in order to test it? If you can, formulate a specific hypothesis for testing.

Unit
A5

SEEKING EXPLANATIONS FOR THE FACTS

Your list of possible explanations for the findings in Epiville (*Question A4–1*) may include a wide variety of factors that could have led to an increase in the number of cases of gastroenteritis—a worsening of sanitary conditions, changes in infant feeding practices, an increase in population size, and so on. However long or short the list of possible causes, it is important, nevertheless, that "noncausal" explanations also be considered.

First, it is possible that the occurrence of the disease did *not* actually increase; the rise may be not a fact but an *artifact*, attributable to a flaw in study methods. The increase may, for example, have been only in the number of cases that were *identified*, rather than in the number that *occurred*. This might be due to an improvement in the completeness of clinical records, to an increase in the public's readiness to use medical services, and so forth.

Second, consideration should also be given to the possibility that the apparent upward trend is due solely to *chance*. We possess data for 7 of the 31 years in the period from 1955 to 1985. It is possible that the number of cases varied randomly from year to year during this period, with no upward trend, but that merely by chance the particular seven observations that were selected show a rise. Most other sets of seven observations might have shown no rise. We cannot completely exclude this possibility. But common sense suggests that it is extremely unlikely, and we would probably decide that we can safely ignore it. If we are in doubt, we can do a test of *statistical significance* to help us make a decision. Actually, an appropriate significance test reveals that if in fact there is no increase in the number of cases with time, the probability that a sample of seven observations would display a monotonic increase is only 2 in 10,000 ("$P = .0002$"). This probability is so low that we would certainly decide to regard the finding as *nonfortuitous* (i.e., not due to chance).

These two questions—*Is the finding actual or artifactual?* and *Can the finding safely be regarded as nonfortuitous?*—should always be asked, and are often the first ones asked.

Keeping Occam's razor in mind, the first explanation chosen for testing (*Question A4–2*) should be one that, if confirmed, would go a long way toward explaining the findings. The explanation should also be a testable one; there is little point in selecting it for testing—however cogent the reasons may be—if the requisite data cannot be obtained. Use these two criteria in appraising your choice of an explanation for testing.

In this instance, most epidemiologists would probably agree that the chief possible explanation for the increase in cases of gastroenteritis in this town in a developing region is that the population increased between 1955 and 1985, so that there was a rise in the number of individuals who were at risk of incurring the disease. This possibility should probably be explored before serious consideration is given to *any* other explanation.

One way of doing this is to examine data on the size of the population in the period under consideration. This is what we will do in the following exercise. Another method—the one usually used—is to calculate and compare gastroenteritis rates per (say) 1,000 population. We will do this in a subsequent exercise.

TESTING EXPLANATIONS

To test an explanation we usually require additional information, drawn from the same study or from another one. We can then see whether the new facts are consistent with the explanation. If they are, our explanation may be (but is not necessarily) correct; if they are not, we can rule out the explanation.

When we seek new information, we should know *why* we want it and *how* we will use it. This enables us to be selective both in seeking and in appraising information. In the present instance, if we can pinpoint the population findings that would explain the increase in cases, we will know exactly what to look for. Our hypothesis is that the population has grown in the same way as has the number of cases. The specific hypotheses are therefore that

1. There was a monotonic increase in the size of the population.
2. There was a threefold increase between 1955 and 1985. (We specify a *relative* increase, since we can assume that a tripling of the number of cases would be associated with a tripling of population size.)
3. The trend in population size changed in the same way as did the

trend in the number of cases; that is, there was a rapid increase in earlier years and a slow increase in later years.

If these specific hypotheses are not confirmed, population growth cannot be the sole explanation for the increase in cases.

To appraise your formulation of a specific hypothesis (in your answer to *Question A4–2*), ask whether it is testable and whether, having obtained the new information you requested, you would be able to come to a clear decision as to whether your explanation is tenable. Can the new information refute the hypothesis?

EXERCISE A5

Table A5–1 provides information about population size. You may assume that the figures are accurate. The table shows the average population of Epiville in the given year—that is, the mean of the population at the beginning and end of the year.

Question A5–1

Summarize the facts in Table A5–1.

Question A5–2

Can the increase in cases of gastroenteritis in Epiville be completely explained by the change in population size?

Question A5–3

Choking on food is an important cause of accidental deaths in infancy. Information about deaths from this cause in England and Wales is shown in *Table A5–2* (data from Roper and David, 1987).

Table A5–1. Population of Epiville in Selected Years, 1955–1985

Year	Population
1955	20,000
1960	30,000
1965	40,000
1970	45,000
1975	50,000
1980	55,000
1985	60,000

Table A5-2. Deaths From Choking on Food* in Infants Aged Under One Year, England and Wales, 1974–1984

Year	Number of Deaths
1974	126
1975	93
1976	97
1977	97
1978	90
1979	110
1980	74
1981	62
1982	41
1983	29
1984	30

*"Inhalation and ingestion of food causing obstruction or suffocation," code E911 in the International Classification of Diseases.

Summarize the facts, list the possible explanations for the decrease between 1979 and 1984, select one explanation for testing, and state how you would test it.

Unit
A6

THE BASIC SCIENTIFIC PROCESS

The sequence we are following is the one we should adopt whenever we examine a table or graph: first, determine and summarize the facts; then, formulate possible explanations; and then, decide what additional information is needed to test the explanation (or for other reasons). There is often a temptation to start by saying "These data tell me nothing, because I don't have information on such-and-such" (e.g., "because I don't have information about population size"). It is generally more helpful, however, if we first see precisely what the data *do* tell us and only then decide what extra information to seek.

It may be helpful to look at this procedure in the context of the process of scientific inquiry as it is used in epidemiology (Note A6–1). There are two basic approaches. The *inductive* approach, which moves from the particular to the general, starts with observed facts, which form the basis for inferences; whereas the *deductive* approach, which moves from general to the specific, starts with a theory or hypothesis that can be proved false by observed facts. In practice (and despite philosophical objections), consistent failure to find facts that falsify a hypothesis may be taken as support for its validity—that is, as verification.

Combining these two approaches, the basic scientific process is:

- If there is no hypothesis:

  Observe and consider the facts.
  Formulate hypotheses that explain them.

- If there is a hypothesis (which may be derived from the facts):

  Seek information that can refute it.
  Observe and consider the new facts.
  See whether they refute or conform with the hypothesis.

- If the hypothesis is refuted, or if there are new ideas (which may be derived from the new facts):

Formulate new or modified hypotheses.
Seek information that can refute them.
Observe and consider the new facts.
See whether they refute or conform with the hypotheses.

and so on.

The procedure we have been following (determine the facts, then formulate possible explanations, and then decide what additional information is needed) is the one to be used whenever we "observe and consider the facts."

To test whether the increase in cases of gastroenteritis in Epiville is explained by a change in population size, we formulated three specific hypotheses, or refutable predictions, and obtained new facts to test them (*Question A5–1*). The new facts show that the changes in population size paralleled the changes in the occurrence of cases. The increase was monotonic, the overall increase was three fold, and the relative changes in successive five-year periods were identical with those observed for gastroenteritis (percentage changes of 50%, 33%, 12.5%, 11%, 10%, and 9%, respectively). You may have drawn a graph to show the change in population size. If you used the same logarithmic scale as you used for cases of gastroenteritis (Question A3–2), you obtained a curve parallel to the previous one, showing that the trends of relative change were identical.

In answer to *Question A5–2*, therefore, the change in population size can completely explain the increase in cases. The explanation is not refuted.

The data on infant deaths in Table A5–2 are real, and do not display the smooth trends that characterize fictional data. Your summary (*Question A5–3*) should include the fact that the annual number of deaths from choking on food declined monotonically between 1979 and 1983, and remained low in 1984. The annual numbers in 1980–1984 were lower than in previous years, and in 1983 and 1984 they were less than one-third of those in any year between 1974 and 1979. You may also have mentioned the stability of the annual number between 1975 and 1978, and the sharp peaks in 1974 and 1979.

Possible explanations for the decline after 1979 include

1. A decrease in the annual number of births. This explanation can be tested by seeing whether there was a decline in births, paralleling the change in deaths from choking. Alternatively, we could examine *rates*, rather than numbers, of deaths from choking. The specific hypothesis (or refutable prediction) would be that the rate did not decline during this period; if it did, the decrease in deaths cannot be attributed solely to this cause.
2. A change in doctors' habits of death certification. In recent years

there has been a rise in reported deaths due to sudden infant death syndrome (SIDS), and possibly deaths are assigned to SIDS that would previously have been attributed to choking. We might examine the annual numbers of deaths from both these causes (combined), to see whether the overall number decreased.
3. Chance variation. This seems an unlikely explanation, but if we wish we can do a test of statistical significance.
4. Changes in infant feeding practices. This is the most important possibility, as it may point the way to preventive measures; but serious consideration should not be given to it until the above "noncausal" explanations have been refuted.

In a discussion of these findings, Roper and David (1987) conclude that the fall in deaths is not merely a reflection of the decline in births, as the infant mortality rate attributable to choking fell in this time from 0.23 to 0.05 per 1,000 live births in boys, and from 0.16 to 0.05 in girls. They point out that the pattern of change of SIDS deaths has been different, reaching a peak in 1982 and declining slightly in 1983 and 1984. The explanation they favor is a change in infant feeding practices; they point out that since the early 1970s, when it was recommended that the early introduction of solid food should be avoided, there has been a decrease in the proportion of infants receiving solid foods before the age of three months. According to surveys in England and Wales, this proportion was 85% in 1975 and 55% in 1980.

RATES

Information about the frequency of an event or attribute in a group or population is commonly summarized by calculating a *rate*. The number of events, or the number of individuals with the characteristic (the *numerator* of the rate) is divided by a suitable *denominator* (e.g., the number of people in the population) and multiplied by 100, 1,000, or another convenient figure. This controls for the effect of population size on the frequency of the event or attribute.

Incidence rates measure the frequency of events, such as episodes of acute disease, that occur during a specified period. An *incidence rate (spells)* is based on the number of episodes of disease in the period; and an *incidence rate (persons)*, on the number of people who incur the disease in a given period (each person can appear in the numerator only once). *Death rates* are incidence rates that measure the frequency of deaths. The *infant mortality rate* is the number of infant deaths (under the age of one year) divided by the number of live births during the same period.

EXERCISE A6

Question A6–1

You will be asked to calculate the annual rates of gastroenteritis per 1,000 population in Epiville between 1955 and 1985. Before you do so, can you say what findings you would expect if the increase in cases of gastroenteritis is completely explained by the increase in population? In other words, formulate a specific hypothesis for testing.

Question A6–2

Calculate the annual incidence rates of gastroenteritis per 1,000 population in Epiville between 1955 and 1985, using the numbers of episodes (Table A1) as numerators and the average population figures (Table A5–1) as denominators. The formula is

$$\frac{\text{Number of episodes}}{\text{Average population}} \times 1,000$$

Question A6–3

Can you draw an inference about the risk of acute gastroenteritis for an individual in Epiville during this time? (If you want definitions of "risk," see Note A6–2.)

Question A6–4

Is there any possibility that the risk of incurring acute gastroenteritis for an individual in Epiville actually *decreased* between 1955 and 1985? Is there any way in which this kind of confusion could occur? (In answering this question, you may assume that the information on incidence and population size is accurate.)

Question A6–5

In a given year the incidence rate (persons) of acute gastroenteritis was 10 cases per 100 population in region A, and 5 per 100 population in region B. The population size was 10,000 in region A and 5,000 in region B. Which (if any) of the following statements are true?

1. There were the same numbers of cases in both regions.
2. There were twice as many cases in region A as in region B.

3. There were four times as many cases in region A as in region B.
4. The risk of incurring the disease during the year was about the same for individuals in the two regions.
5. The risk of incurring the disease during the year was twice as high for individuals in region A as for those in region B.
6. The risk of incurring the disease during the year was four times as high for individuals in region A as for those in region B.
7. The incidence rate in the total area (A and B combined) was 7.5 per 100 population.
8. The incidence rate in the total area (A and B combined) was 15 per 100 population.

NOTES

A6–1.   For a debate on the philosophical principles of epidemiological research, centering on the logic of Popper (1968), who argued that science advances by the process of deduction alone, see Buck (1975), Davies (1975), Smith (1975), Jacobsen (1976), and Susser (1986), or a collection of readings on causal inference (including most of the above) assembled by Greenland (1987a), or a set of essays on competing philosophies presented by Rothman (1988).

A6–2.   *"Risk.* A probability that an event will occur, e.g., that an individual will become ill or die within a stated period of time or age. Also, a nontechnical term encompassing a variety of measures of the probability of a (generally) unfavorable outcome"— *Dictionary of Epidemiology* (Last, 1983). "Risk is defined as the probability of a disease-free individual's developing a given disease over a specified period, conditional on that individual's not dying from any other disease during the period" (Kleinbaum et al., 1982).

Unit

A7

RATES (CONTINUED)

In answer to *Question A6–1*, if the increase in gastroenteritis is completely explained by the increase in population, we would expect the incidence rate to be the same each year. The specific hypothesis for testing is that there was no change in the annual incidence rate between 1955 and 1985. When you calculated the rates (*Question A6–2*), you found that each year the rate was 20 per 1,000, in accordance with this hypothesis.

The rate of incidence of an event in a population is an estimate of the risk (on average) for its individual members. As the rate was 20 episodes of gastroenteritis per 1,000 population per year, individuals in Epiville had a 20 in 1,000 (or 2%) risk of having an episode in each of the years for which data were available (*Question A6–3*).

We will return to *Question A6–4* at a later stage.

To answer *Question A6–5*, the numbers of cases in the two regions must be calculated. This is easily done:

$$\text{Rate per } 100 = \frac{\text{Number of cases}}{\text{Population}} \times 100$$

Hence,

$$\text{Number of cases} = \frac{(\text{Rate per } 100) \times \text{Population}}{100}$$

31

Thus

$$\text{Number of cases in region A} = (10 \times 10,000)/100 = 1,000$$

$$\text{Number of cases in region B} = (5 \times 5,000)/100 = 250$$

Statements (1) and (2) are therefore false; statement (3) is true.

As the annual incidence rate in region A was double that in region B, the risk for individuals was twice as high in region A. Statement (5) is therefore true, and statements (4) and (6) are untrue.

In the total area (regions A and B combined), the number of cases was $(1,000 + 250) = 1,250$. The total population was $(10,000 + 5,000) = 15,000$. The overall rate was therefore $(1,250/15,000) \times 100$, or 8.33 per 100. Statements (7) and (8) are thus both untrue. Statement (7) uses the simple average (mean) of the two rates, and statement (8) uses the sum of the rates. The overall rate is actually the *weighted mean* (see Note A7) of the two separate rates, using the population sizes as weights. *The contribution of a subpopulation to the findings in a total population depends on the relative size of the subpopulation.* This may be a truism, but as we will see later, it has important implications.

INSPECTING A TWO-DIMENSIONAL TABLE

Age is a variable whose role should be considered in all epidemiological studies, since health status is probably more strongly related to age than to any other personal characteristic. In the next exercise, we will therefore look at the age composition of the population of Epiville and exam-

Table A7–1. Population* by Age in Selected Years (1955–1985)

Year	Age (Years) 0–4	5–14	15–44	≥45	Total
1955	1,400	3,000	8,000	7,600	20,000
1960	2,700	5,000	12,000	10,300	30,000
1965	4,600	9,000	15,000	11,400	40,000
1970	6,000	11,000	16,500	11,500	45,000
1975	8,000	12,000	18,000	12,000	50,000
1980	10,000	13,500	19,000	12,500	55,000
1985	11,500	15,000	20,500	13,000	60,000

*The average population in the given year is shown—that is, the mean of the population in the specific age group at the beginning and end of the year.

ine its changes over the years. To do this we require a two-dimensional table (or cross-tabulation), in which population figures are shown both by age and by calendar year (Table A7–1).

When inspecting a table of this sort in order to determine and summarize the facts, it is generally advisable to do at least the following (not necessarily in this order):

- Examine each row (horizontal line) of figures.

- Compare the rows (look for similarities and differences).

- Examine each column.

- Compare the columns.

Here, each column represents the time trend in a specific age category. When examining the columns, you may use the same procedures that you used previously to examine the time trends in the population as a whole.

Each row shows the frequency distribution, by age, of the population in a given year. When examining frequency distributions it is generally helpful to calculate percentages, using the total (the row total) as the denominator. In the first row, for example, 1,400 is 7% of 20,000, 3,000 is 15%, and so on. These percentage distributions are shown in Table A7–2. In such a table it is helpful if "100%" is shown in the appropriate places, in order to show what totals were used as denominators. Note that in one instance the percentages do not add up to precisely 100%; this discrepancy is caused by rounding-off, and is acceptable.

When we compare the columns in Table A7–2, we are examining time trends with respect to the *percentage* of the population in each age category. This overcomes the effect of the changes in the total size of the population.

Table A7–2. Percentage Distribution of Population of Epiville by Age in Selected Years (1955–1985)

Year	Age (Years)				Total
	0–4	*5–14*	*15–44*	*≥45*	
1955	7.0	15.0	40.0	38.0	100.0
1960	9.0	16.7	40.0	34.3	100.0
1965	11.5	22.5	37.5	28.5	100.0
1970	13.3	24.4	36.7	25.6	100.0
1975	16.0	24.0	36.0	24.0	100.0
1980	18.2	24.5	34.5	22.7	100.0
1985	19.2	25.0	34.1	21.7	100.0

EXERCISE A7

Question A7–1

Summarize the facts shown in Tables A7–1 and A7–2.

Question A7–2

What is the most plausible explanation for these changes in the age composition of the population? You may assume that the information is accurate.

Question A7–3

Could the changes in the age composition of the population of Epiville have influenced the incidence rate of acute gastroenteritis in the town?

NOTE

A7.   The formula for the weighted mean M of a set of values x_i, where x_i is the value for group i, the size of which is N_i, is

$$M = \frac{\Sigma(x_i \cdot N_i)}{\Sigma N_i}$$

The symbol Σ (the Greek capital letter "sigma") means "the sum of the values of." In the present instance,

$$M = [(10 \times 10{,}000) + (5 \times 5{,}000)]/(10{,}000 + 5{,}000) = 8.33$$

U n i t
A8

INSPECTING A TWO-DIMENSIONAL
TABLE
(CONTINUED)

In answer to *Question A7–1*, we want to examine both the age composition of the population in different years (the rows), and the time trends in population size in different age groups (the columns). Examining the rows, we see that both the absolute numbers (in Table A7–1) and the percentage distribution (in Table A7–2) changed from year to year. The only consistent features seen in Table A7–2 are that the 0–4 age group was the smallest category each year, and the 15–44 age group was the largest.

When we inspect the columns in Table A7–1, we see that in each age group there was a monotonic increase between 1955 and 1985. The relative increase during this period varied with age, being largest in children aged 0–4 years and smallest in the oldest group. The ratios of the 1985 figures to the 1955 ones in Table A7–1 were: 0–4 years, 8.2; 5–14 years, 5.0; 15–44 years, 2.6; and ≥45 years, 1.7. You may have summarized these findings by drawing a graph, using a logarithmic scale. Such a graph would clearly show the difference between the time trends in different age groups. It would also show that in each age group the trend of relative increase was steeper in 1955–1965 than in subsequent years.

Inspection of the columns in Table A7–2 shows very different time trends in the different age groups. The percentages in the 0–4 and 5–14 age groups tended to increase, whereas the percentages in the older groups decreased monotonically.

Note that the columns in Tables A7–1 and A7–2 show different relative changes. For the 0–4 age group, for example, the ratio of the 1985 figure to the 1955 one was 11,500/1,400 = 8.2 in Table A7–1, and only 19.2%/7.0% = 2.7 in Table A7–2. For the ≥45 year age group, the corresponding ratios were 1.7 and 0.6. Can you suggest a reason for these discrepancies? (For answer, see Note A8.)

Changes in age composition may be due to aging, inward or outward movements, births, and deaths. The most plausible explanation for the extreme change observed in this growing community is selective immigration (*Question A7–2*). A high proportion of the added population apparently consisted of families with young children, born before or after entry into the town.

In answer to *Question A7–3*, we have previously seen that the overall rate in a population is a weighted mean of the rates in its constituent subpopulations, and that the relative size of each subpopulation determines its contribution to the findings in the total population (see Question A6–5). We now know that the age composition of Epiville changed with time. This may well have influenced the incidence of gastroenteritis in the town. If, for example, the incidence of the disease was especially high in young children, the rise in the percentage of young children must have increased the overall incidence. The next exercise will make this clear.

At this stage, you may like to reconsider your answer to Question A6–4.

EXERCISE A8

The incidence rates we have been using are based on the occurrence of gastroenteritis in the total population; such rates are termed *crude* rates. We can clarify matters by using the gastroenteritis rates in different age groups—that is, *age-specific* rates. A specific rate is one whose numerator and denominator refer to the same defined category: for example, children aged 0–4 (an age-specific rate), or males (a sex-specific rate), or boys aged 0–4 (an age- and sex-specific rate).

Table A8–1. Numbers of Cases of Acute Gastroenteritis in Epiville in Selected Years (1955–1985) by Age

Year	Age (Years)				Total
	0–4	*5–14*	*15–44*	*≥45*	
1955	350	50	0	0	400
1960	540	60	0	0	600
1965	690	110	0	0	800
1970	780	120	0	0	900
1975	880	120	0	0	1,000
1980	970	130	0	0	1,100
1985	1,060	140	0	0	1,200

Table A8–2. Incidence Rates of Acute Gastroenteritis in Epiville in Selected Years (1955–1985) by Age (Episodes per 100 Population of Specified Age)

Year	Age (Years)				
	0–4	5–14	15–44	≥45	Total
1955	25.0	1.7	0	0	2.0
1960	20.0	1.2	0	0	2.0
1965	15.0	1.2	0	0	2.0
1970	13.0	1.1	0	0	2.0
1975	11.0	1.0	0	0	2.0
1980	9.7	1.0	0	0	2.0
1985	9.2	0.9	0	0	2.0

We can calculate age-specific rates if we know the age distribution both of the population (Table A7–1) and of the cases of gastroenteritis. If we know that in 1955, for example, there were 350 episodes in 1,400 children aged 0–4 years, the specific rate for this group in 1955 was $(350/1,400) \times 100 = 25$ per 100.

The age distribution of the cases is shown in Table A8–1, and the age-specific rates are listed in Table A8–2. Check the calculation of some of the rates, to be sure you know how they were obtained.

Question A8–1

Summarize the facts shown in Table A8–2.

Question A8–2

Did the risk of incurring acute gastroenteritis in Epiville change between 1955 and 1985? (In answering this question, you may assume that the data on incidence and population size are accurate.) Refer to your reply to Question A6–4.

Question A8–3

How can we reconcile the changing incidence rate observed in the children with the unchanging rate seen in the population as a whole?

NOTE

A8.   There is no reason why the columns in Tables A7–1 and A7–2 should show identical trends. Each column in Table A7–1 shows the trends in the *number* of individuals in a given age group, whereas each column in Table A7–2 shows the trends in the *percentage* of the age group. The percentage depends not only on the number in the given age group, but also on the numbers in other groups. The reason for the decrease in the percentage of older people, for example (Table A7–2), despite the increase in their absolute number (Table A7–1), was the marked increase in the number of younger residents.

Unit
A9

INSPECTING A TWO-DIMENSIONAL
TABLE
(CONTINUED)

Inspecting the rows in Table A8–2, we find that the rates were consistently much higher in the 0–4 than in the 5–14 age group. The differences (in absolute or relative terms) between these age groups were larger in 1955 and 1960 than in subsequent years. The rates in the 15–44 and ≥45 age groups were consistently zero. This, incidentally, might be due to absence of the disease, failure of adults with the disease to request medical care, or a tendency to use other diagnostic labels (enteritis, dysentery, food poisoning) for adult patients; but in fact, it was due merely to a wish to simplify the exercise.

When we examine the columns, we find that in both the 0–4 and 5–14 age groups there was a monotonic decrease between 1955 and 1985. In the older groups, the rate was consistently zero, and we already know that in the total population it was consistently 2.0 per 100. The relative decrease was greater in the 0–4 than in the 5–14 age group, the ratios of the 1985 to the 1955 rates being, respectively, 0.37 and 0.53 (if you think these are misprints, see Note A9–1). In both age groups, the drop was steeper between 1955 and 1970 than between 1970 and 1985. (You may have shown this graphically. If you wish, calculate the relative changes in these two periods; for answers, see Note A9–2.) In both of the 15-year periods, the decrease was steeper in the 0–4 than in the 5–14 age group.

The salient facts then, in answer to *Question A8–1*, are that the rate was consistently higher in younger than in older children; that there were no adult cases; and that between 1955 and 1985 the rates in children fell steeply, especially in children under 5 years, and especially in the first half of this period.

We may infer that for children—who were the only ones to get the disease—the risk of incurring acute gastroenteritis declined markedly between 1955 and 1985 (*Question A8–2*). Our previous inference—based on the constancy of the crude rates—that the risk of incurring the illness did not change turns out to be misleading.

The disparity has an obvious explanation. As we have seen, the incidence rate varied markedly with age. In a previous exercise (see Unit A7), we saw that the crude (overall) rate of a disease in a population is a weighted mean of the specific rates in the population's subgroups, the weights being the sizes of the subgroups. In other words, a subgroup's contribution to the rate in a total population depends on the relative size of the subgroup. The relative size of the child population of Epiville increased with time (Table A7–2), and the contribution of this high-incidence age group to the overall incidence therefore also increased with time. This increased weight was just enough to cancel out the effect of the decreasing risk of gastroenteritis in children, so that the crude rates remained constant. The average risk for residents of Epiville remained constant, but only because of the increased chance that the resident was a child. If the child population had grown even more, the crude gastroenteritis rates would have shown a rising trend—and this despite the decline in the risk of the disease! (By hindsight, we now see that the correct answer to Question A6–4 was yes, and the above circumstances explain why.)

What we have seen is an example of *confounding* of an association. Before looking at this important phenomenon in more detail, let us consider what is meant by an "association."

ASSOCIATIONS

An association (or "statistical dependence") between two variables is said to be present if the probability that one variable will occur or be present, or the quantity of the variable, depends on the occurrence, presence, or quantity of the other variable.

If 30% of bald men are ugly and 30% of hairy men are ugly, being bald does not alter the probability of being ugly, and there is thus no association between baldness and ugliness. If the prevalence of ugliness differs in bald and hairy men, there is an association between alopecia and ugliness. The detection of associations is usually based on comparisons of this sort. A difference means there is an association.

The association between two variables is called positive if they "go together"—that is, if one event or characteristic, or high values of one variable, are associated with the presence or occurrence of another event or characteristic or with high values of a second variable. The association is negative if they "go in opposite directions"—for example, if the presence of one characteristic is associated with the absence of another. If we know that 30% of men are bald and 40% of men are ugly, and if being bald does not alter the probability of being ugly (no association), we would expect 40% of bald men to be ugly; that is, 30% × 40%, or 12%, of men would be both bald and ugly. If we find that the proportion of bald ugly men in the population is above or below 12%, we can say that these two attributes are associated. If the proportion is above 12%, they are positively associated; and if it is less than 12%, they are negatively (or inversely) associated—that is, they occur together *less* frequently than we would expect.

An association does not necessarily imply a causal relationship. Associations may be artifacts caused by flaws in study methods, or they may arise by chance, or they may be attributable to confounding effects.

Conditional associations are associations that are observed in defined conditions (e.g., in specific population groups). For example, a positive association between baldness and self-appraised ugliness—that is, bald people regarding themselves as ugly—might be found in one ethnic group and not in another, or in one sex and not the other. A negative association between these variables—that is, bald people regarding themselves as attractive—might be found in another ethnic group or in the other sex. An association may be present in one group and not another, or may be stronger in one group than in another, or may be opposite in direction in different groups. When we examined the columns in Table A8–2, we looked at the conditional associations between gastroenteritis incidence and time in the 0- to 4- and 5- to 14-year age groups.

EXERCISE A9

State whether the following statements are true or false.

1. If you find that 60% of students who develop infectious mononucleosis (the "kissing" disease) are habitual smokers, this shows the presence of an association between the disease and smoking.
2. If you find that 5% of students who smoke develop infectious mononucleosis during a one-year follow-up period, this shows the presence of an association between the disease and smoking.
3. If 60% of a large sample of male students and 30% of a large sample of female students smoke, there is an association between sex and smoking.
4. If, in a class of five male and five female students, none of the males smoke and all of the females smoke, there is an association between sex and smoking.
5. If 75% of the smokers in a college are males and 25% are females, there is an association between sex and smoking.
6. If over half the adults in a neighborhood have sedentary occupations and over half the residents have recurrent low back pain, there is an association between sedentary work and low back pain.
7. If adults with low body weights tend to have lower blood pressures

than adults with high body weights, there is an inverse association between body weight and blood pressure.
8. If during an influenza epidemic there is a higher incidence rate of the disease among smokers than among nonsmokers, there is an association between smoking and influenza.
9. If during an influenza epidemic there is a lower incidence of the disease among smokers than among nonsmokers, there is no association between smoking and influenza.
10. If during an influenza epidemic there is a lower incidence rate among people who had influenza shots than among people who did not have shots, there is a positive association between influenza shots and incidence of the disease.
11. If you compare children of four ethnic groups and find that they differ in their mean hemoglobin levels, there is an association between ethnic group and hemoglobin level. The association is neither positive nor negative.
12. If the incidence rate of gastroenteritis is higher in infants than in older children, there is a positive association between gastroenteritis and age.
13. If a follow-up study shows relatively high mortality rates among people with very low and very high blood cholesterol levels, and a relatively low mortality rate among people with intermediate cholesterol levels, there is no association between blood cholesterol and mortality.
14. If a comparison of countries shows that the more video cassette recorders there are per 100 population, the higher the mortality rate from coronary heart disease, this shows an association between the prevalence of VCRs and coronary mortality.

NOTE

A9–1. Some readers have been surprised to encounter ratios that are less than 1. A ratio is the number of times that one number contains another, and is calculated by dividing the one number by the other. The ratio of 25 to 9.2 is 2.72 (or 2.72 to 1, or 2.72:1), and the ratio of 9.2 to 25 is 0.37 (which is the reciprocal of 2.72; i.e., it is 1 divided by 2.72). If the numbers are equal, the ratio is 1.

A9–2. According to Table A8–2, the percentage decrease in the 0–4 year group was $(25 - 13)/25 \times 100 = 48\%$ in 1955–1970, and 29% in 1970–1985. In the 5–14 age group, the corresponding figures were 35% and 18%. Or (using ratios): in the 0–4 age group the ratio of the 1970 rate to the 1955 rate was $13/25 = 0.52$, and the ratio of the 1985 rate to the 1970 rate was $9.2/13 = 0.71$; in the 5–14 age group the corresponding ratios were 0.65 and 0.82.

U n i t
A10

ASSOCIATIONS (CONTINUED)

Here are the answers to the true–false questions (Exercise A9):

1. False. We must have a comparison before we can conclude that there is an association. It is not enough to know the smoking habits of students who develop the disease; we must also know the smoking habits of students who do not develop the disease. If we find a difference between the proportions who smoke, we have an association. This is called a "retrospective" approach, because we move from the postulated outcome to the postulated cause.
2. False. Without a comparison we cannot conclude that there is an association. It is not enough to know the incidence rate of the disease in smokers; we must also know the incidence rate in nonsmokers. If the incidence rates are different, there is an association. This is called a "prospective" approach, because we move from the putative cause to the putative outcome.
3. True. There is a difference; therefore, there is an association.
4. True. There is a difference; therefore, there is an association. In such a small sample, there is a high likelihood that the association is fortuitous, but it certainly exists.
5. False. We have no comparison and hence can draw no conclusion about an association. It is possible that among nonsmokers also, 75% are males.
6. False. We have no comparison, for example, between the proportion of sedentary workers who had back pain and the proportion of nonsedentary workers who had back pain. You may have thought of an association at a population (not necessarily individual) level, because sedentary work and low back pain seem to "go together" in the same neighborhood. But here too we have no comparison. What were the proportions with back pain in neighborhoods with fewer or more sedentary workers? We have no data for other neighborhoods, and cannot draw a conclusion about the presence of an

43

association: the rate of low back pain may be the same in populations with more active occupations.

7. False. The association is a positive one. Low body weights hang together with low blood pressures; that is, the variables tend to go in the same direction.

8. True. There is a positive association between smoking and influenza.

9. False. If smoking is linked with a low incidence of influenza, there is a negative association between these two variables.

10. False. If influenza shots are associated with a low incidence rate—that is, the presence of one characteristic is linked with low values of another—the association is a negative one.

11. True. There is a difference; therefore, there is an association. As ethnic categories do not fall into a natural order (there are no "high" or "low" values), we cannot call the association positive or negative.

12. False. The association is a negative one. Low age goes together with a high incidence of gastroenteritis.

13. False. There is an association, but it is not a simple "linear" (straight-line) one. If plotted on a graph, the mortality rates would form a U-shaped curve, or maybe a J-shaped or reverse J-shaped one.

14. True. But the association is, of course, not necessarily a causal one. The association exists at a group or population level (this is sometimes called an "ecological" association), but it does not necessarily exist at an individual level; individuals who possess or use VCRs do not necessarily have an increased risk of dying of coronary heart disease.

CONFOUNDING

Let us return to Epiville and the distorted picture we obtained of the time trend in the incidence of gastroenteritis.

We were interested in the association between two variables: time (the independent variable) and the occurrence of the disease (the dependent variable) (Fig. A10–1); specifically, we were interested in the effect of time on the occurrence of the disease. When we looked at the crude rates (in Question A6–2), we found no association between these variables. But when (in Question A8–1) we introduced a third variable, age, we found clear evidence of an association; the age-specific rates showed

Figure A10–1. Causal association between two variables.

Figure A10–2. Conditions for confounding of *A–B* association by *C*.

a strong downward trend in both the age groups in which the disease occurred.

This distortion occurred because the crude data reflected the mingled effects of time and age on incidence. Age was strongly associated with both time and the incidence of the disease; that is, the age composition of the population varied with time, and the incidence of gastroenteritis varied with age. This is shown schematically in Fig. A10–2, where A is time, B is the occurrence of the disease, and C is age.

The essential elements are that C must affect B (hence the arrow in the diagram), and that A and C must be associated with each other. The association between A and C need not be causal (hence no arrow), but C can affect A. A, however, must not affect C. When this constellation exists, it may be difficult to separate whatever effect A may have on B from the effect of C on B; the interplay of the associations may distort the picture of the A–B relationship. C is a *potential confounder* of the association between A and B (from the Latin *confundere*, "to mix together"). If distortion of the A–B relationship actually happens, as in our Epiville example, C is a *confounder* (confounding factor, confounding variable).

It should be noted that only if the associations between the confounder and the other variables are strong ones can there be a confounding effect of any importance: The confounding effect is "only a relatively weak echo" (Note A10–1). If distortion is slight, it can usually be ignored.

If confounding occurs, we can obtain an undistorted picture only if we control the effects of the confounding variable (C), as we did by looking at each age group separately.

In Epiville, age was a factor that distorted the relationship between time and gastroenteritis incidence. In this instance the confounder *masked* the association. In other instances a confounder may *diminish*, *reverse*, or *exaggerate* an association. Commonly, it *produces an apparent association* when none really exists.

If the relationships pictured in Fig. A10–2 are present or suspected to be present, the variable denoted by "C" may be considered a potential confounder. This is a simple operational method for the selection of possible confounders, satisfactory in most situations, and the only one used by many epidemiologists. When this model is used, should age be considered a possible confounder in a study of the effect of smoking on stomach cancer? (See Note A10–2.)

This simple model, while generally adequate, does not give full expression to the complexity of the requirements for confounding (see Note A10–3). Here is a somewhat more complete formulation (which you may prefer to skip). If we are interested in appraising the causal influence of variable A (independent) on variable B (dependent) and wish to identify possible confounders, the requirements are:

1. The potential confounder (C) must be causally related to B; it must be a variable that (according to prior knowledge or theory) influences B or is a stand-in for a variable that influences B. That is, it may itself be a cause of B or may cause a change in B, or it may be an indicator of a known or unknown correlated factor (or set of factors)—other than A—that affects B. Age, for example, may be considered a potential confounder because it is a surrogate for age-related causal factors. If B is a disease, C (or what it represents) may influence the likelihood of its diagnosis, not only the risk of its occurrence. If C is affected by B, or if it is a manifestation of B, it is not (in this context) a potential confounder. It is not essential to demonstrate an association between C and B in the data; but failure to find the expected association in the data may point to an inadequacy in prior knowledge.
2. C must be associated with A in the study sample. Prior knowledge may be a better guide than the data in some study designs, especially if numbers are small (Miettinen and Cook 1981), but it is seldom available. C is not a potential confounder (in this context) if the reason for the association is that (according to prior knowledge or theory) A influences C. We return to this important requirement in a later unit.
3. Although the selection of possible confounders is commonly based on the existence of simple associations between C and the other variables, it is actually the conditional associations (see Unit A9) with A and B that matter: The association with A must exist when B is held constant, and vice versa. If the independent variable (A) is exposure to a supposed etioligic factor, a criterion commonly used is that the association between C and B must occur even in the absence of exposure to the causal factor. If B is a disease, the association between C and A should be apparent in the source population from which the cases are derived, or in controls representative of that population.

Decisions about possible confounding effects can clearly not be made in an offhand way. They demand prior knowledge or assumptions about causal processes, may need examination of the data, and require the application of judgment.

When we try to explain an association between two variables, we should not seriously consider the possibility that it is a cause–effect relationship until we have asked three questions: *Is the association an artifact? Can it be regarded as nonfortuitous?* And, *is it produced by confounding?*

EXERCISE A10

Question A10–1

These questions refer to the sharp decline in the incidence rate of gastroenteritis in children aged 0–4 years in Epiville between 1955 and 1985 (Table A8–2). In trying to explain this decline, how would you decide whether sex should be considered as a possible confounder? You may assume that the time trend is not an artifact, and is not due to chance.

Question A10–2

How would you decide whether sex is *actually* (not *potentially*) a confounder?

Question A10–3

If sex should turn out to be a confounder, how could you control (i.e., neutralize or eliminate) its effect?

Question A10–4

What (if any) are the important confounders to be considered in trying to explain the decline in gastroenteritis incidence seen in children aged 0–4 years in Table A8–2?

NOTES

A10–1.   For numerical examples showing that the confounding effect is weak unless the associations with the confounder are strong, see Breslow and Day (1980, p. 96) and Bross (1966, 1967).

A10–2.   The required association between C and B is present, since the risk of stomach cancer varies with age. The required association between C and A is also present, since smoking habits vary with age, and this is not because smoking affects age. Age is therefore a potential confounder of the causal association between smoking and stomach cancer.

A10–3.   For fuller simple descriptions of confounding, see Rothman (1986, pp. 89–94) and Hennekens and Buring (1987, pp. 287–293). Finer points and controversial issues are discussed in papers (not all of them easy to read) by Fisher and Patil (1974), Miettinen and Cook (1981), Boivin and Wacholder (1985),

Greenland and Robins (1986), Grayson (1987, 1989), Greenland et al. (1989), and Weinberg (1993). Confounding has diverse definitions; the working definition used in this text is that the ratio of rates (or whatever measure of the association is used) is different when the confounder is ignored and when the effects of the confounder are held constant by stratification, standardization, or other methods.

Unit
A11

CONFOUNDING (CONTINUED)

In answer to *Question A10–1*, sex can have a confounding effect on the association between time and gastroenteritis incidence only if it is associated with both the latter variables. Gastroenteritis incidence may well have differed in the two sexes, as does the incidence of many other diseases; but there is no reason to believe that the sex composition of the child population changed appreciably during this period. We are therefore probably safe in concluding that sex need *not* be regarded as a possible confounder.

To determine whether a confounding effect actually exists (*Question A10–2*), we must compare what we see in the crude data with what we see when we neutralize or eliminate the effect of the suspected confounder. Is there an important difference in the findings? One way of doing this is to look separately at the data for each category (or "stratum") of the suspected confounder. It was by using this *stratification* procedure that we detected the confounding effect of age: we compared the time trend shown by the crude incidence rates with the time trends shown by age-specific incidence rates. We can now repeat this procedure, for sex. We can "control for sex" by calculating sex-specific rates (for children aged 0–4 years), and seeing whether the time trend shown by the crude data for these children is a satisfactory reflection of the time trends seen in the two sexes.

By using stratified data, such as age- or sex-specific rates, we eliminate the effects of the stratifying variable (age or sex) on the associations that interest us (*Question A10–3*). We could also control these effects in other ways—for example, by standardization (which we will deal with later). Whatever method is used, two birds can be killed with one stone: the same procedure can both demonstrate the existence of a confounding effect and neutralize it.

The variables that are candidates for inclusion in a list of possible confounders (*Question A10–4*) are those that are known or suspected to affect the dependent variable. Any of these that is known or believed to

49

be associated with the independent variable as well, but is not affected by it, may be listed as a possible confounder. It must be remembered that there can be an important confounding effect only if the associations are strong. There are a number of variables that are so often of relevance in epidemiological studies that consideration should always be given to their inclusion. These "universal variables" include age, sex, parity, ethnic group, religion, marital status, social class, and its components (occupation, education, income), rural or urban residence, and geographical mobility.

In Epiville, where we know that the population has grown extensively because of immigration, and where we have found that a change in its age composition has distorted the time trends in gastroenteritis incidence, we should give serious consideration to the possibility that selective immigration has resulted in changes in other demographic characteristics as well, resulting in other confounding effects. For example, the composition of the population may also have changed with respect to ethnic group or social class. If we know or suspect that such changes occurred, and if we believe that these variables may influence gastroenteritis incidence, we should investigate the possibility that they are confounders.

EFFECT MODIFICATION

In a previous exercise we extended our understanding of the association between two variables (gastroenteritis incidence and time) by investigating the influence of another variable (age) on the association. This, a very common analytic procedure, may be termed *elaboration* of the association. Stratification according to the categories of the other variable is the simplest way of doing this.

When we compared the associations seen in Table A8–2, which showed incidence rates by year and age, we observed two kinds of discrepancy. First, there were differences between the associations shown by the specific and crude rates; this was our evidence for the confounding effect of age. Second, there were discrepancies between the findings in the various specific strata—a striking decline in children aged 0–4, a less marked decline in older children, and no change in adults. The conditional associations (see Unit A9) between gastroenteritis incidence and time were different. This phenomenon may be termed the *modifying effect* of age on the association between gastroenteritis incidence and time. Age turned out to be both a confounder (because the time trends shown by the crude and age-specific rates differed) and a modifier (because the time trends in the various age strata differed from one another). The same stratification procedure demonstrated both effects.

Table A11. Incidence Rate of
Gastroenteritis Among Children Aged
0–4 Years in Epiville in Selected Years,
1955–1985

Year	Incidence Rate per 100
1955	25.0
1960	20.0
1965	15.0
1970	13.0
1975	11.0
1980	9.7
1985	9.2

EXERCISE A11

Question A11–1

For your convenience, the decline in gastroenteritis incidence among
children aged 0–4 in Epiville is again shown in Table A11. Do you think
it might be advantageous to use narrower age categories, and if so, why?

Question A11–2

Suppose you suspect that social class has a confounding effect on the
association seen in Table A11, as a result of selective immigration with
regard to social class. You propose to examine this possibility by using
stratification. Construct a skeleton table (a table with captions, but without figures) to accommodate the new data you require for this purpose;
provide space both for the raw figures and for whatever summary statistics are needed. For simplicity, use two social classes ("high" and
"low") in this exercise.

Question A11–3

What else—with specific reference to associations between variables—
might you learn from the new figures you hope to put in the skeleton
table?

Unit
A12

REFINEMENT

In answer to *Question A11–1*, it might be useful to use narrower age categories, in order to discover whether the incidence of gastroenteritis varies *within* the categories we have so far used. In the 0–4 age group in particular, are the rates higher in the first six months, in the second six months, in the second year, or in the third, fourth, or fifth year of life? This knowledge might help to pinpoint groups that are at high risk and need special preventive care, and might also provide useful clues to the causation of gastroenteritis in this community.

The use of finer instead of broad categories is an example of a procedure termed *refinement*, which is often used in order to throw added light on an association. This procedure also sometimes reveals associations that were not previously apparent. We may refine a crude scale of measurement, as in the instance of age, or we may refine the variable itself. For example, instead of regarding acute gastroenteritis as a single entity, we might calculate the rates of acute gastroenteritis associated with various specific microorganisms.

SKELETON TABLES

The drawing of a skeleton table to accommodate new information is often a challenge that serves to clarify one's thinking and translate a fuzzy idea of "what I would like to know" into a clear-cut need for well-defined facts.

A skeleton table may be meant for raw data, for summary measures (such as rates, percentages, and means), or for both. Designing the table may necessitate decisions about the selection of variables, of categories, and of summary measures, and about the arrangement of variables (e.g., in cross-tabulations) so as to provide information on the associations of interest. Sometimes the table serves to draw attention to prac-

Table A12–1. Incidence of Gastroenteritis in Children Aged 0–4 in Epiville in Selected Years (1955–1985) by Social Class

					Social Class							
		High			Low			Unknown			Total	
Year	Pop.	No. of Cases	Rate per 100	Pop.	No. of Cases	Rate per 100	Pop.	No. of Cases	Rate per 100	Pop.	No. of Cases	Rate per 100
1955												
1960												
1965												
1970												
1975												
1980												
1985												

53

tical difficulties that have been overlooked; only when the requirements for data are clearly stipulated may it be realized that they cannot be met.

A skeleton table need not be prepared with obsessive attention to detail, but it should meet the basic requirements for a well-constructed table. It should include column and row captions. If categorical scales are used, they should be comprehensive and their categories should be mutually exclusive. Allowance should be made for "unknowns"; if there are many cases with missing data, it may be difficult to draw useful conclusions from the findings. If the figures are to be provided by a computer with the use of a ready-made package of programs, the arrangement of the table should conform to one of the formats offered by these programs.

The skeleton table requested in *Question A11–2* should look something like Table A12–1. It should show year-by-year incidence rates for each social class, together with the raw data (population figures and numbers of cases) required for calculating these rates.

ELABORATING AN ASSOCIATION

In answer to *Question A11–3*, the figures inserted in the skeleton table would not only help us to detect and control for possible confounding by social class, it would also tell us about:

1. The association between social class and time. Did the social class distribution of the population change?
2. The association between social class and gastroenteritis incidence. Did the rates in the social classes differ?
3. The modifying effect of social class on the association between gastroenteritis incidence and time. Did the time trends differ in the social classes?
4. As a corollary to (3), we would also learn about the modifying effect of time on the association between gastroenteritis incidence and social class. (Did the social class differences in incidence vary at different times?) These two modifying effects—(3) and (4)—are different expressions of the same phenomenon; one cannot exist without the other.

As we will see later, elaboration of an association can also help us to test the possibility that the added variable is an *intermediate cause*—that is, a link in the chain of causation between the independent and dependent variables.

Table A12-2. Incidence of
Gastroenteritis in Children Aged 0-4
Years in Epiville in Selected Years
(1955-1985) by Social Class:
Rates per 100

| Year | Social Class | | Total |
	High	Low	
1955	14.6	31.9	25.0
1960	13.0	24.7	20.0
1965	11.1	17.6	15.0
1970	10.1	14.9	13.0
1975	9.1	12.3	11.0
1980	8.4	10.6	9.7
1985	8.2	10.5	9.2

EXERCISE A12

Let us assume that there were no children whose social class was unknown. The incidence rates in children aged 0-4 are shown in Table
A12-2, separately for each social class and for the age group as a whole.

Question A12-1

Summarize the facts shown in Table A12-2. In your summary, state
what associations are shown.

Question A12-2

Does social class have a modifying effect on the association between
gastroenteritis incidence and time?

Question A12-3

Does social class have a confounding effect on this association?

Question A12-4

What would be the importance of finding a modifying effect?

Question A12-5

What would be the importance of finding a confounding effect?

MODIFYING AND CONFOUNDING
EFFECTS

To answer *Question A12–1*, we should inspect the table's columns and rows. Each column shows a monotonic decrease in gastroenteritis incidence with time. The ratio of the 1985 to the 1955 rate was 0.37 in the 0–4 age group as a whole, 0.56 in the high social class, and 0.33 in the low social class. The absolute differences between the rates in 1985 and 1955 were 15.8, 6.4, and 21.4 per 100 in the total group and in the children of high and low social class, respectively. The decline with time was thus much steeper in the low social class.

In each row we see a negative association between social class and gastroenteritis incidence—the rate is consistently higher in the low than in the high social class. The difference was biggest in 1955, when the absolute difference was 17.3 per 100 and the ratio (low : high) was 2.2. The difference became progressively less, but was still apparent in 1980, when the absolute difference was 2.3 per 100 and the ratio was 1.3. In each year, the rate in the total group was intermediate between those in the two social classes.

In answer to *Question A12–2*, social class is clearly a modifier of the association between gastroenteritis incidence and time; the time trends in the social classes differ.

To determine whether social class has a confounding effect on the association between gastroenteritis incidence and time (*Question A12–3*), we may compare the trends seen in the total group with those in the specific strata (social classes). The comparison is difficult because of the difference between the trends in the social classes, and the answer is not clear-cut. There is no basic difference between the trend in the total group, as expressed by either the rate ratio or the rate difference, and the trends observed in the separate social classes; the direction of change is the same in each instance, and the values of the separate social classes straddle those in the total group. The rate ratio in the total group, however (unlike the rate difference), is much closer to the rate ratio in the

Figure A13–1. Effect modification; the modifier (C) has three categories.

low social class than to that in the high social class, possibly as a result of confounding. We might conclude that the picture provided by the crude data (without controlling for social class) is not distorted enough to matter, and that there is no confounding effect of any importance: controlling the effect of social class (by stratifying) does not alter the conclusion that over the years there has been an appreciable decrease in the incidence rate of gastroenteritis.

Effect modification is pictured in two different ways in Figs. A13–1 and A13–2, where C modifies the association between A (an independent variable) and B (the dependent variable). This means that the effect of A (in our example, time) on B (incidence) varies, depending on C (social class). It also always means (as a corollary) that the effect of C (social class) on B (incidence) varies, depending on A (time). It is the specific combination of A and C that determines the value of B. This may also be referred to as *interaction* between the two independent variables, A and C, in their association with B. Figure A13–1 is appropriate if C has two or more categories (e.g., different social classes); it highlights the fact that there is a different A–B association for each category of C. Figure A13–2 emphasizes the interaction between A and C, and is appropriate even if the modifier does not have separate categories (e.g., if C is weight in kilograms or height in inches).

When we detect a modifying effect (*Question A12–4*), we gain new information that may have important theoretical and practical implications. In Epiville, the fact that gastroenteritis declined more steeply in low-social-class children may help us in our search for the reasons for the decline. It is a clue that may help us to formulate appropriate hypotheses for testing. We may also use a different viewpoint: not only did the time trend in gastroenteritis incidence differ in the two social classes, but the difference between the rates in the social classes altered with time. This fact, too, may give us food for thought, and we may wish to explore it further. Third (at a simpler level), until we detected

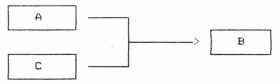

Figure A13–2. Effect modification (interaction).

the modifying effect, we may not have known that social class was associated with incidence. As the diagram shows, a modifier is always associated with the dependent variable; in fact, it can usually be regarded as a cause or determinant. We may wish to go on to formulate and test possible explanations for the association between social class and gastroenteritis incidence.

The discovery of effect modification may also have practical implications. If A and C were sex and social class, for example, we would be able to identify children (say, boys in a low social class) who are especially likely to benefit from preventive intervention.

The importance of finding a confounding effect (*Question A12–5*) depends on whether it was previously known that the confounder influences the dependent variable. If this effect was already known (as is usually the case), discovery of the confounding effect leads only to a realization that the conclusions drawn from the crude data are misleading and require revision, by controlling for this "nuisance variable." Sometimes, however, a search for a confounder leads to new etiological insights—the fact that C affects B (or maybe both A and B) may be a new finding, and C may turn out to be a key factor in the causal processes.

A variable may be neither a modifier nor a confounder, or both, or a confounder and not a modifier, or a modifier with no material confounding effect. If the modifying effect is extremely strong, it is arguable that the confounding effect becomes irrelevant. Suppose, for example, that the incidence of gastroenteritis had risen sharply in one social class and had fallen steeply in the other. With such wide divergence, it would be so important to pay separate attention to the social classes that there might be little interest in the overall change in the town, confounded or not.

EXERCISE A13

In Table A12–2 we saw a strong association between gastroenteritis incidence and social class in children aged 0–4 in 1955. The rates in the two classes were 31.9 and 14.6 per 100. We now stratify the data in accordance with the mother's duration of residence in Epiville, and obtain the results shown in Table A13–1.

Question A13–1

Summarize the facts concerning the association between gastroenteritis incidence and social class. How would you explain the discrepancy between the associations shown by the crude and specific rates? Does mother's duration of residence in Epiville modify the association between gastroenteritis and social class?

Table A13–1. Incidence of Gastroenteritis Among Children Aged 0–4 Years 02.10lin Epiville in 1955, by Social Class and Mother's Duration of Residence in Epiville

Mother's Duration of Residence in Epiville	Social Class					
	High			Low		
	Pop.	No of Cases	Rate per 100	Pop.	No of Cases	Rate per 100
Over 5 years	280	14	5.0	179	9	5.0
2–4 years	240	48	20.0	239	48	20.1
Under 2 years	40	20	50.0	422	211	50.0
Total	560	82	14.6	840	268	31.9

Question A13–2

Let us suppose that when we stratify the data in accordance with the children's nutritional status (measured before the onset of gastroenteritis), we obtain the results shown in Table A13–2. Summarize the facts concerning the association between gastroenteritis incidence and social class. How would you explain the discrepancy between the associations shown by the crude and specific rates?

Table A13–2. Incidence of Gastroenteritis Among Children Aged 0–4 Years in Epiville in 1955, by Social Class and Nutritional Status

Nutritional Status	Social Class					
	High			Low		
	Pop.	No of Cases	Rate per 100	Pop.	No of Cases	Rate per 100
Well nourished	280	14	5.0	179	9	5.0
Slightly malnourished	240	48	20.0	239	48	20.1
Markedly malnourished	40	20	50.0	422	211	50.0
Total	560	82	14.6	840	268	31.9

Unit
A14

ELABORATING AN ASSOCIATION
(CONTINUED)

The association between gastroenteritis incidence and social class is elaborated in Table A13–1, where the data are stratified according to mother's duration of residence in Epiville. In answer to *Question A13–1*, the crude rates (in the bottom row of the table) show a strong association between gastroenteritis and social class. The ratio of the incidence rate in the low social class to that in the high social class is 31.9 : 14.6—or 2.2. But when mother's duration of residence is held constant, the association disappears; in each "duration of residence" category, the specific incidence rates in the two social classes are almost identical (the ratio of the rates is 1.0).

We can attribute this discrepancy between the associations shown by the crude and specific rates to the confounding effect of mother's duration of residence. The relationship with social class can be explained by the relationship with mother's duration of residence. As the table shows, recency of immigration is strongly associated both with social class and with gastroenteritis incidence. (What is the evidence for these associations? For answer, see Note A14.) We may conclude that social class can be disregarded as a determinant of the occurrence of the disease.

Mother's duration of residence in Epiville does not modify the relationship between gastroenteritis incidence and social class. The ratio of rates is the same (1.0) in each "duration of residence" category.

The figures in Table A13–2 are identical with those in Table A13–1. Here too, the stratifying variable (nutritional status) is strongly associated both with gastroenteritis and with social class; and here too, the crude rates show an association with social class whereas the specific rates do not. Yet the interpretation of the facts is different. We cannot conclude that social class has no role in the causation of gastroenteritis, since nutritional status may well be a link in the chain of causation

Figure A14-1. Intermediate cause.

between social class and gastroenteritis. We cannot regard nutritional status as just a confounder whose effect misled us to think that social class might play a causal role. Rather, we might infer that nutritional status is the intervening cause that accounts for the difference in incidence between the social classes: we could regard the association between social class and gastroenteritis as a meaningful one that might be explained by the effects on nutritional status of behavioral, economic, environmental, or other characteristics connected with social class.

This example carries an important message. The prerequisites for a confounding effect, as stated in Unit A10, were shown schematically in Fig. A10–2. A and C must both have an effect on B, and A and C must be associated with each other. The association between A and C may be noncausal. But if it is causal, with A affecting C, C is an intermediate link in the chain of causation between A and B (Fig. A14–1). It is then not a potential confounder, but an intermediate or intervening cause. Just as with a confounder, the associations seen in the crude data may differ from those seen when stratification or some other procedure is used to "hold C constant." However, although the statistical findings may be the same, their interpretation is different, as we have just seen in the Epiville example. If the association between A and C is a causal one with C affecting A (Fig. A14–2), C is a potential confounder and not an intermediate cause.

Figure A14-2. Confounding by a common cause.

The above considerations apply not only if C is an intermediate cause, but also if it is a stand-in for an intermediate cause—for example, if it is a manifestation or result of some factor (known or unknown) that is affected by A and affects B. Variable C should then not be treated as a confounder. In the above instance, stratifying by skin dryness (an expression of nutritional status, but not a cause of gastroenteritis) might (like stratifying by nutritional status) have misled us to believe that social class has no role in the causation of gastroenteritis. It has been suggested that no variable that is determined, even in part, by A should be treated as a confounder (Weinberg 1993).

A dilemma arises if the causal processes are unclear, and it is not certain whether C is determined by A or not. There is also a dilemma if C is partly caused by A, and partly a marker for some quite different variable. In such circumstances it may be advisable to do parallel analyses, one treating *C* as a potential confounder, and one not, and reach alternative conclusions about the *A–B* association (if so-and-so then so-and-so, and if such-and-such then such-and-such). The two approaches may lead to similar conclusions.

Emphasis has been given in this unit and in Unit A10 to the conditions that must be met before a variable can be regarded as a potential confounder of a causal association and therefore held constant in the analysis. This does not mean, however, that a variable should not be held constant unless these conditions are met. There may be other reasons for doing so. We might, for example, have the notion that the social class differences in gastroenteritis are only partly accounted for by differences in nutritional status, and test this hypothesis by holding nutritional status constant, as in Table A13–2; if we then found an association between social class and gastroenteritis (which we did not find in Table 13–2), this would support our notion.

EXERCISE A14

Question A14–1

The effects of a confounding variable may be controlled by stratification and by other techniques that we have not yet discussed. What technique, other than stratification, have we used for this purpose in these exercises? This may be regarded as a trick question, since the technique is a widely used one that is often applied in a routine manner, without specific thought as to its function in controlling for confounding.

Question A14–2

The incidence rate of gastroenteritis is twice as high in Epiville as in Shlepiville. Can the data shown in Table A14 explain this difference?

Table A14. Population Size and Incidence of Gastroenteritis in Two Towns, 1986

	Epiville	Shlepiville
Total population	60,000	30,000
Cases of gastroenteritis per 1,000 population	20	10

Question A14–3

This question deals with the formulation and testing of causal explanations. To avoid confusion, let us move to fresh pastures—the town of

Zepiville, where there is a strong association between ethnic group (Easterners or Westerners) and the incidence of gastroenteritis in children aged 0–4. The incidence rate is much higher among Easterners than among Westerners in this town.

As far as we can tell, this association is not an artifact, and a test of statistical significance shows that we can safely regard it as nonfortuitous. We have looked for evidence of confounding and have found none. Of course, we cannot be sure (one never can) that there is no confounding by some variable that we have not measured, tested, or maybe even thought of; however, we have decided that for practical purposes we will reject the possibility that the association is caused by confounding. In the course of the analysis, we found no evidence that the association was modified by sex, social class, mother's age, or mother's duration of residence; the association of incidence with ethnic group was apparent in each category of these variables.

List all the possible causal explanations you can think of for the difference in incidence between Easterners and Westerners (forget Occam's razor).

NOTE

A14. In Table A13–1, a strong association between recency of immigration and social class is shown by the striking difference between the two frequency distributions of mother's duration of residence (280, 240, and 40 in the high social class and 179, 239, and 422 in the low social class). The differences between the gastroenteritis incidence rates in the "duration of residence" groups (5, 20, and 50 per 100) show an association between recency of immigration and the disease.

Unit
A15

THE USE OF RATES

At the outset of this series of exercises, we saw (in Table A1) that the annual number of cases of gastroenteritis in Epiville rose markedly between 1955 and 1985. We subsequently found that this rise could be attributed to the increase in population. The association between the number of cases and time was in fact due to the confounding effect of population size, a variable that was strongly associated with both the dependent variable (number of cases) and the independent variable (time). When we calculated incidence rates, we found no time trend: the rate was the same each year (20 per 1,000). The time trend disappeared because we used the rate—the number of cases per 1,000 population—as our dependent variable, rather than just the number of cases. By using rates, we were able to hold the effect of population size constant in the comparison.

This, of course, is one reason why rates are used. In answer to *Question A14–1*, when we compare the occurrence of a disease in two populations we are aware that a difference in the numbers of cases may be due mainly to a difference in population size. We therefore use rates rather than numbers of cases. This controls for the confounding effect of population size. Percentages and other ratios are also used for this purpose. When we wished to see whether the age composition of the population of Epiville changed between 1955 and 1985, we used percentages (Table A7–2) so as to neutralize the effect of differences in population size.

The use of rates and proportions is probably the most widely used method of controlling for confounding. The basic principle is replacement of the dependent variable by another variable, which is defined in such a way that it incorporates, and neutralizes the effect of, the confounder—for example, "cases per 1,000 population" instead of "cases." This technique may be used to deal with confounders other than population size. When one compares body weights, for example, the confounding effect of height can be controlled by using a weight–height index, such as the ratio of weight to height or to the square of height; or a relative weight can be used, calculated by expressing the observed weight as a percentage of the "standard" weight of people of the same age, sex, height, and so forth, in order to neutralize the effects of these variables; or weight can be replaced by a weight percentile that expresses the child's position in relation to the weights of other children of the same age and sex. Another common example is the use of an intelligence quotient or developmental quotient that expresses a test score as a percentage of the average score of children of the same age.

In answer to *Question A14–2*, the data shown in Table A14 *cannot* explain the difference in gastroenteritis rates. The difference in population size cannot explain the difference in gastroenteritis rates, since its effect is neutralized by the use of rates. There were (20/1,000) × 60,000 = 1,200 cases in Epiville, and (10/1,000) × 30,000 = 300 in Shlepiville. There was a fourfold difference in cases, which is reduced to a twofold difference (20:10) when we control for population size by using rates.

CAUSAL EXPLANATIONS

In thinking of causal explanations for an association, it may be helpful to use an epidemiological model, such as the well-known host–agent– environment triangle (Fig. A15–1) or the model suggested by Kark (1974), which features the interrelationships between (a) the state of health of a population or group (in terms of diseases, disabilities, and deaths, and somatic and psychological characteristics); (b) the biological, social, and cultural attributes of the population or group; (c) the environment (natural, human, and man-made) and material resources of the population or group; and (d) the health care system (Fig. A15–2).

Associations with "universal variables" (see Unit A11), such as sex or ethnic group, usually have a variety of possible explanations. Members of different ethnic groups may differ not only in their culture (and hence in their habitual dietary, smoking, and other practices), but in their genetically determined characteristics, in their environmental exposures, in the availability of medical services, and in other respects.

Causes are always multiple. When we list possible causal explanations, we are not generally trying to suggest a set of alternatives, one of

Figure A15–1. The epidemiological triangle.

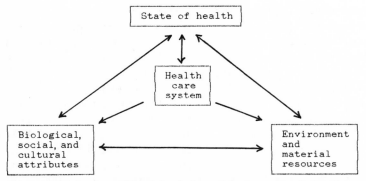

Figure A15–2. An epidemiological model of causal relationships.

which will turn out to be the sole cause. We are enumerating various factors that may each contribute in some degree to the phenomenon we are studying, exerting its effect in a direct or indirect manner, separately or in combination with other factors. The causes we list need not be "necessary" ones for the outcome to occur, or "sufficient" to produce the outcome. They may be causes that might be described (if we wished to use such terms) as "predisposing," "enabling," "precipitating," "reinforcing," "concomitant," or "intermediate." Any factor whose modification may be expected to modify the frequency or quality of another may be regarded as a causal factor (see Note A15–1).

There is, of course, no "correct answer" to *Question A14–3.* Your list of possible explanations for the ethnic difference in gastroenteritis may (inter alia) include differences in infant feeding practices, differences in nutritional status, differences in the hygiene of foodstuffs or food utensils, and differences in hand-washing practices. You may have thought of more elaborate explanations, such as the possibility that differences in family size may lead to differences between ethnic groups in the amount of contact with other children, resulting in differences in the incidence of respiratory infections, and, as a consequence, differences in susceptibility to gastroenteritis. You may have also included factors (such as the way that mild diarrhea is treated at home) that may affect the severity rather than the occurrence of illness, on the grounds that differences in the reported incidence rate may be due to differences in the proportion of cases who have subclinical and mild illnesses that are not detected or do not meet the criteria required for definition as a "case."

TESTING CAUSAL EXPLANATIONS

The basic way of testing a causal explanation is to seek new facts and see whether these fit in with what we might expect to find if the explanation was correct. If they do not, the explanation can be discarded; if they do, they provide supportive evidence for the explanation. This procedure may not really "prove" causality; but if enough new facts that could refute the explanation are sought and they persistently uphold a causal interpretation, they can constitute proof that is strong enough to provide a basis for decision and action.

Testing is best done by first formulating refutable predictions—statements of what findings may be expected if the causal explanation is correct. These statements are specific *"research hypotheses,"* which can then be tested by seeking the appropriate empirical facts. They are generally positive declarations, and not the "null hypotheses" required for tests of statistical significance (see Note A15–2).

To be useful, the hypothesis must be testable. It must be formulated in very specific terms, leaving no doubt as to what information is needed to test it; and obtaining this information must be feasible.

EXERCISE A15

Question A15–1

In the last exercise you suggested a number of possible explanations for the difference between Easterners and Westerners in the incidence of gastroenteritis in children in Zepiville. Now choose one of these explanations for testing (remember Occam's razor).

Question A15–2

Formulate an appropriate specific hypothesis (or hypotheses) that will test the explanation you have chosen.

Question A15–3

Construct a skeleton table (or tables) to accommodate the information you require for this purpose.

NOTES

A15–1. A causal association may be defined as an association between two categories of events in which a change in the frequency or quality of one is observed to follow alteration in the other. In certain instances the possibility of alteration may be presumed and a presumptive classification of an association as causal may be justified. (MacMahon et al., 1960)

In medicine and public health, it would appear reasonable to adopt a pragmatic concept of causality. A causal relationship would be recognized to exist whenever evidence indicates that the factors form part of a complex of circumstances that increases the probability of occurrence of a disease and that a diminution of one or more of these factors decreases the frequency of that disease. (Lilienfeld and Lilienfeld, 1980, p. 295)

A15–2. Statistical testing requires a *null hypothesis*, which is a negative declaration such as: "There is no correlation between birth weight and the incidence of gastroenteritis," or "There is no positive correlation between birth weight and the incidence of gastroenteritis." The test indicates whether we can confidently reject this null hypothesis. What we have called the research hypothesis (e.g., "There *is* a correlation" or "There *is* a positive correlation") is generally what statisticians call *"the alternative to the null hypothesis."* The precise formulation of the null hypothesis and its alternative depends on the kind of data available and the kind of statistical test used.

Unit
A16

TESTING CAUSAL EXPLANATIONS
(CONTINUED)

In accordance with Occam's razor, the explanation chosen for examination should preferably be a likely one that, if true, would go a long way toward explaining the phenomenon we are studying (the ethnic difference in gastroenteritis incidence). It should also be a testable one. There is little point in selecting an explanation for testing—however cogent the reasons—if the information required for this purpose cannot be obtained. The explanation you chose in your answer to *Question A15–1* should meet these requirements.

Appraise your formulation of specific hypotheses (*Question A15–2*) by seeing whether the following criteria are satisfied:

- The hypothesis should be one that can meet its purpose; can observed facts refute the causal explanation?

- The hypothesis should be stated in clear, operational terms, so that there is no doubt as to what information is needed for testing it.

- Collection of the required information should be practicable.

As an illustration, suppose that the explanation selected for testing is that a difference in infant feeding practices caused the ethnic difference in gastroenteritis incidence. In phrasing a specific hypothesis for testing, we would start by eliminating the word "caused." Except maybe in strictly experimental situations, it is not possible to test hypotheses containing such words as "produces," "causes," "results in," "influences," "reduces," "increases," or "affects." These are useful terms when we draw inferences or consider possible explanations for findings, but when we formulate specific hypotheses for testing, we should rather speak of associations (positive or negative), differences, and changes—for which empirical evidence may be available.

We might accordingly decide to test the hypotheses (a) that ethnic

group is associated with infant feeding practices in this population, or
(b) that infant feeding practices are associated with the occurrence of
gastroenteritis. Alternatively, our hypothesis might be that if differences
in infant feeding practices are controlled in the analysis, the difference
between Easterners and Westerners in the incidence of gastroenteritis
will be lessened. If any of these statements turns out to be untrue, we
can reject our causal explanation.

   These hypotheses are useful formulations but are not really specific
enough to be operational: they do not tell us precisely what information
we require. For example, what exactly is meant by "infant feeding practices"? Also, do we want information about all children, or about samples of children of different ethnic groups, or with different feeding
histories or different experience of acute gastroenteritis? How do age
and other variables enter into the hypotheses? and so forth. We might,
for example, make the hypothesis more specific by postulating that differences in the mean duration of lactation and the mean age of introduction of fruit juices, cereals, eggs, and other specified food items will be
found when Eastern children are compared with Western children; or
our hypothesis might be that such differences will be found when children with two or more episodes of gastroenteritis in their third year of
life are compared with age-matched controls with no episodes of the
illness in their third year. We might sharpen these hypotheses by stating
the direction of the expected differences.

   If the hypotheses you drafted do not meet the criteria listed above,
you may wish to try your hand again.

   Skeleton tables can be properly constructed only if decisions have
been made about the information to be collected. In answering *Question
A15–3*, you may have found that constructing the tables helped you to
clarify your thinking about the formulation of hypotheses. Appraise the
table by asking whether the figures (when they are entered) will enable
you to test your hypothesis, and whether the requirements for table
construction (see Unit A12) are satisfied.

   We will return to the topic of causality and its appraisal in Section E.

BASIC PROCEDURE FOR APPRAISAL OF DATA

As we may be in danger of losing sight of the wood for the trees, it will
probably be helpful if we now review the basic procedure for the
appraisal of data. This will bring together the highlights of what we have
done and discussed so far. This review includes references to the units
in which the topics were dealt with, so that you can refer to them if
necessary.

When we examine a table or graph, or a more substantial body of data, we should consider three questions:

- What are the facts?

- What are the possible explanations?

- What additional information is required, for its own sake or to test these explanations?

Usually all three of these questions are asked, but sometimes the second or third or both are omitted. We may need to know nothing but the facts themselves and be uninterested in explanations, or we may be able to draw simple inferences from the facts—for example, about the individual's risk (Unit A7)—that require no testing.

Figure A16 emphasizes the cyclic nature of the process of data appraisal.

1. What Are the Facts?

To answer this question, we must first ensure that we know what the numbers represent and how they were obtained or calculated (Unit A2). If the data are tabulated, we should carefully examine and compare the rows and columns of figures (Unit A7). We should not regard inferences as facts. We will generally need to summarize the findings; for this purpose we may have to calculate rates (Unit A6), percentages, or other summary statistics, and it may be helpful to draw a diagram (Unit A4). We should see whether there are associations between variables (Units A9 and A10). If so, we should summarize the features of the associations

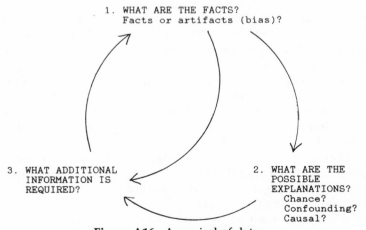

Figure A16. Appraisal of data.

not only in qualitative terms (direction, linearity, monotonicity), but in quantitative ones, using suitable measures of their strength (such as the difference between rates or proportions, or the ratio of rates or proportions). The data may tell us whether associations are consistent, or whether they differ in different strata.

Before or immediately after determining what the findings are, we should consider the possibility that shortcomings in the methods of gathering the data may have produced distortions. The findings may be biased (Note A16–1), and the ostensible facts may not be true ones (Unit A5). Apparent associations, or their absence, may be artifactual rather than actual. We may need to seek additional information that will enable us to decide whether these problems exist, and whether and how we can make allowance for them. The better our understanding of the basic techniques of study design and data collection (Note A16–2), the more likely we are to detect possible artifacts.

2. What Are the Possible Explanations?

Explanations of four kinds should be considered:

- artifactual effects (see above)
- chance occurrence
- confounding (Units A10 and A11)
- causal explanations (Unit A15)

We may be concerned with explaining the facts we have just observed, or facts observed previously as well. In considering possible explanations, we should take account of what we already know, as well as of the facts we have just observed.

A test of statistical significance may be needed to enable us to decide whether we can safely regard the finding as nonfortuitous (Unit A5). Sometimes simple inspection of the data (the "eye test") will enable us to make this decision.

We should list possible confounders that may have affected the associations that interest us. The variables to be considered as possible confounders are those that we know or suspect to be causally related to the disease or other dependent variable, and that are also related to (but not determined by) the other variable involved in the association (see Fig. A10–2). The confounding effect can be important only if the confounder is strongly associated with the other variables. The "universal variables" (age, sex, social class, etc.) are usually candidates for consideration as possible confounders (Unit A11).

Causal explanations can be given serious attention only when we have decided that we can safely ignore the possibility that the association is artifactual, due to chance, or distorted by confounding. We can then consider likely causal explanations (using an appropriate epidemiological model to help us if we wish), select the one we want to test, and frame a hypothesis for testing.

3. What Additional Information Is Required?

If we suspect distortions due to flawed methods, we may need extra information about how the data were obtained and the accuracy of the methods used. (We will return to this topic in later exercises.)

If confounding is suspected, we may require new data that will enable us to detect its presence and control its effects, using stratification (Unit A11) or other procedures.

To appraise causal explanations, we will require whatever data are needed to test specific hypotheses.

We may also be interested in additional information for other purposes, not to test explanations for the facts we have, but to add in other ways to our understanding of the phenomenon we are studying. We may be interested in knowing whether an association is consistent in different categories of people or in different circumstances: is there effect modification (Units A11 and A13)? Or we may think that refinement of variables (Unit A12) may give us useful new knowledge; or we may be led by association of ideas to an interest in information about other variables.

New information may serve more than one purpose. Elaborating an association by stratification, for example, may reveal effect modification as well as testing the possibility that a variable is a confounder or an intervening cause (Units A12 and A14).

Whatever new information we require, we should be able to explain precisely why we want it.

Constructing a skeleton table (Unit A12) will often assist us to crystallize our thoughts about the additional data needed.

EXERCISE A16

This simple exercise, the last in this series, deals with the *uses* of epidemiological data. We now go to another town, where we find that the incidence of acute gastroenteritis is much higher than in the other places we have visited. We will leave the town nameless, so as not to upset the residents.

Question A16–1

We learn that the annual incidence rate (persons) in children aged 0–4 in this town is 60 per 100. What are the possible uses that can be made of this information?

Question A16–2

We also learn that the rate differs in the two ethnic groups. It is 90 per
100 in Easterners and 30 per 100 in Westerners. What are the possible
uses of this additional information?

Question A16–3

If the ethnic difference disappears when social class is controlled in the
analysis, how would this alter your answer (to Question A16–2) about
the possible uses of the information that the rate differs in the two ethnic
groups?

Question A16–4

Suppose that stratification reveals that the ethnic difference in incidence
is not attributable to confounding by social class, but is *modified* by social
class. How would this affect the use of the data?

NOTES

A16–1. *"Bias.* Any effect at any stage of investigation or inference
tending to produce results that depart systematically from the
true values . . . The term 'bias' does not necessarily carry an
imputation of prejudice or other subjective factor, such as the
experimenter's desire for a particular outcome. . ."—*A Dictionary of Epidemiology* (Last, 1983). In this definition, "systematically" means "in a specific direction," for example, in the
direction of a higher value than the true one.

A16–2. Investigative methods are discussed briefly in most epidemiology textbooks, and more fully by Abramson (1990) and Holland et al. (1991).

Unit

A17

USES OF EPIDEMIOLOGICAL DATA

Epidemiological data may be used for a variety of purposes (Note A17–1), depending on the interests of the user. Users fall into three main categories: First, in instances where the data relate to a defined community or population, there are users who have a practical concern with the specific community. These include practitioners of public health and community medicine, planners and administrators, physicians and other health professionals, community leaders, and citizens and others with a special interest in the health status or health care of the community. They may be interested in health and health care at the community level, or they may have a responsibility for the care of individuals who belong to the community; or they may be practitioners of community-oriented primary care (Note A17–2), who are concerned with health care at both the community and individual levels.

Second, there are other "pragmatic" users of epidemiological findings, who have no special concern with the community or sample that was studied, but wish to take what can be learned from the data and apply it in a practical way in their own work, wherever it is. They include practitioners of public health and community medicine, administrators, and others who are interested in health care on a broad scale, as well as physicians and other professionals who provide care for individual patients.

Third, there are users whose basic interest is in "research," who seek knowledge of general interest, without reference to a special local situation or immediate practical applications. This may relate to etiological processes, the natural history of diseases, growth and development, and other topics.

To this list we may add people who use epidemiological data for teaching and learning purposes. The same user may of course fall into more than one category.

The information on the incidence of gastroenteritis in a specific town

75

(*Question A16–1*) may thus have a variety of uses. It is of obvious interest
to those who have a specific concern with the town. It becomes part of a
community diagnosis that provides a factual basis for decisions on the
planning and provision of health care. The incidence rate is a measure of
the magnitude of the problem, and may help to determine what importance should be attached to the disease, and what priority it should be
given in relation to other problems: does it warrant further investigation, and should intervention be undertaken? The rate indicates the
extent of the need for primary and secondary preventive activities (Note
A17–3). It may also be used as an indicator of the effectiveness (or
ineffectiveness) with which the existing health services prevent the disease. If a decision is made to develop an active program, the present
level of the rate may be used to determine a practical target for primary
prevention: to what level is it hoped to reduce the rate within the first
year or the first five years of the program? Knowledge of the incidence
may help in the design of a detailed operational plan: what resources
will be needed, in terms of time or manpower, oral rehydration salts,
antibiotics, etc.? The incidence rate also provides a baseline for the measurement of change, and hence for evaluating the effectiveness of future
efforts in primary prevention.

For physicians, workers in maternal and child health services, and
others who provide care at the individual level in the town, the incidence rate provides an estimate of individual risk. Children aged 0–4
have a 60% risk of developing acute gastroenteritis each year. This
knowledge may well influence the care and counseling that are given,
both in health and in illness.

The incidence rate in this town is unlikely to be of practical interest to
practitioners elsewhere, unless they have good reason to believe that
their own population is so similar that the findings can validly be
applied to it.

Finally, there is a slim possibility that the incidence rate in this town
may be of interest to researchers who, by making comparisons with the
rates in other populations, may develop interesting new hypotheses to
explain the differences.

For users interested in this town, the information about the ethnic
difference in incidence (*Question A16–2*) amplifies the community diagnosis. It identifies a population group at especially high risk, and may
lead to decisions about the allocation of resources and concentration of
attention on a high-risk target group. The ethnic difference may also
provide clues to etiology, possibly leading to a better understanding of
the major causes of the disease in this town, so that suitable strategies
and procedures can be selected, and the disease can be more effectively
prevented.

For the clinician practicing in the town, the extra information provides a better way of identifying individual children who are at high risk, so that he or she can give them the preventive care they deserve.

For the researcher, there is a possibility (although maybe a slim one) that an exploration of the ethnic difference in incidence may yield new knowledge about etiology, not relevant to this town only.

Pending these discoveries, the only value the ethnic difference in this town is likely to have for practitioners elsewhere is that it may lead them to an interest in the possibility that similar differences may exist in their own populations.

The information that the ethnic difference is attributable to confounding by social class (*Question A16–3*) need *not* affect the use of ethnic group as an indicator of risk, at either the population or the individual level. Whatever the reason for the ethnic difference in incidence, this difference remains a fact. Easterners are at higher risk, even if this association is not due to ethnic factors themselves but rather to interrelationships with social class. When exploring the causes of gastroenteritis, however, we need no longer consider causes that are specifically connected with ethnicity. The ethnic difference provides no clues to etiology. The social class difference, however, may do so.

The information that the ethnic difference in incidence varies in different social classes (*Question A16–4*) brings two important benefits. First, it can sharpen the estimates of risk. The stratified data provide us with a specific incidence rate—and hence an estimate of individual risk—for each combination of ethnic group and social class. We now have a more effective way of identifying groups and individuals who are at special risk. Second, comparisons of the incidence rates for different combinations of these variables, and examination of the possible reasons, may lead us to a better understanding of causal factors.

NOTES

A17–1. In his book *Uses of Epidemiology*, Morris (1975) describes these uses under seven chapter headings: "Historical study," "Community diagnosis: community health," "Working of health services," "Individual chances and risks," "Identification of syndromes," "Completing the clinical picture," and "In search of causes." Specific uses that are discussed in detail in various monographs include: applications in health policy and planning (Ibrahim, 1985; Knox, 1979); community medicine (Kark, 1974); applications in clinical medicine (Fletcher et al., 1982; Roberts, 1977; Sackett et al., 1985; Wright and MacAdam, 1979); and epidemiologic research (Kelsey et al., 1986; Kleinbaum et al., 1982; Miettinen, 1985).

A17–2. Community-oriented primary care (COPC) combines two ele-
         ments, the health care of individuals in the community and the
         health care of the community as a whole, in a single integrated
         practice (Kark, 1981; Connor and Mullan, 1983; Kark and
         Abramson, 1983; Kark and Kark, 1983; Nutting, 1987). Physi-
         cians and other clinical workers are responsible both for indi-
         vidual care and for programs that deal in a systematic way with
         the community's main health problems. Epidemiologic data
         provide the basis for the planning, implementation, monitor-
         ing, and evaluation of these programs (Abramson et al., 1983;
         Abramson, 1990).

A17–3. *"Prevention.* The goals of medicine are to promote health, to
         preserve health, to restore health when it is impaired, and to
         minimize suffering and distress. These goals are embodied in
         the word 'prevention' . . ."—*A Dictionary of Epidemiology*
         (Last, 1983). A distinction is usually made between different
         "levels" of prevention; these do not have universally agreed
         definitions, and their boundaries are not clear-cut. Primary,
         secondary, and tertiary prevention should not be confused
         with primary, secondary, and tertiary care. *Primary prevention*
         refers to the promotion of health (e.g., by improving nutri-
         tional status, physical fitness, and emotional well-being and by
         making the environment salubrious), and to the prevention of
         specific disorders (e.g., by immunization). *Secondary prevention*
         refers to the early detection of diseases and other departures
         from good health, and to prompt and effective intervention
         to correct them. *Tertiary prevention* refers to the avoidance or
         reduction of complications, impairments, disability, and suf-
         fering caused by existing (irremediable) disorders, and to the
         promotion of the patient's adjustment to such conditions
         (sometimes termed *quaternary prevention*).

Unit A18

TEST YOURSELF (A)

Now that you have completed this series of exercises, you should be able to do everything included in the following list. Go through the list carefully. If there is anything you think you may not be able to do, return to the relevant unit, which is indicated in parentheses.

You should be able to do the following:

- Describe, and use, the basic procedure for appraising data (A16).

- Determine and summarize the facts shown by a table (A2, A7).

- Determine the facts shown by line diagrams that use (a) arithmetic and (b) logarithmic scales (A4).

- State what condition must be met if graphs are to be used for comparing rates of change (A4).

- Explain the difference between a bar diagram and a histogram (A4).

- Draw

  a line diagram using an arithmetic scale (A3).
  a line diagram using a logarithmic scale (Note A3–2).
  a bar diagram (A4).
  a histogram (A4).
  a pie chart (A4).
  a frequency polygon (A4).

- Explain how graphs can deceive (A4).

- Formulate possible explanations for the facts shown in a table (A5, A11, A14, A16).

- State what criteria should be used in choosing an explanation for testing (A5, A16).

- Construct a skeleton table (A12).

79

- Explain what is meant by

  an association (A9, A10).
  a dependent variable (Note A3–1).
  positive and negative (inverse) associations (A9).
  an "ecological" association (A10).
  an artifactual association (A5).

- Calculate absolute and relative differences (A2).

- Compare the uses of absolute and relative differences (A3).

- Specify two ways of measuring the strength of an association (A16).

- Explain (in general terms)

  when and why statistical significance tests are done (A5).
  what is meant by a null hypothesis (Note A15–2).
  what is meant by "the alternative to the null hypothesis" (Note A15–2).
  the difference between inductive and deductive reasoning (A6).

- Explain what is meant by elaboration of an association (A11).

- Use stratification to elaborate an association (A11).

- State what new information may be provided by stratification (A13, A14).

- Explain (in general terms) what is meant by confounding (A10).

- State what effects confounding may have on an association (A10).

- Explain how to identify possible confounders (A10).

- Detect confounding (A11).

- Describe at least two methods of controlling for confounding (A11).

- Explain what is meant by effect modification (A11).

- Explain what is meant by interaction between variables (A13).

- Detect effect modification (A11, A13).

- Explain the value of detecting effect modification (A13, A17).

- Explain what is meant by

  a causal relationship (Note A15–1).
  an intermediate or intervening cause (A14).

- Describe two epidemiological models of causal relationships (A15).

- Test a causal explanation (A15, A16).

- Formulate a specific research hypothesis (A–17, A–18).

- State the criteria that should be met by a specific research hypothesis (A16).

- Explain

  what is meant by a rate (A6).
  why comparisons should be based on rates rather than on absolute numbers of cases (A15).
  the difference between crude and specific rates (A8).
  the difference between an incidence rate (spells) and an incidence rate (persons) (A6).

- Calculate

  an incidence rate (A6).
  an age-specific incidence rate (A8).
  a weighted mean (Note A7).

- Explain what is meant by

  risk (Note A6).
  bias (Note A16–1).
  "universal variables" (A11).
  statistical dependence (A9).
  refinement of variables (A12).
  Occam's razor (A4).
  monotonicity (Note A2–1).
  primary, secondary, and tertiary prevention (Note A17–3).
  community-oriented primary care (Note A17–3).

- State the main uses of epidemiological data (A17).

- State how epidemiological findings can be used for estimating individual risk (A7, A17).

When you feel that you have nothing more to learn from Section A take a (brief) rest, and proceed to Section B.

SECTION
B

Rates and Other Measures

"Can you do Addition?" the White Queen asked. "What's one and one and one and one and one and one and one and one and one and one?"

"I don't know," said Alice. "I lost count."

(Carroll, 1872)

Unit
B1

INTRODUCTION

Section B deals with rates and other simple summary measures that express the amount of a disease or other characteristic in a group or population. Its purposes are to ensure that you will be able to make sense of these measures when you encounter them, and use them to summarize your own data. The main topics are

- how rates of different kinds are calculated

- the questions to be asked if we want to know exactly what information a rate gives us

- sources of bias

- the uses to which rates, averages, and other measures may be put by practitioners of public health and community medicine, clinicians, and researchers

We will start with prevalence rates, and will then deal with incidence rates, odds, odds ratios, averages, and other measures, and with standardized rates and the pros and cons of their use for detecting and controlling confounding effects.

Real data are used in these and most subsequent exercises. If imaginary numbers are used or the facts have been modified so as to simplify the exercise, you will be told so.

WHAT IS A RATE?

The term "rate" is commonly used for a wide variety of measures of the frequency of a disease or other phenomenon, in relation to the size of a population or some other quantity. Most rates are prevalence rates, which measure the presence of a disease or other attribute in a group or population, or incidence rates, which measure the occurrence of new cases of a disease or other events. All rates are ratios, calculated by dividing a numerator (e.g., the number of deaths in a given period) by a denominator (e.g., the average population during this period). The result is usually multiplied by 100, 1,000, or some other convenient figure, and expressed as a rate per 100, per 1,000, and so on. Some rates are proportions; that is, the numerator is contained within the denominator.

The correct use of the term "rate" has unfortunately become controversial. For simplicity's sake we will ignore this controversy, and will use the term "rate" for all measures that are commonly called rates, even in instances where some epidemiologists regard this as incorrect; alternative terms will be mentioned, so that you can use them if you prefer. Some authors restrict the use of the term to ratios that reflect the relative changes (actual or potential) in two quantities, and others restrict it further, to ratios that represent change over time; in this usage, a prevalence rate is not a "true" rate.

PREVALENCE RATES

A prevalence rate tells us what proportion of individuals have a given disease or other attribute at a given time. It is a measure of what *exists*, unlike an incidence rate, which is a measure of what *happens*.

A *point prevalence rate* refers to a specific point of time. The number of people with the disease at that time is divided by the size of the group or population. The numerator contains people who developed the disease before the specified point of time, and were alive and in the population at that time. The rate depends on the incidence rate and the mean duration of the disease, until recovery or death.

A *period prevalence rate* is the proportion of the population with the disease at any time during a specified period (usually a year). The numerator comprises people who developed the disease before and during the period, including those who left, died, or recovered during the period.

A *lifetime prevalence rate* is the proportion of people who have had the disease at any time in their lives, generally until a specified age, sometimes until death.

When used without qualification, "prevalence" usually refers to point prevalence.

EXERCISE B1

Question B1–1

(Skip this question if you are quite sure you know how to calculate prevalence and incidence rates.)

A health center needs information for use in planning a home care program for people who are too disabled to leave their houses: for example, how many cases can be expected to be under care at any given time, how many new cases can be expected each year, and what is the total number of cases that will be treated during a year? The following information is obtained from an agency that has a program in a similar neighborhood. At the beginning of 1987 the population size was 24,000, and at the end of the year it was 26,000. At the beginning of 1987 there were 96 house-bound patients; 20 of these died during 1987, and 4 moved elsewhere. Another 40 people became housebound during 1987, and 8 of them died during the year. (The actual numbers have been altered.)

Calculate the point prevalence rates at the beginning and end of 1987, the period prevalence rate in 1987, and the incidence rate in 1987.

Question B1–2

A survey provides point prevalence rates of inguinal hernia in men of different ages. Are these lifetime prevalence rates?

Question B1–3

The prevalence of congenital anomalies was measured in a follow-up study of all the children born alive in a defined place and period. The numerator of the rate included children whose anomalies were detected at birth or only later in their lives, or (in some cases) only when they died. The denominator consisted of all the children studied. Is this a point or period prevalence rate?

Question B1–4

In a health survey in a city neighborhood (Note B1), 52 of 431 people aged 65 or more were found to have congestive heart failure, yielding a prevalence rate of 12.1 per 100. Each person was examined once, but the examinations were staggered over a period of two years. Is the rate a point or period prevalence rate? Is it a crude or age-specific rate?

Question B1–5

In recent years there has been a marked increase in the prevalence rate of pulmonary tuberculosis in the imaginary Pepi region, and a marked decrease in the equally imaginary Quepi region. Assuming that these are true changes (not artifacts due to changes in case-finding, migration, etc., and not caused by confounding), what are the main explanations you would consider, with special reference to changes in the effectiveness of health care?

Question B1–6

In the survey referred to in Question B1–4, the prevalence rate of congestive heart failure at 65–74 years was 6.6 per 100, and at ≥75 years of age it was 23.9 per 100. What is the probable explanation for this positive association with age?

Question B1–7

According to the U.S. National Health Interview Survey, in 1985 the prevalence rate of diabetes per 1,000 was 109 in the 65–74 age group and 95 in the ≥75 age group (Moss and Parsons, 1986). What are the possible explanations for this negative association with age?

This is a continuing nationwide health survey based on interviews. The sample (which included over 90,000 people in 1985) is representative of the total civilian noninstitutionalized population of the United States.

NOTE

B1.   The figures refer to the presence of "probable congestive heart failure," based on the presence of characteristic symptoms and physical signs (Kark et al., 1979; Gofin et al., 1981).

U n i t
B2

PREVALENCE RATES (CONTINUED)

In answer to *Question B1–1*, the point prevalence rate per 1,000 was
(96/24,000) × 1,000, or 4, at the beginning of 1987 and [(96 + 40 − 20 − 4
− 8)/26,000] × 1,000, or 4, at the end of the year also. The denominator
usually used for period prevalence and ordinary incidence rates is the
average population during the period; the midyear population may be
used, or the numbers at the beginning and end may be averaged. The
average population was (24,000 + 26,000)/2, or 25,000. The period prevalence rate per 1,000 was therefore (96 + 40)/25,000, or 5.44, and the
incidence rate was 40/25,000, or 1.6.

Point prevalence rates of inguinal hernia (*Question B1–2*) can be regarded as lifetime prevalence rates only in populations where hernias
are never repaired. The numerator of a lifetime prevalence rate should
include people who report hernia operations or (preferably) have her-
niorrhaphy scars.

In *Question B1–3*, the rate of congenital anomalies may be regarded as
a point prevalence rate, the point of time being the individual's moment
of birth—a single point of time for each individual, although the calendar time differs. The anomalies are present at birth but come to light
only later. Fuller ascertainment of cases requires long-term follow-up.

A rate based on staggered examinations (*Question B1–4*) may also be
regarded as a point prevalence rate—a single point of time for each
individual, although the calendar time differs. A rate whose numerator
and denominator refer to the same age group is, of course, an age-
specific rate.

The prevalence of a disease depends on incidence and on the mean
duration of the disease. The rise in the prevalence of tuberculosis in the
Pepi region (*Question B1–5*) can therefore be attributed to a rise in incidence, an increase in mean duration, or both these factors. The increase
in mean duration might be due to a decrease in the chance of recovery or
to a decrease in the risk of dying. Conversely, the declining prevalence

in the Quepi region may be due to a drop in incidence, an improved chance of healing, or an increased risk of dying. Improved health care may reduce prevalence (fewer new cases, more cures) or may raise it (fewer deaths). A worsening of health care may raise prevalence (more new cases, fewer cures) or may reduce it (more deaths). Hence no clear conclusion can be reached about the effectiveness of health care in the two regions.

The most obvious explanation for a rise with age in the prevalence of a disease like congestive heart failure (*Question B1–6*) is the continued accrual of new cases. If the incidence of new cases exceeds the loss of old ones by death or (less likely) recovery, cases accumulate and the prevalence rate rises.

Question B1–7 deals with the paradoxical finding that the prevalence of diabetes was found to be lower at >75 years than at 65–74 years, although diabetes is regarded as a condition that does not disappear. There are a number of possible explanations for this negative association with age, apart from the possibility that it happened by chance in this particular sample. First, the data were obtained by interviewing, and it is possible that there was more underreporting of diabetes in the older age group. Second, the sample was drawn from people living at home. If people with diabetes (which is often associated with other disorders) are more prone to be in an institution, this will mean that people living at home have a relatively low prevalence rate; and this effect is likely to be most marked in those aged ≥75, whose risk of being in an institution is highest. Third—and this is the most obvious explanation for a lower prevalence of a long-term disease in older people—the disease may reduce the chance of surviving to an advanced age. This selective survival will tend to reduce the rate in older people. The rate may become lower than in younger people, unless the loss of cases is counterbalanced by an accrual of new ones. Furthermore, the incidence of new cases may decline in old age; most of the people who were "going to get" the disease may have got it when they were younger.

Fourth, there may be *confounding*. Especially in changing populations, people of different ages may differ in their ethnic group, social class, or other characteristics, and these differences may confound associations with age. And fifth, it must be remembered that the age groups represent the survivors of separate birth cohorts (people born at different times), who have lived through different experiences and may have been exposed to different risks. Age-related variation in disease prevalence may be expressions of this *birth cohort effect* (Note B2): older people in the United States may have been less exposed in their earlier lives to whatever environmental or behavioral factors contribute to the development of diabetes, and this—rather than their more advanced age—may account for their lower prevalence of diabetes.

The difference observed in the U.S. National Health Survey was in

fact not statistically significant. We need not not give serious consideration to any of the above explanations, unless we obtain confirmatory
evidence of the association in other studies or other samples.

EXERCISE B2

When we are presented with a prevalence rate, we must make sure we
know exactly what the figure represents ("What are the facts?"), and
appraise its accuracy, before making use of it.

In a paper entitled "Varicose veins and chronic venous insufficiency
in Brazil: prevalence among 1755 inhabitants of a country town" (Maffei
et al., 1986), we are told that the prevalence rate of varicose veins in
adults was 47.6%.

List the questions that you would want answered in order to ensure
that you know exactly what information you have been given.

NOTE

B2.   A *cohort effect* or *generation effect* refers to "variation in health status
      that arises from the different causal factors to which each birth
      cohort in the population is exposed as the environment and society
      change. Each consecutive birth cohort is exposed to a unique en-
      vironment that coincides with its life span"—*A Dictionary of Epi-
      demiology* (Last, 1983).

Unit B3

QUESTIONS ABOUT A RATE

To know what information a rate provides (*Exercise B2*), we need to ask four basic questions: What kind of rate is it? What is it a rate *of*? To what population or group does it refer? And, how was the information obtained? (These questions may be asked about any kind of rate, not only prevalence rates.)

1. What Kind of Rate Is It?

We might, for example, want to know whether it is a point or period prevalence rate.

2. Of What Is It a Rate?

How was the disease (or other attribute) defined? Was the same definition used in all instances? Most diseases exhibit a wide spectrum of abnormality, ranging from extremely mild to severe conditions, and different cutting-points might be used for deciding whether the disease is present or absent. Or, as often happens, does nobody know what the diagnostic criteria were? This is especially likely to occur if the diagnostic information is obtained secondhand, from clinical records, or from the subjects themselves.

3. To What Population or Group Does the Rate Refer?

The population should be defined with respect to *place, time,* and sometimes *personal characteristics.* (Who? Where? When?) In the present instance we have some information about the place (a country town in Brazil), but we do not yet know when the study was done, or what precisely is meant by "adults."

4. How Was the Information Obtained?

Was the whole of the target population or group studied? If only part was studied, how was it selected? (Who were the 1,755 people who were studied?) Was the sample a representative one, chosen by acceptable methods (see Note B3–1)? If not, the rate may be biased (see Note A16). Were many members of the population or sample excluded because they refused, could not be located, or for other reasons? If so, this may have biased the rate. (Is anything known about the characteristics of those who were excluded?) If a sample was studied, how big was it? The smaller it was, the greater the chance that the findings in the sample may differ from those in the population as a whole (sampling variation; see Note B3–2). How was the numerator information obtained? By observation (e.g., clinical or laboratory examinations), or by asking questions, or from documentary sources? If by observation, what methods were used (and were they standardized and tested)? If by asking questions, what was asked, who did the asking, and was a standard wording used? If from documentary sources, what records were used? Whatever methods were used, what is known about their accuracy? To understand what the rate of varicose veins tells us, we need answers to all these questions (and will probably find them if we carefully peruse the paper describing the survey). In some instances we may also need to ask how information was obtained about the size of the denominator.

EXERCISE B3

In this exercise you are asked to consider possible sources of inaccuracy in prevalence studies. In each of the following instances, suggest one possible source of bias, and (if you can) specify the direction of the bias. ("Bias" was defined in Note A16.)

1. What bias would you suspect in a survey of the prevalence of disability in the elderly population of a city, based on an investigation of members of old people's clubs?
2. What bias would you suspect in a household survey to determine the prevalence of senile dementia in a city?
3. What bias would you suspect in a survey of the prevalence of various electrocardiographic abnormalities after an acute myocardial infarction, conducted by examining all the patients treated for this condition in hospitals in the city?
4. What bias would you suspect in a community survey of mental illness in which 30% of the study sample refused to be interviewed or examined?
5. What bias would you suspect in a survey of the prevalence of

diabetes in a city, based on the use of the question "Has a doctor ever told you that you have diabetes?"

6. What bias would you expect in a survey of the prevalence of drug abuse?

7. What bias would you suspect in a survey of the prevalence of cigarette smoking, based on questions put to people who had been exposed to intensive antismoking education?

8. What bias would you expect in a survey of the prevalence of peptic ulcer, based on questions about the occurrence of typical ulcer pain?

9. What bias would you suspect in a survey of the prevalence of congestive heart failure based on one-time examinations?

10. What bias would you suspect in a survey of the prevalence of hypertension based on one-time measurements of blood pressure?

11. According to the U.S. National Health Interview Survey (see Question B1–7), the prevalence rate of diabetes in people aged 45–64 years was 51.4 per 1,000 in 1985, with a 95% confidence interval of 42.8 to 61.0. Can these findings be applied to the United Kingdom? Do you know what a confidence interval is?

NOTES

B3–1.   A sample selected by *strictly random* methods—that is, by drawing lots or by using tables of random numbers—can be regarded as a representative one. The population may first be divided into groups, and a random sample selected from each group (*stratified random sampling*). The sampling units need not be individuals, but may be households, schools, or other aggregations (*cluster sampling*). A *systematic sample* (e.g., taking every third individual in a list) may often be regarded as equivalent to a random sample. Haphazard methods, not based on strictly random selection or a predetermined system, are sometimes misreported   as   "random,"   but   do   not   guarantee representativeness.

B3–2.   Chance differences may be expected between the findings in different random samples drawn from the same population, and the findings in any specific sample may differ from those in the whole population. This is called *random sampling variation* or, more simply, "sampling variation" or "sampling error."

Unit
B4

SOURCES OF BIAS

Exercise B3 illustrates two kinds of bias: selection bias and information bias. *Selection bias* occurs if the individuals for whom data are available are not representative of the target population (the population we wish to investigate). *Information bias* is caused by shortcomings in the way that information is obtained or handled.

Questions (1) to (4) provide examples of possible selection bias. In (1), old people who are active enough to be members of clubs are not representative of the elderly population, and the prevalence of disability is therefore likely to be underestimated. In (2), people living at home (and not in institutions) are not representative of the elderly population of the city, and the prevalence of senile dementia is probably underestimated. In (3), patients treated in hospital for myocardial infarction are not representative of all patients with this condition, since those with very mild lesions or very severe ones (so serious that there is a strong chance of dying before reaching hospital) will tend to be excluded from the study; the direction of the bias with respect to electrocardiographic abnormalities is difficult to predict. In (4), the high nonresponse rate may well lead to a biased picture of the prevalence of mental illness, but it is difficult to guess the direction of the bias: mentally ill people may have been particularly eager, or particularly reluctant, to participate in the study.

Questions (5) to (10) provide simple illustrations of possible information bias. The use of questions is likely to yield underestimates of the prevalence of diabetes (many people with diabetes do not know they have it), and of drug abuse and smoking, because people tend to give answers they think are socially acceptable; a study in Holland has shown that a question-based survey of alcoholism would miss over half the known problem drinkers (Mulder and Garretsen, 1983). On the other hand, the use of questions is likely to overestimate the prevalence of peptic ulcer, since most people with typical symptoms do not have

ulcers on x-ray. If the definition of congestive heart failure includes
patients who are temporarily in remission, one-time examinations may
yield an underestimate of prevalence. On the other hand, if hypertension is defined as sustained hypertension, one-time measurements of
blood pressure will provide an overestimate of prevalence.

In (11), the prevalence of diabetes was studied in a sample of the
population of the United States, and we have no good reason to believe
that we can apply the findings to the United Kingdom. The confidence
interval (see below) does not help us in this respect.

CONFIDENCE INTERVAL

Because of random sampling variation (see Note B3–2), the findings in a
random sample may not accurately reflect the situation in the target
population from which the sample was drawn. The confidence interval
tells us within what range we can assume the true value in the target
population to lie, with a specified degree of confidence (see Note B4). A
narrower range (for a given degree of confidence) means a more precise
estimate. The larger the sample, the more precise the estimate will be.

In Exercise B3 (11) we are told that the true prevalence rate of diabetes
in people aged 46–64 years in the United States, as measured by the
methods used in the National Health Interview Survey, is probably
between 42.8 per 1,000 (the lower confidence limit) and 61.0 per 1,000
(the upper confidence limit). This interval has a 95% probability of including the true value.

It can be calculated that if a sample four times bigger had been studied, the 95% confidence interval would have been 47.2–56.6 per 1,000. If
a sample had been one-quarter the size, the confidence interval would
have been 33.8–70.0 per 1,000.

Confidence intervals are sometimes used when it is wished to gener-
alize the findings to a broad reference population, even though a random sample of this population was not studied. We are then estimating
what findings might be expected in a hypothetical large population of
which the study population was a random sample. This use of confidence intervals is open to question. In the present instance we have no
reason to assume that the United States is representative of the world,
and it would be wrong to use the confidence interval as an estimate of
the probable prevalence rate in people (of this age) in general.

VALIDITY

Exercise B3 can be used to illustrate the uses of the term "validity" (from
the Latin *validus*, meaning "strong"). The term is used in three main
ways.

First, it may be applied to a method for measuring a specific characteristic. The *validity of a measure* refers to the adequacy with which the
method of measurement does its job; how well does it measure what we
want to study? When we suspected information bias in Exercises B3 (5)
to (10), we were expressing doubt about the validity of the measures.

Second, the term may be applied to a study as whole (*study validity*) or
to the inferences drawn from a study. Inferences about causal associations, for example, are not well-founded if due attention has not been
paid to possible artifacts, chance effects, and confounding; and a study
is not valid if it cannot provide accurate information, or cannot enable
well-founded inferences to be drawn concerning the target population
that was studied. This is sometimes termed the *internal validity of the
study*. A study's validity may be impaired by selection bias, information
bias, uncontrolled confounding, an unduly small sample, or other shortcomings.

Third, the term may be applied to generalizations to a broader reference population, beyond the target population that was studied. This is
the *external validity of the study*. When we doubted that the findings of the
U.S. Health Interview Survey could be applied to the United Kingdom or
to people in general, we were questioning the study's external validity.

EXERCISE B4

In this exercise you are asked to consider the uses of prevalence data.
(You may wish to review Unit A17, which dealt with uses of incidence
data.)

The prevalence of infection with *Schistosoma mansoni*, the parasite that
causes intestinal bilharzia, was investigated in a rural district of Zambia
(Sukwa et al., 1986). A sample of villages was selected (cluster sampling—see Note B3–1), and the parasite's eggs were sought in stool
specimens from the residents of these villages. You may assume that
there was no selection bias and that the methods of study were valid.
The figures shown in Table B4 were calculated from the published
findings.

Question B4–1

How would the facts shown in Table B4 help you if you were a doctor
providing clinical care in this region of Zambia?

Question B4–2

What uses could you make of these facts if you were responsible for
planning and organizing health services in this region? Give considera-

Table B4. Prevalence of *Schistosoma Mansoni* Infection, Zambian Villages, by Age

Age (yr)	Rate per 100*
5–9	66 (59–73)
10–14	80 (72–86)
15–19	75 (61–85)
20–39	69 (60–76)
≥40	62 (54–70)
Total (≥5)	69 (66–73)

*95% confidence intervals shown in parentheses.

tion to the possible use of prevalence data in evaluating the effectiveness of health services.

Question B4–3

Can facts like those shown in the table, or facts on the prevalence of infection in relation to characteristics other than age, be used to identify groups or individuals who have an especially high risk of becoming infected?

Question B4–4

Assuming that we knew very little about the causation of bilharzia, could the prevalence data provide clues to etiology? If we had a similar table for another region of Zambia, showing much lower rates, how would this help? What reservations might you have in making this kind of use of prevalence data?

NOTE

B4. More strictly, the 95% confidence interval is the interval calculated from a random sample by a procedure which, if applied to an infinite number of random samples of the same size, would, in 95% of instances, contain the true value in the population. To unravel this and to learn how to determine a confidence interval, consult a statistics textbook.

Unit
B5

USES OF PREVALENCE DATA

In answer to *Question B4–1*, the prevalence rate of a disease tells a clinician what probability he or she can assign to the presence of the disease in an individual patient, before interviewing and examining that patient. This "pretest probability" can help the clinician decide what diagnoses to explore and what tests to perform. Doctors who are aware that the prevalence rate of *Schistosoma mansoni* is well above 50% (from the age of 5 years) would know that every one of their patients (from the age of 5 years) is more likely than not to have this infection. Thus a physician could decide to do specific diagnostic tests as a routine, or (if treatment is safe) to skip the tests and give specific treatment to all patients. The findings might also lead the clinician to undertake preventive activities.

Prevalence rates like those in Table B4 contribute to the community diagnosis that provides a factual basis for decisions on the planning and provision of health care (*Question B4–2*). They indicate the size of the problem and may help in determining priorities; how much effort should be put into investigating and controlling the problem? Prevalence rates may sometimes pinpoint groups requiring special care; but in our instance the rates in all age groups are so high that there seems little justification for giving special attention to older children, although their rate is especially high. The high rates might lead to a decision to undertake a mass chemotherapy campaign, as well as intensive educational and environmental measures.

The prevalence of a condition that (like bilharzia) can be prevented or cured can be used to measure the effectiveness of health care. If an intervention program is in operation or contemplated, its effectiveness may be monitored by repeated measurements of the prevalence rate. It may be difficult to use prevalence data for the evaluation of recent preventive activities, since the prevalence of a long-term condition may be a reflection of what happened long before. In the present instance, however, the high rate (66%) among children aged 5–9 shows that recent preventive activities have not been effective. It is also obvious there is no effective program for the treatment of bilharzia in this region.

In answer to *Question B4–3*, prevalence is not determined solely by the incidence of new cases, and therefore a prevalence rate (unlike an incidence rate) cannot generally be used as an indicator of risk. Prevalence is determined both by incidence and by the mean duration of the condition. Table B4 shows a higher prevalence rate in older than in younger children, but this may not mean that they are at higher risk of becoming infected. Their higher rate may be due solely to the cumulation of cases, and the lower rates in adults may be due to treatment or spontaneous disappearance of the infection. Prevalence rates can be used to indicate risk only if they reflect incidence, as they may do in short-term diseases. If we found a much higher prevalence of influenza in school A than in school B, we could certainly infer a difference in the risk of developing the disease. With respect to most long-term diseases, the prevalence rate of cases of recent onset may also be a useful indicator of risk.

Differences between prevalence rates can sometimes provide clues to etiology (*Question B4–4*), though they may reflect differences in the duration of the condition as well as the effect of etiological factors. The higher prevalence rate in older children may have no etiological significance. But if we knew that the infection was more prevalent in this region than in another, this might provide us with clues to etiology; but we would have to be certain that the difference was not due to a difference in the effectiveness of treatment.

The chance of finding clues to etiology in a prevalence study of a long-term condition may be limited because of the time that has passed since the initiation of the disease. The causal factors may no longer be present, or may be difficult to investigate. Even if interesting associations *are* found, it may be difficult to study time relationships: for example, did the postulated cause precede the postulated effect? It may be easy to find that the prevalence of diabetes is higher in obese people, but it is not so easy to know whether the obesity preceded the diabetes.

INCIDENCE RATES

An incidence rate describes the frequency of an event in a group or population during a given period. The events that may be measured include the onset of a disease or disability, the occurrence of an episode, recurrence, or complication of a disease, the occurrence of seroconversion or other evidence of infection, admissions to hospital, and visits to doctors. A *mortality rate* (death rate) is an incidence rate that describes the frequency of deaths in a group or population during a given period.

The individuals to whom the event may occur—the "population at risk" or "candidate population"—make up the obvious denominator for an incidence rate. This may be a restricted population. If, for example, we want to measure the incidence of recurrences or deaths after a myocardial infarction, the denominator consists of people who have had an infarction.

There are different ways of calculating incidence rates. The method usually used in a city, region, nation, or other changing population—that is, in which there are births, deaths, and movements in and out—is to divide the number of events during a specified period by the average population size and then multiply the result by 100, 1,000, etc. This rate is usually referred to simply as the incidence rate; to avoid confusion, we will refer to it as the "ordinary" incidence rate. The total population (or, for a specific rate, the total population in a specific stratum) is used as the denominator, even when one is calculating the incidence rate of new cases of a chronic disease, although this denominator includes people who already have the disease and are not "at risk" of getting it. (Can you suggest why a correction is not made? See Note B5–1.)

In a longitudinal study in which all members of a cohort (group) are followed up for a specified period, the incidence rate can be calculated by dividing the number of events by the number of people in the cohort at the outset. If we do a follow-up study of a cohort that contains 2,000 initially disease-free people, and find 100 new cases of a chronic disease during a year, the rate in one year is 100/2,000, or 5 per 100 people. This may be called a *cumulative incidence rate*, since the numerator is the number of new cases that accumulate during a defined period. It is a measure of the individual's risk of incurring the disease during this period. Some epidemiologists prefer not to use the term "rate" for this measure, and call it the "cumulative incidence" or "risk."

Another measure of incidence is the *person-time incidence rate* (also called—among other terms—the "incidence density," "average incidence rate," and "interval incidence density"). It is generally used in follow-up studies in which individuals are "at risk" for different periods. This may happen because members of the cohort cease to be candidates for the event being studied: they may move away, refuse to cooperate, get lost, or die, or the end-point event may occur and they are therefore no longer at risk of its occurrence. Individuals may also enter the study cohort at different times. In a study of the incidence of recurrences, complications or death after a myocardial infarction, each subject may enter the study immediately after the infarction, but at different calendar times, and may be followed up for different periods.

A person-time incidence rate is calculated by dividing the total number of events by the sum total of the subjects' periods at risk, measured in person-time units. Each subject's *period at risk* must be calculated—that is, the length of time from the start of follow-up until withdrawal from follow-up (including withdrawals because of occurrence of the end-point event) or until the end of the study. In our one-year follow-up study of 2,000 people, there were 1,900 who remained disease free. Each of these 1,900 was at risk of developing the chronic disease during a whole year, and contributes one person-year to the denominator. The other 100 were at risk for various periods less than a year, from the outset of the study until the onset of the disease, and each contributes a part of a person-year. A subject who became diseased at mid-year, for example, contributes six person-months, or 0.5 person-years. If the total number of person-years at risk was 1,950, the person-time incidence rate would be 100/1,950, or 5.13 per 100 person-years. This rate is not a proportion. (Why not? See Note B5–2.)

There are actually only two main types of incidence rate: the cumulative incidence rate and the person-time incidence rate. The "ordinary" incidence rate is an estimate of the person-time incidence rate, since the average size of the population at risk during a year is an estimate of the number of person-years of risk during that year.

These two kinds of rate generally have very similar values (see Note B5–3), and usually the only important reason for distinguishing between them is that we may not be able to recognize possible sources of bias unless we know what kind of rate it is. If the rate is very high or the follow-up period is very long, however, the cumulative incidence rate— the measure of risk—may be appreciably lower than the person-time rate. If a measure of risk is required and only a person-time incidence rate is available, a simple formula can generally be used to estimate risk (Note B5–4).

Mortality rates are measured in the same way as other incidence rates: there is the "ordinary" mortality rate, the cumulative mortality rate, and the person-time mortality rate.

EXERCISE B5

Question B5–1

For light relief, consider a highly imaginary army base, where there is a complete change of personnel every three months and the total strength is always 1,000. It is found that 2,000 soldiers incur syphilis each year. This gives an annual incidence rate (persons) of 200%. Is this a satisfactory measure of risk? If not, what measure do you suggest?

Question B5–2

You learn that the incidence rate of gonorrhea in the United States in 1984 was 375 per 100,000 population (National Center for Health Statistics, 1986). What questions would you ask in order to ensure that you know exactly what this figure represents ("What are the facts?")?

NOTES

B5–1.   People who already have a chronic disease are not generally removed from the denominator when an "ordinary" incidence rate is calculated, for two reasons: the data are seldom available; and the correction makes a negligible difference, unless the prior prevalence is higher than it generally is. If the prevalence is 5 per 100, the correction will change the incidence rate by about 5% of its value.

B5–2.   A proportion is a ratio whose numerator is contained in its denominator. The numerator of a person-time incidence rate (the number of events) is not contained in the denominator (person-time).

B5–3.   Person-time incidence rates and cumulative incidence, and the mathematical relationships between them, are explained in detail by Kleinbaum et al. (1982, chap. 6). The cumulative incidence rate during t years is approximately equal to PTI·t if PTI·t is small (say, less than 0.1), where PTI is the incidence rate per person-year. If occurrence of the event we are studying does not remove the subject from the population at risk (e.g., when we measure the incidence of headaches or short spells of a disease), the person-time and cumulative incidence rates are identical. The "ordinary" incidence rate is an estimate of the person-time incidence rate, since the average size of the population at risk during a year is an estimate of the number of person-years of risk during that year. The estimate is a good one if the population did not change much in size or composition during the study period—that is, if individuals who left were replaced by others who were similar to them in their chance of occurrence of disease, death, or whatever other event was measured.

B5–4.   The cumulative incidence rate (risk) can easily be estimated from the person-time incidence rate, provided that the latter rate does not vary during the period we are interested in. The simplest formula is

$$CI = \frac{PTI \cdot t}{(PTI \cdot t/2) + 1}$$

where CI is the cumulative incidence rate during t time units (e.g., years), and PTI is the rate per person-time unit. [Another formula is: $CI = 1 - \exp(-PTI \cdot t)$.] As an example, if PTI = 5.13 per 100 person-years, the estimated CI after one year is

$$\frac{0.0513 \times 1}{(0.0513 \times 1/2) + 1} = 0.05$$

that is, 5 per 100 persons. On the assumption that the PTI remains constant over a five-year period, the estimated CI after five years ($t = 5$) is 22.7 per 100 persons. The reverse formula, for estimating the PTI per person-time unit from the CI after t time units, is

$$PTI = \frac{CI}{(1 - CI/2) \cdot t}$$

Unit
B6

INCIDENCE RATES (CONTINUED)

In *Question B5–1* a new cohort of 1,000 soldiers enters the army camp every three months and is followed up for three months. The simple and obvious way of measuring the risk of incurring syphilis is to calculate the cumulative incidence rate during a three-month stay in the base.

This is easy to do. During a year there are 4,000 soldiers who are followed up for three months, and 2,000 of them contract syphilis. The cumulative incidence rate after three months in the base is therefore 2,000/4,000, or 50 cases per 100 soldiers. This rate, 50%, expresses the individual's risk of developing the disease during three months of service in the base. Our data do not enable us to estimate what the risk would be if soldiers remained in the base for a whole year. It might be anything from 50% to 100%.

The annual incidence rate of 200% is an "ordinary" incidence rate, with the average size of the population used as its denominator. It is therefore an estimate of the person-time incidence rate, and may be expressed as 200 cases per 100 person-years. The person-time incidence rate is not a proportion (see Note B5–2) and may therefore exceed 100%; a rate of 200 per 100 person-years is quite acceptable. We can express this rate in terms of person-months: 200 cases per 100 person-years is the same as 200 cases per 1,200 person-months, or 16.7 cases per 100 person months, or 0.167 case per person-month.

The person-time incidence rate is not a direct measure of risk. When incidence is high, as in the present instance, the person-time incidence and cumulative incidence rates may differ appreciably. If we wish, we can calculate the estimated risk that corresponds to an incidence rate of 200 cases per 100 person-years (using the formula in Note B5–4). But we may hesitate to do this, on the grounds that in this instance the "ordinary" incidence rate is probably not a good estimate of the person-time incidence rate: there were many soldiers who contracted syphilis but remained in the denominator of the rate, although they stopped being at risk. This may have produced an appreciable downward bias of the rate, so that the rate underestimates the true risk. If we nevertheless calculate the risk from this rate (for the computation, see Note B6–1), we will find that the estimated risk of contracting the disease in three months is 40%; this is lower than the true value of 50%.

If you want practice in the calculation of a person-time incidence rate, assume that in each three-monthly batch of 1,000 soldiers there were 250 who contracted the disease after precisely one month—on payday?—and another 250 who did so after precisely two months. Calculate the sum total of the soldiers' periods of exposure to risk, for use as a denominator, and calculate the person-time incidence rate. (For solution, see Note B6–2.)

In answer to *Question B5–2*, the same questions may be asked about an incidence rate as those we previously asked about a prevalence rate (Unit B3): What kind of rate is it? (It may not really be an incidence rate; not everyone knows the difference between incidence and prevalence.) What is it a rate *of*? To what population or group does it refer? And, how was the information obtained? In this instance, there seems no need to ask what kind of rate it is; it is obviously an "ordinary" incidence rate, based on spells of gonorrhea. When the incidence is as low as this, the difference between person-time and cumulative incidence rates is, in any case, negligible. We may be surprised to learn (from a footnote) that this rate refers to the civilian population only; servicemen are excluded. The most important questions are about the numerator: How were the cases identified? How was gonorrhea defined? Were standard diagnostic criteria used? The data are in fact based on reporting of notifiable diseases to State health departments. We can be sure that the rate is an underestimate of the true incidence.

EXERCISE B6

In each of the following instances, state the main possible source of bias. If you can, specify the direction of the suspected bias. (The illustrations are fictional unless a reference is cited.)

1. In a study to determine the incidence of a chronic disease, 150 people were examined at the end of a defined follow-up period. Twelve cases were found, giving a cumulative incidence rate of 8%. Fifty other members of the initial cohort could not be examined, 20 of them because they had died.
2. In a study of a random sample of adults in Los Angeles County, the presence of depression was determined by asking a set of questions (which you may assume were satisfactory for this purpose). The sample included 809 people who were not depressed; the incidence

of depression was measured by interviewing them again after a defined period. Among 729 who were reinterviewed, 83 (11.4%) were found to be depressed; 80 others refused to be interviewed or could not be contacted (Clark et al., 1983).

3. Some children have convulsions when they are feverish. In order to determine what risk these children have of becoming epileptic, a series of children with febrile convulsions who had medical care at a university hospital were followed up for a period of many years. It was found that 40% became epileptic (Ellenberg and Nelson, 1980).

4. In a study of the incidence of headaches and other disorders for which medical care is usually sought only if they are severe, use was made of diaries in which the subjects recorded the symptoms they experienced, day by day for two months.

5. In order to determine the incidence of episodes of asthma in adults, detailed records of illnesses and reasons for absence from work were maintained by all the occupational health services in a city.

6. In order to study the incidence of impotence as a side effect of drug treatment for hypertension, patients were questioned after a year of treatment. They were not told the reason for asking the question.

7. In a similar study, the patients were told the reason for asking the question about impotence.

8. In a third study, in which the patients were not told why they were asked about impotence, two physicians reported very different rates of incidence of this symptom although they had very similar patients and used identical treatment schedules.

9. A two-stage case-finding procedure was used in a study of the incidence of pulmonary tuberculosis. All participants were subjected to mass miniature radiography, and all those with positive results were then given a complete diagnostic work-up. What would you like to know in order to appraise the extent of the possible bias?

10. The annual incidence rate of pulmonary tuberculosis in the Quepi region was similar each year from 1970 to 1984. In 1985, it was five times as high.

11. The annual incidence rate of malaria in the United States decreased steeply between 1946 and 1949. The number of cases reported annually fell from 48,610 in 1946, through 17,317 and 9,797, to 4,239 in 1949 (Mainland, 1964).

12. According to death certificate data, the rate of mortality due to diabetes in the United States in 1984 was 9.5 per 100,000 (National Center for Health Statistics, 1986).

13. According to death certificate data, the death rate for motor vehicle accidents in the United States in 1984 was 19.6 per 100,000 (National Center for Health Statistics, 1986).

14. The incidence rate of road accident injuries in the Emirate of Sharjah was 810 per 100,000 in 1977, according to hospital records. Patients

with these injuries have to be reported to the police, and are therefore specifically identified in the records (Weddell and McDougall,
1981).

15. The incidence rate of road accident injuries in the United States in
1985 was 3.1 per 100 person-years, according to the National Health
Interview Survey (Moss and Parsons, 1986).

NOTES

B6–1.   By use of the formula in Note B5–4, the estimated cumulative
incidence rate in three months ($t = 3$), calculated from the rate of
0.167 per person-month, is $(0.167 \times 3)/[(0.167 \times 3/2) + 1] = 0.4$
$= 40\%$.

B6–2.   In each cohort of 1,000 soldiers, there are 250 who are at risk for
one month (until they contract the disease), 250 who are at risk
for two months, and 500 who are at risk for the full three
months, without developing the disease. Each batch is therefore
exposed to risk for $(250 \times 1) + (250 \times 2) + (500 \times 3) = 2,250$
person-months. This is the denominator. The numerator (the
number of cases) is 500. The rate is therefore 500 per 2,250 person-months $= 0.222$ per person-month. This rate is based on a
follow-up period of three months, and we have no information
whatever about what would happen after a longer period in the
base. If we wish to estimate individual risk, we can safely do so
only for a three-month period. We may say that the rate is 0.67
(i.e., 67%) per three person-months, and use this as a rough
indication of a soldier's risk of incurring syphilis during three
months at the base. Because the rate is high, it would be preferable, however, to calculate the corresponding cumulative incidence rate, which is a more direct measure of risk. The conver-
sion formula (Note B5–4) gives us an estimated cumulative
incidence rate of 0.50 (i.e., 50%).

Unit
B7

BIAS IN INCIDENCE STUDIES

In *Exercise B6*, studies (1) to (4) provide examples of possible selection bias.

Losses to follow-up are a common source of bias. In (1), the incidence rate of 8% is likely to be an underestimate if having the disease increases the chance of dying. We can "play it safe" by calculating an extreme range: what would the rate have been if (a) none of or (b) all of the lost subjects had incurred the disease? In the former instance the rate would have been $12/(150 + 50) = 6\%$, and in the latter $(12 + 50)/(150 + 50) = 31\%$; thus the rate may be between 6% and 31%. This range is so wide (even without allowing for sampling variation) that we might well decide not to use the results. In (2), where the direction of the bias is hard to guess, the possible range is from 10.3% to 20.1% (83/809 to 163/809); on the basis of their knowledge of the nonrespondents' characteristics, the researchers estimated that the true incidence rate was 10.4%.

In (3), the results may have been biased by the fact that the children were a selected group treated at a teaching hospital, which they may have reached because their convulsions were especially severe or frequent. Such children may be particularly likely to become epileptic. For physicians at this hospital, the finding may indeed by a useful prognostic indicator. But the external validity (see Unit B4) of the finding may be questioned; the rate may overestimate the risk of the average child with febrile convulsions. In fact, a literature search revealed 11 other studies of children treated at hospital clinics or specialty referral clinics, showing rates of subsequent epilepsy that ranged from 6% to 42%; whereas in five studies that tried to identify and follow up all children in a clearly defined population who experienced febrile seizures, the epilepsy rates ranged from 1.5% to 4.6%. Ellenberg and Nelson (1980) concluded that their findings are "probably generalizable to other common and frequently benign conditions . . . Clinicians eval-

uating the need for therapeutic intervention should consider that studies from clinic-based populations may overestimate the frequency of
unfavorable sequelae." This kind of bias has been called *referral filter bias*
(Note B7–1).

In a study of symptoms based on diaries (4), there is a strong possibility of selection bias: people who are prepared to maintain diaries of
this kind are not necessarily representative of the general population.
Those who have symptoms and are concerned about their health may be
more willing to cooperate. This is a kind of "volunteer bias." In some
populations, literacy may also be a factor. There is also a possibility of
information bias: there is likely to be underrecording, especially toward
the end of the study period.

In study (5), the incidence of asthma episodes among workers may
not be a valid reflection of their incidence in the total adult population,
since people with troublesome asthma may be less likely to be in
employment. This is sometimes called the "healthy worker effect."

In studies (6) to (15), there is possible information bias.

In (6), impotence is a symptom that people may prefer to keep to
themselves, and underreporting may be suspected. In (7), where subjects were told that impotence was a possible side effect of the treatment
they were getting, the direction of possible bias is difficult to guess. The
patient's response to a question about impotence may be colored by his
global attitude to his treatment. In (8), there is a possibility that the
apparent variation in incidence is due to differences in the way the
physicians questioned their patients: what phrasing they used, what
their manner was, whether or not they suggested that an answer of a
particular kind was expected, and how insistent they were. The results
may reflect the physicians' prior opinions about the hazards of
treatment.

When a screening test is used, as in (9), the possibility must be considered that the test may miss some cases. It would be helpful to know the
validity of the test. In particular, what proportion of cases does it miss?
What is its false negative rate?

In (10) and (11), the sudden change in incidence strongly suggests
that there were changes in case-finding methods or diagnostic criteria.
The rise in tuberculosis incidence may have been due to an organized
effort to detect cases. The striking apparent decline in malaria incidence
in the United States was largely due to a change in diagnostic methods;
certain health authorities started to require demonstration of the malaria
parasite in the blood before accepting a diagnosis of the disease (Mainland, 1964).

Statistics based on death certificates (study 12) usually grossly underestimate the incidence of deaths attributable to diabetes. The reason is
that each death is assigned to a single underlying cause of death, and
deaths are seldom assigned to diabetes if another disease appears in the
certificate, even if the diabetes contributed to this other disease. Mor-

tality rates are two to three times higher in diabetics, but only 10–20% of the death certificates of diabetics assign diabetes as the underlying cause of death. Despite the relatively low mortality rates (according to conventional statistics), diabetes is a leading cause of death in developed countries and many developing countries. "Excess mortality attributable to diabetes has, in the past decade, caused more deaths than all wars combined" (WHO Expert Committee on Diabetes Mellitus, 1980).

Each of the listed methods of studying the incidence of injuries caused by road accidents is likely to yield an underestimate. Death certificates (13) may have little bias as a source of information on fatal injuries; but if we are interested in all injuries caused by road accidents, they clearly provide only a partial picture. If reliance is placed on clinical records (14), only the injuries that received medical care will be ascertained, and then only if there are good records, including a statement of the cause of the injury. When information about accidental injuries is based on questions (15), there is a possibility that mild injuries will not be remembered or reported ("recall bias"); fatal injuries can obviously not be ascertained in this way. As with many other disorders, single sources of information are likely to yield incomplete data; the more sources that are used, the fuller the picture.

EXERCISE B7

This exercise deals with specific aspects of the use of incidence rates. The uses of incidence rates are covered in a more general way in Unit A17 (with reference to gastroenteritis in Epiville).

Question B7–1

It is sometimes said that incidence rates are used for acute (short-term) diseases and prevalence rates for chronic ones. Would you accept this as a recommendation? What use might be made of prevalence data for acute illnesses, or of incidence data for chronic ones?

Question B7–2

Incidence rates are often used for evaluating the effectiveness of health care, both in clinical trials of medical treatments and in evaluative studies of health programs directed at communities. What are the kinds of events whose incidence may tell us something about the effectiveness of care?

Question B7–3

A visit to a large (imaginary) hospital, during which a bed-by-bed survey is conducted, reveals that 10% of patients who have undergone surgical procedures have definite evidence of wound infection. Can you estimate the average risk of wound infection, for patients who underwent surgery in this hospital in the recent past?

Question B7–4

Follow-up studies of women with breast cancer, based on data for 1977–1982 in cancer registries maintained in nine states of the United States, show that 26% died in the first five years after the diagnosis of the disease (National Center for Health Statistics, 1986). Is this a cumulative mortality rate or a person-time mortality rate? Is it a case fatality rate? (For definition, see Note B7–2.) For patients with this neoplasm, what is the probability of surviving for at least five years after diagnosis? What is the probability of surviving for at least one year? What is the probability of surviving for at least ten years?

Question B7–5

A report on a series of 40 patients who were given a revolutionary new treatment for a previously incurable disease in a (make-believe) teaching hospital states that the cure rate (the cumulative incidence rate of complete recovery) was 50% in the first year, 50% in the second year, and 75% in the total two-year period. Can these rates be correct?

Question B7–6

A hypothetical study of 1,000 children, all of whom were carefully followed up for a year, yielded the findings shown in Table B7. According

Table B7. Number of Spells of Acute Gastroenteritis During a Year: Frequency Distribution

No. of Spells per Child	No. of Children
0	700
1	200
2	80
3	10
4	5
5	2
6	0
7	0
8	0
9	0
10	3
Total	1,000

to these data, what is the average child's risk of contracting gastroenteritis during a year? What is his or her risk of having two or more spells
of the disease? How many spells may the average child be expected to
have in a year?

NOTES

B7–1. *"Referral filter bias.* As a group of ill are referred from primary to
secondary to tertiary care, the concentration of rare causes, multiple diagnoses and 'hopeless cases' may increase" (Sackett,
1979).

B7–2. The *case fatality rate* is usually defined as the proportion of individuals with a specified disease who die of it during a stated
period.

USES OF INCIDENCE RATES

In answer to *Question B7–1*, incidence and prevalence rates can be used for both acute and chronic diseases. For acute diseases, use is generally made of incidence rather than prevalence rates, for all purposes for which rates are employed. However, the prevalence of an acute disease is also sometimes of interest. During a cholera epidemic, for example, the health authorities may want to know not only how many new cases occur each day, but also how many cases are currently under treatment.

For chronic disorders, prevalence rates provide a basis for inferences about needs for curative and rehabilitative care and may provide clinicians with a useful guide to the probability of a diagnosis; they are less useful than incidence rates for other purposes. The rate of incidence of new cases of a chronic disease provides an indication of the present or recent activity of causal factors. Incidence rates may thus point to a need for primary prevention and may also identify the groups in which this need is most marked. A change in the incidence rate of new cases may be a measure of the effectiveness of primary prevention, and changes in the incidence of complications and other outcomes may be used to measure the effectiveness of curative and rehabilitative care. For the clinician, the incidence rate of new cases provides an estimate of individual risk, and the incidence rates of subsequent outcomes give an indication of the prognosis. For the researcher, the incidence rates of various outcomes may provide an understanding of the natural history and clinical course of the disease, and comparisons of rates (of new cases or of outcomes) may throw light on etiological processes.

In answer to *Question B7–2*, the occurrence of any event that health care aims to prevent, or any desirable or undesirable effect of health care, may be used as an indication of the effectiveness of care. The goals of health care include the promotion, preservation, and restoration of health (see Note A17–3). Events whose incidence may be measured in clinical trials and other studies of the effectiveness of care thus include the occurrence of infection and other precursors of disease; the occurrence of the disease itself; and the occurrence of subsequent events, such as recovery, remission, complications, recurrences, various signs and symptoms, biochemical and immunological changes, return to work, incapacitation, and death. The occurrence of side effects of treatment may also be measured. In evaluative studies of health educational programs, the main events that are measured are changes in habitual practices, such as the commencement or cessation of cigarette smoking.

If we wish to know the risk of incurring a disease or the probabilities of various outcomes, it is essential to have incidence data. The prevalence data provided in *Question B7–3* cannot tell us the risk of wound infection. The point prevalence rate of such infections among postoperative patients, 10%, tells us nothing about risk. Like all prevalence rates, it is a reflection not only of incidence, but also of average duration; the longer the duration of the disorder, the higher the point prevalence. In this instance, the length of stay in hospital also plays a part: Are patients with wound infections kept in this hospital longer? Or, are they perhaps discharged especially early, to prevent their continued exposure to hospital pathogens or to reduce the hazard to other patients? All we can be sure of is that there *is* a risk of wound infection in this hospital, but we cannot say how big it is.

In *Question B7–4*, we are told that 26% of women died in the first five years after diagnosis of breast cancer. This is a cumulative mortality rate, not a person-time mortality rate; the denominator is the number of patients in the cohort at the beginning of the follow-up period, that is, at the time of diagnosis. This rate may exceed the case fatality rate (Note B7–2), since some patients may have died of other causes.

The probability of remaining alive for a given time can be calculated by subtracting the risk of dying during that time (the cumulative mortality rate, expressed as a percentage) from 100%. This is called the *cumulative survival rate*, or just the *survival rate*. These terms are sometimes used with reference not only to remaining alive, but to staying free of a particular disease, complication, or other end-point event. A survival rate is thus the complement of (i.e., 100% minus) a cumulative incidence or mortality rate.

In *Question B7–4*, we are told that the cumulative mortality rate for a five-year period is 26%. The individual patient's probability of surviving for five years is thus 74%. We can easily find the theoretical probability of surviving for one year after diagnosis, by computing the person-time mortality rate during the five-year period, which is the average rate at which patients die, and using this to calculate the expected survival after one year (see Note B8). This procedure can be correct, however, only if the rate at which patients die during the five-year period is a constant one. We have no certainty that this is so: all the patients who die within five years may do so in the first year, or all may die after the first year.

We therefore cannot estimate the probability of surviving for one year. Similarly, we cannot estimate the ten-year survival rate; we have no reason to assume that the rate of dying in the second five years will be the same as in the first five years.

The rates cited in *Question B7–5* may look wrong, but they are correct. The follow-up study started with a cohort of 40 patients; 20 were cured in the first year (cure rate, 50%); of the 20 who were still ill at the end of the first year, 10 were cured in the second year (cure rate in the second year, 50%). In the total two-year period, 30 of the 40 were cured (cure rate, 75%). The method used to combine cumulative incidence (or mortality) rates for separate periods, so as to obtain the rate for the total period, is simple: calculate the survival rates for each period, multiply them together to obtain the survival rate for the total period, and subtract this from 100%. In this study, the cure rate (the cumulative incidence rate of cures) was 50% each year; the survival rate ("freedom from cure") was therefore (100 − 50)%, that is, also 50%, each year. The survival rate in the two-year period was 50% × 50%, that is 25%, and the cumulative incidence rate of cures in the two-year period was (100 − 25)%, or 75%.

In the cohort study described in *Question B7–6*, there were 700 children who survived the year without contracting gastroenteritis, and 300 who had one or more spells during the year. The cumulative incidence rate (persons) was therefore 30%, and the risk for the average child was therefore 30%. There were 100 children who had two or more spells, and the risk of having two or more spells was therefore 10%. To know the number of spells a child can expect during a year, we must calculate the mean number of spells per child, by dividing the total number of spells by the total number of children. The total number of spells is (200 × 1) + (80 × 2) + (10 × 3) + (5 × 4) + (2 × 5) + (3 × 10) = 450, and the mean number of spells per child in the population is 450/1,000 = 0.45. This is also the annual incidence rate (spells).

EXERCISE B8

Incidence rates of fractures of the proximal femur ("fracture of neck of femur," "fractured hip") in women in Oxford, England, in 1983 are presented in Table B8 (Boyce and Vessey, 1985). The information, which came from hospital records, refers to "nonpathological" fractures of the neck of the femur, not caused by tumors or other local bone diseases. Census figures were used as denominators. For the purpose of this exercise, you may assume that only patients with a first fracture were included, and that very few of these failed to reach the hospitals that were studied.

Table B8. Annual Age-Specific
Incidence of Fractured Neck of Femur
in Women, Oxford, 1983

Age (yr)	Rate per 10,000
0–34	0
35–54	2
55–64	9
65–74	22
75–84	112
85–94	322

Data from Boyce and Vessey (1985).

Question B8–1

Summarize the facts shown in the table. What kind of incidence rate was used?

Question B8–2

What are the possible explanations for the association with age?

Question B8–3

What risk does a woman aged 75 in Oxford have of sustaining a fracture of the neck of her femur within the next year? Do you have any reservations about your answer?

Question B8–4

What is the risk that she will have such a fracture during the next ten years (if she lives that long)?

Question B8–5

Can you guess (or, if you are that way inclined, can you calculate) the probability that a woman in Oxford will sustain a fracture of the neck of the femur during her lifetime, if she lives to the age of 95. Is it about 1%, 2%, 3%, 4%, 5%, 20%, 40%, or more?

Question B8–6

Can the findings be generalized to men in Oxford?

Question B8–7

Can they be generalized to women who live elsewhere?

NOTE

B8.   Using the formulae in Note B5–4, the person-time mortality rate that corresponds to a cumulative mortality rate of 0.26 after five years is 0.06 per person-year, and the estimated cumulative mortality rate after one year is 0.058, or 5.8%. The one-year survival rate (on the unlikely assumption of a constant rate of dying during the five-year period of observation) is therefore (100 − 5.8)% = 94.2%.

Unit
B9

ESTIMATING THE INDIVIDUAL'S CHANCES

The rates in Table B8 (*Question B8–1*) show a steep monotonic rise in incidence with increasing age. Looking at the differences between the rates, we see that the rise becomes steeper with increasing age. The rates are based on census figures; they are therefore "ordinary" incidence rates—that is, estimates of person-time incidence rates (see Unit B5). As they refer to patients with first fractures only, they are incidence rates (persons).

We have no reason to suspect that the association with age is an artifact, and it is very unlikely to be due to chance. It is also extremely unlikely that there can be any confounding factor strongly enough associated with both age and fractures of the femur to produce an age trend as strong as the one shown in the table. The main possibility, therefore (*Question B8–2*), is that the trend is caused by biological aging or some concomitant of aging, such as increased brittleness of the bones or a tendency to fall or to be involved in accidents of other sorts. We might tentatively suggest that a birth cohort effect (Unit B2) may also play a part: older women may be particularly prone to this fracture because they belong to a generation whose bones are especially brittle in old age because of nutritional inadequacies at a younger age.

Incidence rates provide an indication of the average risk of an individual. Because the annual rate for women aged 75–84 was 112 per 10,000, we can infer that for a woman aged 75, the risk of having a first fracture within the next year (*Question B8–3*) is about 1.1%. The rates are not cumulative incidence rates, which would be direct measures of risk; however, they are so low that over short periods they are almost equivalent to the corresponding cumulative incidence rates. (If we use the formula in Note B5–4, the highest annual rate in the table—322 per 10,000—is equivalent to a cumulative incidence of 317 per 10,000.) A more important reservation is that the rate we are using, 112 per 10,000,

119

applies to a ten-year age group. In view of the steep rise in incidence with age, there is a strong possibility that for women aged 75, who are at the lower margin of the 75–84 age span, the annual incidence rate is lower than 1.1% (and for women aged 84, it is higher).

The risk that a woman aged 75 will have a fracture during the next ten years (*Question B8–4*) is about 11%. The average annual rate at 75–84 years is 1.1%, so that if we follow up a cohort of women aged 75, we can expect about 1.1% to sustain a fracture each year, and ten times this proportion, or 11%, in ten years.

The same approach can be used to obtain a rough idea of the lifetime probability of a fracture (*Question B8–5*). If we follow up a cohort from birth, we can expect few fractures below the age of 75; then about 1.1% of women will have a fracture in each of the next ten years (11% in all), and another 3.2% will have a fracture each year in the next ten years (another 32%), making the total lifetime probability about 43%.

This method is obviously not accurate, since women who sustain a fracture—who (as we have just seen) are numerous—are not removed from the denominator. A better method is the one described in Unit B8 (see comment on Question B7–5): calculate the cumulative incidence rate for each year of life (using the formula in Note B5–4), subtract it from 100% to obtain the corresponding survival rate (the rate of freedom from a fracture), multiply all the survival rates together to obtain the survival rate for the total period, and subtract this from 100%. If we do this, we obtain an estimated lifetime probability (to age 95) of 37%. This laborious but straightforward actuarial procedure is called *life table analysis*. Because it is based on "current" rates—that is, on incidence rates observed at a particular time (1983)—it is termed *current life table analysis*.

We must not forget that this estimate is a theoretical expectation, not derived from actual observations of a cohort. It is based on the assumption that the incidence rates observed in 1983 held good, and will continue to hold good, throughout the life-span of the women in question. This is not necessarily true. In fact, the age-specific incidence rates of fractures of the neck of the femur in Oxford were about twice as high in 1983 as they were 27 years earlier (Note B9–1), and we have no idea of what they will be 27 years later. For women who were old in 1983, the lifetime probability that we calculated is an overestimate of the risk they actually experienced during their lives. For women who were young in 1983, we do not yet know what their risk will be.

(Can you suggest a quite different way, conceptually simple although not necessarily feasible, of measuring the lifetime probability of incurring a fracture of the femur? A clue: it has something to do with information about people who die. For answer, see Note B9–2.)

In answer to *Question B8–6*, we should hesitate to apply the findings to men, unless we know from studies elsewhere that the incidence of fractures of the femur does not vary much with sex. In fact, men in

Oxford had lower rates than women, and their lifetime probability of a fracture by the age of 95 was 19%, as compared with 37% for women. (Can this difference be explained by the confounding effect of age? Above the age of 85, there were more than three times as many women as men in Oxford in 1983. For answer, see Note B9–3.)

We should also query the generalizability of the findings to women elsewhere (*Question B8–7*). As noted above, the rates for women in Oxford itself varied markedly over a 27-year period.

SURVIVAL CURVES

A survival curve plots the survival experience against time. It may start at 100% and show the cumulative survival rate (curve A in Fig. B9–1); or it may start at zero and show the cumulative incidence or mortality rate (curve B in the figure)—which is, of course, the complement of the survival rate. Figure B9–1 shows that 65% of patients were still alive one year after the onset of a particular disease and that 10% were alive five years after the onset.

A survival curve may be drawn as a smooth line or in steps, each step representing a change due to the occurrence of one or more events. As an example, Fig. B9–2 shows the cumulative incidence of hypertension (i.e., blood pressure consistently 160/95 or higher) after the establishment of a diagnosis of borderline hypertension (i.e., systolic pressure consistently 140–159 and/or diastolic pressure 90–94 mm Hg). Confidence intervals may be shown.

Such curves may be based on direct observation of a group of people who are all followed up for the total period covered by the curve. Usually, however, individual members of the cohort are followed up for different periods, generally because of losses to follow-up or because

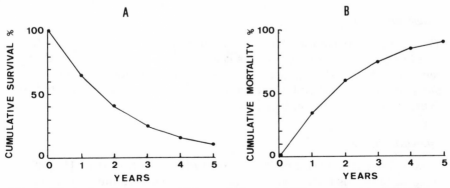

Figure B9–1. Survival curves: (A) cumulative survival rate; (B) cumulative mortality rate.

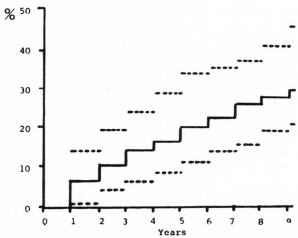

Figure B9-2. Cumulative probability of developing hypertension after establishment of diagnosis of borderline hypertension. Broken lines: 95% confidence limits. *Source:* Abramson et al. (1983), data from Ban and Peritz (1982).

subjects entered the study at different times. Cumulative incidence rates can be obtained from such studies by *cohort life table analysis* (Note B9–4). This is based on a separate computation for each successive period after the start of follow-up, using the experience of those subjects who were actually followed up during that period. The procedure is similar to current life table analysis, but it uses the actual incidence rates observed in a specific cohort.

EXERCISE B9

Question B9–1

The average expectation of life at birth in India in 1982 was 55 years (Last and Foege, 1986). This figure was calculated by the usual method (current life table analysis), using up-to-date age-specific mortality rates. Does this mean that children born in India in 1982 can be expected, on average, to live to the age of 55?

Question B9–2

A survival curve based on a cohort study is portrayed in Fig. B9–1. According to this curve, what is the two-year survival rate? What is the average survival time?

Question B9–3

The median survival time of patients with a certain kind of cancer is five years (i.e., 50% of patients survive for five or more years). Several large-scale studies have shown that when special efforts are made to detect and treat patients early, the median survival time is seven years. What are the main possible explanations for this difference?

Question B9–4

What kind of incidence study will tell us what risk a child has of catching an infectious illness when another member of the family has it?

NOTES

B9–1. The incidence of fracture of the neck of the femur in Oxford in 1983 was twice as high as in 1954–1958. The increase was observed in both sexes and at all ages. Boyce and Vessey (1985), who reported these findings, reexamined the data for 1954–1958, and found no evidence that the increase was an artifact.

B9–2. The simplest way of measuring the lifetime probability of a disease is to determine what proportion of people who die have had the disease during their lifetime, or (if the disease is irreversible) what proportion have it when they die. It may be possible to obtain this information for a sample of decedents by examining clinical records or death certificates, by autopsy, or by questioning relatives or medical attendants. Death certificates alone are not a very good source of information about the prevalence of most diseases at death, even if all the recorded causes of death (underlying and contributory) are taken into account (Abramson et al., 1971).

B9–3. The lifetime probability is calculated from age-specific rates, not crude ones, so they obviously control for effects connected with the number of people in each age group. If males and females have different age distributions in Oxford (as they do), this will not affect the age-specific rates in the two sexes, or the lifetime probabilities. In fact, the use of lifetime probabilities and other indices based on current life table analysis is an accepted method of controlling for the confounding effects of age when we are comparing mortality rates in different populations. If we find that life expectancy alters with time or varies in different countries, we can be sure that these findings are not due to age differences.

B9–4.   The *cohort life table* method is laborious but essentially simple. It is based on a follow-up study of a cohort. A separate cumulative incidence rate is calculated for each successive interval (say, each day, month, or year, or the intervals between successive end-point events), taking account of withdrawals from the study ("censored observations"). These rates are then combined mathematically, to obtain the cumulative incidence rate between any two points of time. For do-it-yourself explanations of the procedure, see Peto et al. (1977) or Kahn and Sempos (1989, chap. 7).

U n i t
B10

ESTIMATING THE INDIVIDUAL'S CHANCES (CONTINUED)

Average life expectancy at birth, calculated by current life table analysis (*Question B9–1*), cannot be used as a measure of the individual's chances. This would require the unwarranted assumption that current age-specific mortality rates were or will be valid throughout the individual's life-span. If mortality rates decrease, the average life-span will be longer. The value of life expectancy statistics is that they provide a way of controlling for the confounding effects of age when comparing populations (Note B9–3).

According to the survival curve (*Question B9–2*), the two-year survival rate is 40%. There are two kinds of average survival time: the *median survival time*, and the mean survival time. The median survival time is the time at which the survival rate becomes 50%. This can be read from the curve; it is about 1.6 years after the onset of the disease. A survival curve does not tell us the mean survival time. To calculate this, we need to know the survival times of all subjects so that we can add them and divide by the number of subjects. This is seldom feasible, as it can be done only after all subjects have incurred the event.

The longer survival time of cancer patients who are detected early, as compared with those detected in the usual way (*Question B9–3*), may be explained in at least three different ways. First, early treatment may be beneficial. Second, the difference may be an artifact, as different starting points are used for measuring survival times in the two groups of patients. If we make a diagnosis earlier in the natural history of the disease, and measure survival from this earlier time, this alone will produce a spuriously longer survival. (This is referred to as *starting time bias* or *lead time bias*.) And third, there may be another kind of bias. Cancers in the preclinical (i.e., asymptomatic, not clinically manifest) phase are a biased sample of all cancers, since slow-growing tumors remain in this phase longer than fast-growing ones, and therefore have a raised prevalence among preclinical cases. The cancers identified by early detection procedures therefore tend to have an overrepresentation of slow-growing tumors, which may continue to grow slowly after detection, resulting in a relatively long median survival time.

To determine a child's risk of catching an infectious disease introduced into his or her family (*Question B9–4*), we need to know the incidence rate of the disease in children exposed to the disease in this way. This can be measured by studying a series of families in which the disease has occurred. The required incidence rate is the *secondary attack rate*. This is a cumulative incidence rate whose denominator is the number of exposed contacts—that is, the total number of individuals (in this instance, children) in these families, excluding the first case (the *index case*) in each family. The numerator is the number of cases (excluding the index cases) that occur within a specified time period. If the disease is one to which some children are immune (as a result of prior disease or immunization), we may want to know the risk of susceptible children; for this purpose, we can restrict the denominator to the susceptible children in the families.

OTHER RATES

You may have to understand or use rates other than those we have so far employed here. *Question B10–1* will test you on some of the following rates. The base (100, 1,000, etc.) is arbitrary. "Per 1,000 population" usually means "per 1,000 in the average (midperiod) population"; for incidence rates the denominator can be person-time units or people, depending on how the information was obtained.

- *Crude birth rate:* live births in a specified period per 1,000 population

- *Fertility rate:* live births in a specified period per 1,000 women aged 15–44

- *Proportional mortality ratio:* deaths assigned to a specific cause in a specified period per 100 total deaths in the period

- *Cause-specific death rate* (or cause-of-death rate): deaths assigned to a specific cause in a specified period per 1,000 population

- *Infant mortality rate:* deaths under the age of one year in a specified period per 1,000 live births in the same period

- *Neonatal mortality rate:* deaths in first 28 days of life in a specified period per 1,000 live births in the same period

- *Postneonatal mortality rate:* deaths in first year of life, excluding first 28 days, in a specified period per 1,000 live births in the same period

- *Fetal mortality rate:* fetal deaths (defined as ≥28 weeks' gestation,

≥20 weeks' gestation, or in some other way) in a specified period per 1,000 total births (live births plus fetal deaths) in the same period

- *Perinatal mortality rate:* fetal deaths plus deaths in the first seven days of life in a specified period per 1,000 total births in the same period

- *Maternal mortality rate:* deaths from complications of pregnancy, childbirth, and the puerperium in a specified period per 100,000 live births in the same period

- *Admission rate:* hospital admissions in a specified period, per 1,000 population

- *Consultation rate:* consultations (usually with a doctor) in a specified period per 1,000 population

WHAT ARE THE ODDS?

Odds may be defined as the ratio of the probability that something is so or will occur, to the probability that it is not so or will not occur. If a follow-up study shows that 30 smokers develop chronic bronchitis and 20 do not, the odds (for smokers) in favor of developing chronic bronchitis are 30 to 20, or 60% to 40%, or 0.6 to 0.4, or 1.5 to one, or—and this is the way they are usually expressed in epidemiology—simply 1.5. This is the odds in favor of future occurrence of the disease (also called the odds that the disease will occur, the odds of the disease, or the *disease odds*). Odds can also refer to the ratio of the probability that something is so in the present (or was so in the past), divided by the probability that it is (or was) not. If, for example, 40 people with chronic bronchitis are smokers and 10 are not, the odds (in these patients) in favor of being a smoker are 4 (to 1); these are the *exposure odds*, because they refer to exposure to a factor that affects health. The odds used in betting on a horse ("3 to 1") are the odds, in the bookmaker's view, *against* the horse's winning—the probability that it will lose, in relation to the probability that it will win.

An *odds ratio* is the ratio of one odds to another. It is a widely used tool in the appraisal of associations. By comparing the odds in favor of a disease in smokers with the corresponding odds in nonsmokers, we can see whether the disease is associated with smoking and measure how strong the association is.

EXERCISE B10

Question B10–1

Calculate the rates specified below, using the following information about the black population of the United States in 1984 (National Center for Health Statistics, 1986; numbers modified to simplify calculations).

Average population 28 million, including 7.2 million women aged 15–44. Live births: 600,000. Fetal deaths: 4,380. Deaths in first week of life: 6,120. Deaths in first 28 days of life (excluding first week): 960. Deaths in first year of life (excluding first 28 days): 3,900. Total deaths: 230,000. Deaths from heart disease: 75,000.

Calculate the following: crude birth rate, fertility rate, crude mortality rate, specific mortality rate for heart disease, proportional mortality ratio for heart disease, fetal mortality rate, infant mortality rate, neonatal mortality rate, postneonatal mortality rate, and perinatal mortality rate.

Question B10–2

If the annual incidence rate of stroke in blacks aged 65–74 in Chicago is 3 per 100 (Ostfeld et al., 1974), what are the odds (in this population) in favor of having a stroke within a year? If 21 out of 75 swimmers who took part in a snorkel race in the Bristol City Docks developed gastrointestinal symptoms during the next week (Philipp et al., 1985), what were the odds that participants would develop these symptoms? Are the odds that an event will occur very different from the probability that it will occur?

Question B10–3

Table B10 shows the relationship between infant feeding and upper respiratory infections (URI) in American Indian children in Arizona. Use odds ratios to appraise this association. First calculate the disease odds (the odds in favor of having one or more episodes of URI) in bottle-fed babies, and the disease odds in breast-fed babies. Then divide the first odds by the second odds. (This ratio of two disease odds is the *disease odds ratio*.) Now calculate the odds in favor of being bottle-fed, first in

Table B10. Distribution of 551 Infants by Feeding Pattern in First Four Months of Life, and Occurrence of Upper Respiratory Infections (URI) in First Four Months of Life

Feeding Pattern	Episodes of URI*		Total
	One or More	None	
Bottle-fed (bottle only, or breast and bottle)	207	238	445
Breast-fed (breast only)	34	72	106
Total	241	310	551

*URI = upper respiratory infection (including otitis media) according to medical (including well-baby clinic) records.
Data from Forman et al. (1984).

the 241 infants with URI and then in the 310 without; divide the one odds by the other to obtain the *exposure odds ratio*. Do you know a short-cut way of calculating odds ratios?

Question B10–4

Now use probability ratios (rate ratios) to appraise the association between infant feeding and URI. First calculate the cumulative incidence rates (persons) of URI in bottle-fed and in breast-fed infants, and divide the first rate by the second. Then calculate the rates of bottle-feeding in children with URI and in children without, and divide the first rate by the second. Compare the rate ratios with the odds ratios.

Question B10–5

In Question B10–3, you calculated the odds ratio showing the association between URI and bottle-feeding. Now calculate the odds ratio showing the association between freedom from URI and breast-feeding—in other words, the ratio of the odds in favor of freedom from URI in breast-fed babies to the same odds in bottle-fed babies. In Question B10–4, you calculated the rate ratio showing the association between URI and bottle-feeding. Now calculate the rate ratio showing the association between freedom from URI and breast-feeding—that is, the ratio of the probabilities of being free from URI in breast-fed and bottle-fed infants. What do you conclude from the results?

Question B10–6

What are the possible explanations for the association between URI and bottle-feeding demonstrated in Table B10?

Question B10–7

What does an odds ratio of 1 mean?

Question B10–8

The odds in favor of disease A are twice as high in vegetarians as in nonvegetarians (i.e., odds ratio = 2). The corresponding odds ratio for disease B is 0.5. Which disease is more strongly associated with eating habits?

OTHER RATES (CONTINUED)

The rates requested in *Question B10–1* are

1. Crude birth rate = 600,000/28,000,000 = 21.4 per 1,000 population.
2. Fertility rate = 600,000/7,200,000 = 83.3 per 1,000 women aged 15–44.
3. Crude mortality rate = 230,000/28,000,000 = 8.2 per 1,000 population.
4. Specific mortality rate for heart disease = 75,000/28,000,000 = 2.7 per 1,000 population.
5. Proportional mortality ratio for heart disease = 75,000/230,000 = 32.6%.
6. Fetal mortality rate = 4,380/(600,000 + 4,380) = 7.2 per 1,000 live births plus fetal deaths.
7. Infant mortality rate = (6,120 + 960 + 3,900)/600,000 = 18.3 per 1,000 live births.
8. Neonatal mortality rate = (6,120 + 960)/600,000 = 11.8 per 1,000 live births.
9. Postneonatal mortality rate = 3,900/600,000 = 6.5 per 1,000 live births.
10. Perinatal mortality rate = (4,380 + 6,120)/(600,000 + 4,380) = 17.4 per 1,000 live births plus fetal deaths.

ODDS RATIO

In answer to *Question B10–2*, the odds in favor of having a stroke were 3% divided by 97%, or 0.031. The odds in favor of developing gastrointestinal symptoms were 21/54, or 0.39. The corresponding probabilities (expressed as decimal fractions) were 0.030 and 21/75, or 0.28. For stroke, the odds and probability are almost identical; but for gastrointestinal symptoms, they are rather different. The reason is that the probability of stroke was low, whereas the probability of tummy upsets was high. The formula is

$$\text{odds} = P/(1 - P)$$

where the probability P is expressed as a decimal fraction. If P is small the denominator is almost 1, so that odds $\approx P$. You may sometimes want to use the reverse formula, which is

$$P = \text{odds}/(1 + \text{odds})$$

In *Question B10–3*, the disease odds are $207/238 = 0.870$ in bottle-fed babies and $34/72 = 0.472$ in breast-fed ones; the disease odds ratio is therefore $0.870/0.472 = 1.84$. The exposure odds are $207/34 = 6.09$ in infants with URI and $238/72 = 3.31$ in infants without; the exposure odds ratio is $6.09/3.31$, which is again 1.84. This is an important advantage of the odds ratio: the answer is the same, whichever way the calculation is done; thus it becomes unnecessary to distinguish between disease and exposure odds ratios, and we can just refer to the "odds ratio" or "relative odds."

A short-cut formula for the odds ratio (without first calculating the separate odds) is ad/bc (see Table B11), where a represents the combined occurrence of the two factors (or categories) whose association we wish to appraise. The figures in the table can be frequencies (numbers of individuals), percentages or other proportions, or rates. The odds ratio is sometimes called the "cross-products" ratio.

If we wish to appraise the association between feeding and URI by comparing rates (*Question B10–4*), we can compare the rates of URI or the rates of bottle-feeding. The rates of URI are $207/445 = 46.5\%$ in bottle-fed babies and $34/106 = 32.1\%$ in breast-fed babies, so that the rate ratio is $46.5/32.1 = 1.45$. This is the ratio of two risks, so we can call it a *risk ratio*, or *relative risk*. The rates of bottle-feeding are $207/241 = 85.9\%$ in the infants with URI, and $238/310 = 76.8\%$ in the infants without. The ratio of these two rates is 1.12. Note that the two rate ratios

Table B11. Odds Ratio*

Factor	Disease	
	Present	*Absent*
Present	a	b
Absent	c	d

*Odds ratio $= ad/bc$.

are different from each other, unlike the two odds ratios. Note also that the odds ratio is quite different from both the rate ratios.

Despite this example, the odds ratio is usually very close to the risk ratio. (Why is this? For answer, see Note B11–1). It is often called the "estimated relative risk."

Question B10–5 draws attention to another feature of the odds ratio. The odds ratio showing the association between URI and bottle-feeding is 1.84, and the odds ratio showing the association between freedom from URI and breast-feeding is (72/34)/(238/207), which is also 1.84. But the rate ratio for the association between URI and bottle-feeding is 1.45, whereas the rate ratio for the association between freedom from URI and breast-feeding is (72/106)/(238/445), which is only 1.27; thus if we look at the same data in another way, the association seems weaker! Fortunately, we seldom look at rates of freedom from disease, so perhaps this paradox should not worry us unduly.

In any case, it is clear that the odds ratio possesses desirable features that the rate ratio lacks: it has the same value whether the disease odds or the exposure odds are compared, and whether emphasis is placed on the presence or absence of the disease. As we will see later, it is sometimes possible to obtain an odds ratio but not a risk ratio. The odds ratio observed in a satisfactory sample is always an estimate of the odds ratio in the population, and, if the disease is rare, it is also an estimate of the relative risk. On the other hand, a rate ratio has the advantage that it is easier to understand. Kahn and Sempos (1989) have summed up the situation:

Since odds are not as much a part of ordinary usage as chance or probability or risk, many people find the concept of an odds ratio less meaningful than a relative risk. We think this is a matter of custom rather than of basic superiority of one method over the other and that odds and odds ratios will be increasingly used by epidemiologists in the future.

Whatever measure of association is used, Table B10 shows a clear positive association between bottle-feeding in the first four months of life and the occurrence of URI in this period. Possible explanations (*Question B10–6*) include (a) chance; (b) the effect of confounding factors (such as mastitis or lactational failure, which may lead both to bottle-feeding and to an increased susceptibility to URI); and (c) causal relationships in either direction: illness may affect the way a child is fed, and bottle-fed babies may be more susceptible to infection or (if infected) to illness—because of what the bottle contains, because of what it lacks, because of the posture in which babies are bottle-fed, because bottle-fed infants have less mothering, or for other reasons. After considering data additional to that shown in Table B10, the authors concluded that their study showed that breast-feeding is beneficial, and reduces the risk of upper respiratory infections not only during the first four months, but up to eight months of age (Forman et al., 1984).

An odds ratio of 1 (*Question B10–7*) means that there is no association; the two odds under comparison are identical. In *Question B10–8*, the odds in favor of disease A are twice as high in vegetarians and the odds in favor of disease B are twice as high in nonvegetarians. The two diseases thus have equally strong associations with eating habits; only the directions differ. An odds ratio tells us both the strength and the direction of an association. If an odds ratio is under 1, it is often easier to understand its meaning if we convert it to its reciprocal (1 divided by the odds ratio).

EXERCISE B11

Rates, percentages and other proportions, and odds are measures of the frequency of an event or attribute. They are used for categorical variables. This exercise is concerned with measures used for noncategorical variables. You should consult a book on statistics if you do not know what standard deviations, standard errors, and percentiles and other quantiles are. You need not be a statistician to make sense of data, but you should know the elements of data summarization and understand the principles underlying basic statistical analyses (see Note B11–2).

Question B11–1

Name some measures that may be used to summarize the central tendency and the spread (dispersion, scatter) of a distribution.

Question B11–2

A study of elderly people with Alzheimer's disease in Finland showed that the concentration of HDL cholesterol in the blood serum was 1.26 ± 0.37 mmol/L (Lehtonen and Luutonen, 1986). What do the numbers mean?

Question B11–3

Examinations were performed of a sample of nonsmoking women living in homes where ten or more cigarettes, cigars, or pipes were smoked daily, and a sample of women not exposed to tobacco smoke in their homes (Brunekreef et al., 1985). The peak flow (a measure of lung function) was lower in the first sample (mean, 6.79 L/sec) than in the second (8.12 L/sec). Is such a difference likely to be due to random sampling variation? If you are not sure, what do you need to know or do in order to answer this question?

Question B11–4

The mean daily caffeine consumption of 2,724 Australian men was 240 mg, with a standard deviation of 145 mg and a standard error of 2.8 mg (Shirlow and Mathers, 1984). Can you calculate the 95% confidence interval (Unit B4)? Assume that the sample was representative, and that caffeine consumption is normally distributed.

Question B11–5

A report on antibodies to poliomyelitis in children in Barbados states that males had slightly higher geometric mean antibody titers than females (Evans et al., 1979). Why were geometric means used instead of ordinary means? (Skip this question if you do not know what titers are.)

Question B11–6

If a study of a large sample demonstrated a bimodal frequency distribution—yielding a curve with two humps, like a Bactrian camel—what explanation would you consider?

NOTES

B11–1.   We have seen that if a probability is low, the odds are very close to the probability. The risk (incidence rate) of most diseases is—fortunately for humanity—low. The disease odds are therefore usually very close to the risk, and the ratio of two disease odds is very close to the risk ratio. This did not occur in Table B10, where the risks were high (46.5% and 32.1%).

B11–2.   There are many good statistics textbooks. If you have studied statistics but need to brush up your knowledge, you may find Kahn and Sempos (1989) particularly helpful; chapter 1 is a brief review of selected elementary statistics.

U n i t
B12

OTHER MEASURES

Measures commonly used to summarize the central tendency of a distribution (*Question B11--1*) are the *mean*, the *median* (which is the value of the middle observation when all the observations are arranged in ascending order), and the *mode* (which is the value that occurs most frequently). Measures of the spread of a distribution include the *range* and, for a normal distribution (one with an approximately bell-shaped curve), the *standard deviation*. The distribution may be described by stating at what points it can be divided into segments containing equal numbers of observations; these may be terciles, quartiles, quintiles, deciles, or percentiles (the 50th percentile is the median). The *interquartile range* between the upper and lower quartiles can be used as a measure of spread.

Question B11–2 tells us that the mean value was 1.26 mmol/L, but we do not know what the 0.37 represents. It may be the standard deviation of the distribution or the standard error of the sample mean. (Actually it is the standard deviation.) The ± convention is best avoided.

Question B11–3 refers to the possibility of random sampling variation (Note B3–2). To know the probability that a difference of the observed size might be found between samples when there is no true difference (between the populations from which the samples were drawn), we must do a significance test. Most physiological attributes are normally distributed, and a *t* test would be appropriate. For this test we need the standard errors of the two sample means, or data from which we can calculate these standard errors—that is, the size of each sample and the standard deviation or variance of each distribution. If a *t* test is not appropriate, we can do a nonparametric significance test like the Mann–Whitney test, which makes no assumptions about the underlying distribution; for this we must know the detailed frequency distribution in each sample.

The 95% confidence interval requested in *Question B11–4* is 234.5–

245.5 mg. It is estimated by multiplying the standard error by 1.96 (or, roughly, 2), and then subtracting the result from the mean (to obtain the lower confidence limit), and adding it to the mean (to obtain the upper limit). The interval is from [240 − (1.96 × 2.8)] to [240 + (1.96 × 2.8)].

An ordinary (arithmetic) mean is the sum of the values, divided by N (the number of observations). The geometric mean (*Question B11–5*) is the Nth root of the product of the values. This is easily calculated by using logs. It is more useful than the ordinary mean for summarizing the central tendency of a series of titers. If we have five blood specimens, for example, with antibody titers of $1:2$, $1:4$, $1:8$, $1:16$, and $1:32$, the median is $1:8$; the arithmetic mean is $(0.5 + 0.25 + 0.125 + 0.0625 + 0.03125)/5$, that is, 0.194, or $1:5.2$; and the geometric mean, the fifth root of $(0.5 × 0.25 × 0.125 × 0.0625 × 0.03125)$, is 0.125, or $1:8$, like the median.

A bimodal curve (*Question B11–6*) may represent the combined findings in samples from two populations that have different but overlapping distributions.

EXERCISE B12

In this exercise we return to fractures of the femur. According to the study described in Exercise B8 (Boyce and Vessey, 1985), the incidence of fractured neck of the femur in women aged 35 or more in Oxford in 1983 was 35.4 per 10,000. We now learn that in Epiville (which, you will remember, is an imaginary town in a developing region) the corresponding rate in 1983 was half this—18.0 per 10,000.

Following our basic procedure for appraising data (Unit A16), we must first consider the possibilities that this apparent difference may be an artifact, a chance finding, or caused by confounding. We are told that the methods of case identification were identical, and valid, in both localities, and that the difference between the rates is highly significant ($P = .0006$). We now wish to explore the possibility that the difference reflects the confounding effect of age.

Question B12–1

The age distributions of the populations of women aged ≥35 in Epiville and Oxford are shown in Table B12. Do these data support the possibility that age may be a confounder?

Question B12–2

One way of controlling for possible confounding is stratification: we could calculate age-specific incidence rates for Epiville and compare

Table B12. Age Distribution of Women Aged ≥35 Years, Epiville and
Oxford: Midyear Populations, 1983

	Epiville		Oxford	
Age (yr)	No.	%	No.	%
35–54	12,000	60.0	10,309	40.1
55–64	5,000	25.0	5,376	20.9
65–74	2,000	10.0	5,558	21.6
75–84	700	3.5	3,400	13.2
≥85	300	1.5	1,055	4.1
Total	20,000	100.0	25,698	100.0

them with those for Oxford. What would be the advantage of using this
method of controlling for age?

Question B12–3

Unfortunately we cannot calculate age-specific rates, as we do not know
the age distribution of the cases in Epiville. Instead, we will use an
indirect way of compensating for the age difference between women in
Epiville and Oxford.

We know the age distributions of both populations (Table B12), and
we know the age-specific incidence rates in Oxford (Table B8). This
enables us to calculate how many cases we would expect to find if the
same age-specific rates occurred in Epiville as in Oxford. We can then
compare the number of cases actually observed in Epiville (which was
36) with the number expected under this assumption. The observed and
expected numbers are both determined by the actual age composition of
the Epiville women, so that the effect of age is neutralized in this comparison. If there is a difference between the observed and expected
numbers, this can be due only to differences between the unknown age-
specific rates in Epiville and the known ones in Oxford.

Calculate the expected number of cases of fracture in Epiville by
applying the Oxford age-specific rates (Table B8) to the women in Epiville, whose age distribution appears in Table B12. Compare the total
expected number with the observed number (36). If there is a difference,
how do you explain it?

Unit B13

INDIRECT STANDARDIZATION

In answer to *Question B12–1*, women in Epiville clearly tend to be young-er than those in Oxford. The percentages in the younger groups are lower in Oxford than in Epiville, and the percentages in the older groups are higher in Oxford. This confirms the possibility of confounding, since age is strongly associated both with fracture of the femur (at least in Oxford) and with place of residence.

The confounding effect of age could be controlled by the use of age-specific incidence rates, which (in answer to *Question B12–2*) would serve additional purposes. They would tell us whether age is an effect modifier (Unit A11)—that is, whether there is a similar difference in incidence between Epiville and Oxford in every age group—and would also, of course, tell us the risks of women in different age groups in Epiville.

On the assumption that the Oxford age-specific rates hold good in Epiville, the expected numbers of cases to be expected in a year in Epiville (*Question B12–2*) are: 35–54 years, $(2/10,000) \times 12,000 = 2.40$ cases; 55–64, $(9/10,000) \times 5,000 = 4.50$ cases; 65–74, 4.40 cases; 75–84, 7.84 cases; and ≥85, 9.66 cases. The total expected number of cases is 28.8.

The observed number of cases in Epiville is 36, and the expected number (if the age-specific rates in Epiville were the same as those in Oxford) is 28.8. Both these numbers are determined by the actual age composition of the Epiville women. The observed number is a reflection of the age-specific incidence rates in Epiville, and the expected number is a reflection of the age-specific incidence rates in Oxford. The dif-ference can mean only that, on balance, the age-specific rates in Epiville are higher than those in Oxford. Controlling for the confounding effect of age, the risk of fractures of the femur is higher in Epiville.

According to the crude rates, however, the incidence in Epiville was only half that in Oxford. We can conclude that this finding was a distortion caused by the confounding effect of age.

This simple method of controlling for a confounding effect is called *indirect standardization*. The ratio of the observed to the expected number of cases is called the *standardized morbidity ratio, or SMR*. It may be used for incidence or prevalence data, or for mortality data, when it is called the *standardized mortality ratio*. In this instance the SMR is 36/28.8, or 1.25.

To calculate the SMR (standardized for age), we require

- the age distribution of the group or population whose SMR is to be calculated

- the age-specific rates in a standard (reference) population; we used the rates of Oxford women for this purpose

The SMR may be used in the same way to control for suspected confounders other than age, or for more than one confounder simultaneously. To control for age and ethnic group, for example, we would need to know the number of people in each age–ethnic category, and must have standard rates for such categories.

The SMR of the reference population is (of course) always 1, since the expected number of cases in this population (using its own specific rates) is the same as the observed number. In our example, the SMR was 1.25 for Epiville and 1 for Oxford.

The process is sometimes taken a step further, by multiplying the SMR by the overall (crude) rate in the standard population, to obtain what is called an *indirectly standardized rate*. (The rationale for this procedure is not simple; see Note B13.) This standardized (or "adjusted") rate is an indication of what the overall rate in the group or population would have been if it had been similar in composition (e.g., with respect to age) to the reference population. In our example, the crude rate in the standard population (Oxford women) was 35.4 per 10,000. If we multiply this by the SMR for Epiville, which is 1.25, we get an indirectly standardized rate of 44.2 per 10,000 for Epiville. The comparable rate for Oxford is, of course, 35.4 per 10,000. This comparison again shows that, controlling for age, the incidence rate was higher in Epiville.

Standardized rates and SMRs are used in the same way. We compare standardized rates or SMRs (based on a common standard) with one another, in order to control for effects connected with the variable(s) we standardized for. Needless to say, SMRs or standardized rates based on different standards should not be compared.

The reference population should be one of the populations we wish to compare, as in the above example, or (less advisedly) some other population can be used as a standard.

Table B13–1. Population Distribution by Age and Annual Age-Specific Incidence of Fractured Neck of Femur in Men, Oxford, 1954–1958

Age (yr)	Midperiod Population	Annual Rate per 10,000
35–54	14,217	1.1
55–64	4,303	6.5
65–74	2,695	6.7
75–84	1,100	21.8
85–94	164	48.8
Total	22,479	4.2

EXERCISE B13

Question B13–1

If you want practice in indirect standardization, calculate SMRs and age-standardized rates for the incidence of fracture of the femur in women aged ≥35 in Epiville and Oxford, using data for men in Oxford in 1954–1958 (Boyce and Vessey, 1985) as the standard. You will find data on the age composition of the two female populations in Table B12, and the facts about the standard population in Table B13–1. The numbers of observed cases in the women were 36 (Epiville) and 91 (Oxford). See if you get the figures shown in Table B13–2. Your results may differ slightly because of rounding-off.

Table B13–2. Crude and Indirectly Age-Standardized Rates (per 10,000) and Standardized Morbidity Ratios (SMR) of Fractured Neck of Femur in Women, Epiville and Oxford, 1983

	Epiville (a)	Oxford (b)	Ratio (a:b)
Crude rate	18.0	35.4	0.5
SMR			
Using Oxford women (1983) as the standard	1.25	1.0	1.25
Using Oxford men (1954–58) as the standard	4.0	4.4	0.9
Indirectly age-standardized rate			
Using Oxford women (1983) as the standard	44.2	35.4	1.25
Using Oxford men (1954–58) as the standard	17.0	18.3	0.9

Question B13–2

Table B13–2 shows the crude rates, SMRs, and indirectly age-standard-ized rates for fracture of the femur in women in Epiville and Oxford. What can we learn from this table?

NOTE

B13.   An indirectly age-standardized rate is calculated by multiplying the observed crude rate by a standardizing factor. This factor is the ratio of the rate S in the standard population to the expected rate E in the population under study (calculated by applying the standard age-specific rates to the age distribution of the latter population). S/E is an expression of the effect of the difference in age composition between the population under study and the standard population. The standardized rate in the study popula-tion is its crude rate O multiplied by S/E. This is the same as the SMR (i.e., O/E) multiplied by S.

Unit
B14

INDIRECT STANDARDIZATION
(CONTINUED)

A basic way of detecting confounding is to compare the association shown by the crude data with the association seen after control of the suspected confounder. We have previously seen that this can be done by ascertaining whether crude and stratified data yield the same conclusions (Unit A11). Another way is to determine whether crude and standardized measures yield the same conclusions.

In this instance (*Question B13–2*), the crude rates clearly yield different conclusions from the SMRs and age-standardized rates; the ratios shown in Table B13–2 are very different. This shows that there was confounding by age.

The table also shows that age-standardized morbidity ratios and indirectly age-standardized rates that use the same standard population yield the same conclusions; the ratios are the same (1.25 or 0.9) in each instance. This of course must be so, since standardized rates (using a given standard population) are calculated by multiplying the SMRs by a constant (the crude rate in the standard population). There is in fact no good reason for using indirectly standardized rates in these comparisons, rather than SMRs.

The table also shows that the use of different standard populations may lead to different conclusions. If we use the women in Oxford as the standard, it appears that (controlling for age) the incidence was higher (ratio, 1.25) in Epiville than in Oxford; whereas when we use men in Oxford as the standard, the rates in the two localities become similar (ratio, 0.9). This is an unfortunate feature of indirect standardization. *The reference population should always be one of the populations we wish to compare.* If it is not, the results may be misleading (Note B14–1): the distortion may be negligible, but it can sometimes be substantial. When rates in different subgroups of a study sample are compared, the combined study sample—or the population from which it was drawn—is often used as a standard, but even then the findings may sometimes be distorted.

Table B13–2 also shows that the level of the standardized rate depends on the choice of a standard population: the two standardized rates for Epiville are 44.2 and 17.0! Indirectly standardized rates have no real-life meaning. Their only use is for comparison with the crude rate in the standard population, or with other age-standardized rates based on the same standard. We might as well use the SMRs.

DIRECT STANDARDIZATION

Directly standardized rates are hypothetical rates based on the fiction that the groups or populations that are compared have a similar composition with respect to whatever confounder is under consideration. A standard population composition is used, not (as in indirect standardization) a standard set of specific rates.

To calculate an age-standardized rate by the direct method, we require

- the age-specific rates in the group whose standardized rate is to be calculated (The denominator in each age category must be large enough to give us a rate we can rely on.)

- the age distribution of a standard (reference) population

The standardized rate is a weighted mean of the stratum-specific rates in the study population, using the sizes of the strata in the standard population as weights (Note B14–2). Direct standardization can be used to control for confounders other than age, or for combinations of confounders. To control for age and sex together, for example, we would need to know the age- and sex-specific rates in the study population, and the size of the various age–sex categories in the standard population.

If two populations have the same age-specific rates, their directly age-standardized rates will always be identical, *whatever standard population is used*. (This is not true for indirectly standardized rates.)

EXERCISE B14

Question B14–1

If you want practice in direct standardization, calculate age-standardized rates for fractures of the femur in women in Epiville and Oxford, using the age distribution of men in Oxford in 1954–1958 as the standard. The age-specific rates you will need are in Table B14–1, and the

Table B14–1. Annual Age-Specific
Incidence of Fractured Neck of Femur in
Women in Oxford and Epiville, 1983:
Rates per 10,000

Age (yr)	Epiville (a)	Oxford (b)	Ratio (a : b)
35–54	1.7	1.9	0.9
55–64	12.0	9.3	1.3
65–74	30.0	21.6	1.4
75–84	142.9	111.8	1.2
85–94	400.0	322.3	1.2

facts about the standard population are in Table B13–1. See if you get the
rates shown in Table B14–2.

Question B14–2

Table B14–2 shows the rates of fracture of the femur in women in Epiville and Oxford, standardized for age by the direct method. Five sets of
rates, using different standards, are shown. Compare the findings with
those shown in Tables B13–2 and B14–1. What are your conclusions
about the use of standardized rates?

Table B14-2. Age-Standardized Rates (per 10,000) of
Fractured Neck of Femur in Women in Epiville and Oxford,
1983 (Standardized by the Direct Method, Using Five
Different Standards)

Standard Population	Epiville (a)	Oxford (b)	Ratio (a : b)
Oxford women (1983)	45.0	35.4*	1.3
Oxford men (1954–58)	16.9	13.4	1.3
European standard population†	24.4	19.3	1.3
African standard population†	11.4	9.3	1.2
World standard population†	18.4	14.6	1.3

*This is the crude rate.
†See Note B14–3.

NOTES

B14–1.   "Indirect standardization is best used only for comparing two groups when one of these groups is the standard." For the mathematical basis for this conclusion, see Anderson et al. (1980). If several groups are being compared and one of them is used as the reference group, it is technically incorrect, although the error is usually negligible, to compare the SMRs of other groups with each other.

B14–2.   A directly standardized rate is a weighted mean (Note A7) of the rates in specific strata. The formula is $\Sigma(s_i r_i)/\Sigma s_i$, where s_i is the size of stratum i in the standard population and r_i is the specific rate in stratum i of the study population. The size of the stratum (s_i) may be an absolute number or a proportion of the total standard population. In the latter instance, $\Sigma s_i = 1$, which simplifies the calculation. If the rates are expressed as 11 per 1,000, 1 per 1,000, and so forth, r_i can be taken as 11 and 1, respectively, for the purposes of the calculation. For detailed explanations of the procedure, consult a statistics textbook. Direct standardization can be applied to statistical measures other than rates, such as means.

B14–3.   The European, African, and world standard populations are hypothetical standard populations for use in direct age standardization. The European population is a relatively old one, with 11% aged ≥65 and 43% aged <30. The African population is a young one, with 3% aged ≥65 and 60% aged <30. For details, see Lilienfeld and Lilienfeld (1980, p. 81).

Unit
B15

THE USE OF STANDARDIZED RATES

In answer to *Question B14–2*, one obvious conclusion to be drawn from the tables is that a standardized rate has little meaning in itself. Table B14–2 shows that the level of a directly standardized rate depends on what standard is used, and Table 13–2 shows the same for indirectly standardized rates. These rates are useful only for comparison with other rates computed in the same way, using the same standard.

Table B14–2 also suggests that the ratio of two directly standardized rates is little affected by the choice of a standard population. In this example, the ratio is consistently 1.2–1.3, which is similar to—and obviously reflects—the ratio of the specific rates in most age categories (Table B14–1). This is an advantage of directly standardized rates; the ratio of indirectly standardized rates or SMRs (Table B13–2) must be treated with circumspection, unless one of the groups compared is used as the standard.

Actually the choice of a standard population can also affect the rate ratio when directly standardized rates are used. This is not shown by our example, because this distortion happens only when the confounder is also a strong effect modifier. In such circumstances—where the associations in different strata are very different—it is arguable, however, that there is little interest in *any* summary measure (crude or standardized) that looks at all the strata together.

Both direct and (if an appropriate standard is used) indirect standardization are useful tools for detecting and controlling confounding effects. The ratio of standardized rates provides a measure of the strength of the association when confounding is controlled. If this differs from the ratio of the crude rates, we know that confounding occurred.

A comparison of standardized rates is not as informative, however, as a comparison of specific ones. The standardized rates tell us that when age is controlled, the overall fracture rate is slightly higher in Epiville than in Oxford. But they cannot tell us that this difference does not occur among younger women (Table 14–1). There is an advantage in examining the specific rates if they are available.

There are, however, at least two good reasons for using standardization. The first is its convenience. A single summary rate is much easier to use than an array of specific rates. This is an especial advantage if two or more confounders are controlled at the same time, so that the number of strata is large. Second, it often happens that specific rates are not available, or the denominators in separate strata may be so small that the specific rates are unreliable; indirect standardization may be used in these instances.

Unit

B16

TEST YOURSELF (B)

Now that you have completed Section B you should be able to do everything in the following list. If you have any doubt, return to the relevant unit.

- Calculate

  point and period prevalence rates (B1, B2).
  ordinary, cumulative, and person-time incidence rates (B5).
  cumulative survival rate (B8).
  crude birth rate and fertility rate (B10).
  cause-specific death rate (B10).
  infant mortality rate (B10).
  fetal and perinatal mortality rates (B10).
  neonatal and postneonatal mortality rates (B10).
  maternal mortality rate (B10).
  hospital admission and consultation rates (B10).
  a confidence interval from a standard error (B12).
  a standardized morbidity or mortality ratio (SMR) (B13).
  an indirectly standardized rate (B13).
  a directly standardized rate (B14).

- Explain the difference between

  prevalence and incidence rates (B1, B5).
  point and period prevalence rates (B1).
  cumulative and person-time incidence rates (B5).
  direct and indirect standardization (B13, B14).

- Explain what is meant by

  lifetime prevalence rate (B1).
  case fatality rate (Note B7–2).
  secondary attack rate (B10).

median survival time (B10).
an odds (B10).
disease odds and exposure odds (B10).
an odds ratio (B10).
a risk ratio (relative risk) (B10).

- State what questions you would ask in order to understand what a rate tells you (B3).

- Appraise the possibility that a rate is biased (B3, B4, B7).

- State possible explanations for

an increase with time in the prevalence of a disease (B2).
a decrease with time in the prevalence of a disease (B2).
an increase with age in the prevalence of a disease (B2).
a decrease with age in the prevalence of a disease (B2).

- Read a survival curve (B9).

- Use incidence rates to appraise the individual's risk (B9).

- Make sense of an odds ratio (B11).

- Compare the uses of prevalence and incidence rates in

the clinical care of individual patients (B5, B8).
the planning and provision of health services (B5, B8).
the evaluation of health care (B5, B8).
the investigation of etiology (B5, B8).

- State why and how standardized rates are used (B13, B15).

- Select an appropriate standard for calculating an indirectly standardized rate (B14).

- State what condition must be met if standardized rates are to be compared (B15).

- Explain the relative advantages of

odds ratios and rate ratios as measures of association (B11).
stratification and standardization as ways of detecting and controlling confounding (B15).
direct and indirect standardization (B15).

- Give a list of

measures of central tendency.
measures of dispersion.

- Explain, in general terms, what is meant by

a birth cohort effect (B2).

selection bias (B4).
information bias (B4).
recall bias (B7).
referral filter bias (Note B7–1).
volunteer bias (B7).
lead time (starting time) bias (B10).
the "healthy worker effect" (B10).
a confidence interval (B4).
validity of a measure (B4).
study validity (B4).
external validity (B4).
current life table analysis (B9).
cohort life table analysis (B9, Note B9–4).
average life expectancy at birth (B10).
random, stratified, cluster, and systematic samples (Note B3–1).
sampling variation (sampling error) (Note B3–2).

SECTION
C

How Good Are the Measures?

"Oh. I know!" exclaimed Alice, "It's a vegetable. It doesn't look like one, but it is."

"I quite agree with you," said the Duchess; "and the moral of that is—'Be what you would seem to be'—or if you'd like to put it more simply—'Never imagine yourself not to be otherwise than what it might appear to others that what you were or might have been was not otherwise than what you had been would have appeared to them to be otherwise.'"

"I think I should understand that better," Alice said very politely, "if I had it written down."

(Carroll, 1865)

Unit
C1

INTRODUCTION

Whether the results we wish to use are our own or those reported by others, we have to judge how accurate they are. The main topic of Section C is the validity of the measures used in the study. The more valid these are, the greater is the validity—both internal and external (Unit B4)—of the study as a whole.

We will consider methods of appraising the validity of measures, the ways in which poor validity can produce biased prevalence and incidence rates and erroneous conclusions about associations, and methods of making allowance for this bias. Other topics are reliability, its appraisal and its implications, and regression toward the mean. The series ends with exercises on the validity of screening and diagnostic tests.

EXERCISE C1

In this exercise you are asked to consider ways of appraising the validity of a measure. We will use a fictional example, to prevent you from being influenced by your prior knowledge about the measure.

TV dementia is an imaginary common disease caused by excessive exposure to television. It is characterized by a long symptom-free period, followed by progressive mental deterioration and culminating in inability to perform activities of daily living unaided. Assume that the diagnosis can be determined with certainty, before or after the development of symptoms, by accurate but costly and elaborate tests.

In a study using a new simple test, imaginatively named test A, the prevalence rate of the disease in a population was found to be 18.4 per 100.

How could you appraise the validity of the test? What kinds of evidence would be helpful? Mention as many possibilities as you can.

Unit
C2

VALIDITY OF A MEASURE

The validity of a measure refers to the degree to which it actually measures what it is designed to measure. The best and most obvious way of appraising validity is to find a criterion (or, in epidemiological jargon, a "gold standard") that we know or believe to be close to the truth, and to compare the results of our measure with this criterion. In this instance (*Exercise C1*) there is an elaborate but completely accurate diagnostic method that could be used for this purpose. This appraisal of *criterion validity* will tell us test A's sensitivity and specificity (see below).

In the absence of this kind of criterion, it would be helpful to know whether follow-up studies show an association between the results of the test and subsequent events (*predictive validity*). In the present instance, for example, are positive results associated with the subsequent development of complete incapacity?

Another possibility is to see whether there are associations with other variables—age, sex, social class, the amount of time spent watching TV—that there is reason to believe should be linked with the variable under study (*construct validity*—see Note C2). These associations provide only weak evidence of validity, but their absence may be strong evidence against validity.

These associations—with a criterion, with an outcome, and with other variables—may be examined in the study population itself, or in other samples.

There are other ways of appraising validity, not based on an examination of associations:

- The high or low validity of the measure may seem obvious (*face validity*). If the information is obtained by questioning, we can see whether the questions are clear and unambiguous; and common sense will tell us the likelihood of recall bias or other forms of bias. On the other hand, it may be obvious that the findings don't "make

154

sense." In this instance, is a prevalence rate of 18% acceptable, in terms of what we know about the disease? If we are dealing with blood pressures, is there "zero preference" (an undue proportion of readings ending in zero)? If so, the readings are obviously inaccurate. Are there very many "unknown" results? If so, the findings cannot tell us the true situation.

- If a set of questions is used, do they cover all the essential components of what they purport to measure (*content validity*)?

- We may also be influenced by the opinions of experts: is there a consensus concerning the validity of the measure (*consensual validity*)?

- It may also be helpful to know whether the measure gives the same result when it is repeated. This is the *reliability* of the measure. If the results are consistent, they are not necessarily valid; but if they are very inconsistent, they can hardly be valid.

SENSITIVITY AND SPECIFICITY

When a test is used to classify individuals as having or not having a specific attribute (say a disease), the *sensitivity* of the measure is the proportion of correct results among people who actually have the attribute, and the *specificity* of the measure is the proportion of correct results among people who are actually free of the attribute. The *false negative rate* is the proportion with incorrect results among people who actually have the disease, and the *false positive rate* is the proportion of incorrect results among people who are free of it.

Using the notation in Tables C2–1 and C2–2, which show the test results in diseased and disease-free people, respectively,

Sensitivity $= a/(a + b)$
False negative rate $= b/(a + b)$
Specificity $= d/(c + d)$
False positive rate $= c/(c + d)$

Table C2–1. Test Results in a Sample of Diseased People

Test Result	Number
Positive	a
Negative	b
Total	a + b

Table C2-2. Test Results in a
Sample of Disease-Free People

Test Result	Number
Positive	c
Negative	d
Total	$c + d$

These values are generally multiplied by 100 and expressed as percentages.

EXERCISE C2

Question C2-1

The validity of test A was measured by applying it to 100 patients known to have TV dementia and 400 people known to be free of this disease; there were 80 positive results in the first group, and eight in the second. What are the sensitivity and specificity of the test, and what are the false negative and false positive rates?

Question C2-2

Is there anything else you would like to know before using these findings?

Question C2-3

If a measure used for determining the prevalence of an attribute has a low sensitivity, how will this affect the prevalence rate?

Question C2-4

If the measure has a low specificity, how will this affect the prevalence rate?

Question C2-5

Can you calculate the prevalence rates that test A will yield in populations (Pepi and Quepi) where the true prevalence rates are 21% and 7%, respectively. If this is too complicated, just guess.

Question C2–6

According to the true prevalence rates in Pepi and Quepi, the rate ratio is 3. If we used the prevalence rates yielded by test A, do you think the rate ratio would be the same, lower, or higher?

NOTE

C2. "Construct validity is concerned with the extent to which a particular measure relates to other measures consistent with theoretically derived hypotheses concerning the concepts (or constructs) that are being measured" (Carmines and Zeller, 1979).

Unit C3

MISCLASSIFICATION

In answer to *Question C2–1*, the sensitivity of test A is 80/100 = 80%. The test's specificity is 392/400 = 98%. The false negative rate is the complement of sensitivity—that is, 100% minus 80%, or 20%—and the false positive rate is the complement of specificity—that is, 2%.

There are at least two things we might want to know before using these results (*Question C2–2*). First, how were the samples for testing validity selected? Many tests are more likely to be positive in full-blown cases of a disease, for example, than in early asymptomatic cases. Was the sensitivity of test A measured in hospital cases of TV dementia? If so, 80% may be an overestimate of its capacity to detect mild cases in the general population. Specificity, on the other hand, may be lower when the test is applied to hospital patients free of the disease under study (because such patients may have other disorders with similar manifestations) than when it is applied to disease-free people in the general population. Second, we might want to know the confidence intervals of the estimates of sensitivity and specificity.

When a measure is used to classify individuals (e.g., as diseased or disease-free), a low validity means that individuals will be misclassified. A low sensitivity (*Question C2–3*) means that people with the disease will be erroneously classified as free of it. This will result in an underestimate of prevalence or incidence. A low specificity, on the other hand (*Question C2–4*) means that there will be individuals who are erroneously classified as having the disease. This will result in an overestimate of prevalence or incidence. In both instances, there is *misclassification bias* (a kind of information bias).

The direction of the bias depends on whether there are more false positive or false negative results. The numbers of these false results are determined both by sensitivity and specificity and by the numbers of diseased and disease-free people in the population. The number of false positives is the false positive rate multiplied by the number free of the

Table C3–1. Expected Results of Test A*
in Relation to Presence of TV Dementia in Pepi
(True Prevalence, 21%)

| Test Result | Disease | | Total |
	Absent	Present	
Positive	158	1,680	1,838
Negative	7,742	420	8,162
Total	7,900	2,100	10,000

*Sensitivity 80%, specificity 98%.

disease, and the number of false negatives is the false negative rate multiplied by the number with the disease.

To answer *Question C2–5*, let us construct Tables C3–1 and C3–2, showing the expected results in Pepi and Quepi. We will assume that the population of each locality is 10,000. First we enter the numbers of diseased and disease-free persons in the bottom lines—2,100 diseased people in Pepi, and 700 in Quepi. Then we calculate the expected numbers with positive tests; for example, in Pepi positive results can be expected in 158 (2%) of the 7,900 disease-free people and in 1,680 (80%) of the 2,100 diseased people. We can then easily complete the tables.

Looking at the right-hand columns, we find that in Pepi, where the true prevalence rate is 21%, test A may be expected to yield a rate of only 1,838/10,000—that is, 18.4%; whereas in Quepi, where the true prevalence rate is 7%, the test will yield a rate of 7.5%.

When the rate of a disease is low (as is generally the case), even a very small rate of false positives can produce enough false positives to outweigh the false negatives, so that surveys that use tests of imperfect validity generally produce overestimates of the true incidence or prevalence rates.

We can use Tables C3–1 and C3–2 to answer *Question C2–6*. Test A

Table C3–2. Expected Results of Test A*
in Relation to Presence of TV Dementia in
Quepi (True Prevalence, 7%)

| Test Result | Disease | | Total |
	Absent	Present	
Positive	186	560	746
Negative	9,114	140	9,254
Total	9,300	700	10,000

*Sensitivity 80%, specificity 98%.

may be expected to yield rates of 18.4% and 7.5%, so that the rate ratio will be 18.4/7.5 = 2.5, instead of the correct value of 3.

This is a typical example. When we compare two groups, using a measure whose sensitivity and specificity are the same in both groups, any misclassification that occurs will *always* reduce the difference between the groups (except in very exceptional circumstances, which we may ignore; see Note C3). If we find a difference, we can therefore be sure that a difference exists, and is actually larger than it seems. The reverse, however, is not true: If we do *not* find a difference we cannot be sure that one does not exist. Misclassification may obscure a true association.

If a measure has the same sensitivity and specificity in both groups— that is, if its validity is *nondifferential*—the consequent misclassification is termed nondifferential. In the next exercise we look at *differential misclassification*—the effect of using a measure with a different validity (sensitivity, specificity, or both) in the groups under comparison.

EXERCISE C3

Question C3–1

Dissatisfied with test A, Dr. B has developed a new test for TV dementia. This test, named test B after its inventor, has a sensitivity of 99% and a specificity of 86%. Test B is now used to measure the prevalence of the disease in Quepi, and the result is compared with the rate (using test A) in Pepi; the latter rate, you will remember, was 18.4%, and the true prevalence rate in Pepi was three times that in Quepi.

Without doing any calculations, can you say whether the ratio of the rate in Pepi (using test A) to the rate in Quepi (using test B) will be more than 3, between 1 and 3, or less than 1?

Question C3–2

If you want to, construct a table (like Table C3–2) to show the expected results when Test B is used in Quepi. You can then supply the rate ratio requested in Question C3–1.

NOTE

C3. If two groups are compared, using a measure whose sensitivity and specificity are the same in both groups, misclassification will always reduce the difference between the groups, unless the measure is wrong more often than it is right, in which case the direction of the association may be reversed. The specific meaning of being "wrong more often than right" is that the false positive rate plus the false negative rate totals over 100%. Measures whose validity is as low as this are unlikely to be used at all, and this possibility can therefore safely be ignored. See Fleiss (1981), pp. 188–211, for full algebraic explanations of the effects of misclassification.

Unit
C4

DIFFERENTIAL MISCLASSIFICATION

The correct answer to *Question C3–1* is no. It is *not* possible, without doing calculations, to say what the rate ratio will be. If misclassification differs in the groups under comparison—that is, if there is a difference in sensitivity, specificity, or both—*bias in any direction may occur*. A true difference may be artificially lessened, obscured, or increased, or its direction may change; a difference may be seen when really there is none. In the present instance, tests with a different validity were used. Misclassification may also differ when a single test is used, if for any reason its validity differs in the groups under comparison.

We happen to know what the true rate was in Quepi. We can therefore construct Table C4 to show the expected results when Test B is used in Quepi (as requested in *Question C3–2*). According to this table, test B can be expected to yield a prevalence rate of 1,995/10,000, or 19.9%. The ratio of the rate in Pepi (using test A) to the rate in Quepi (using test B) is 18.4/19.9, or 0.92. The disease appears to be more prevalent in Quepi!

Table C4. Expected Results of Test B*
in Relation to Presence of TV Dementia in
Quepi (True Prevalence, 7%)

	Disease		
Test Result	Absent	Present	Total
Positive	1,302	693	1,995
Negative	7,998	7	8,005
Total	9,300	700	10,000

*Sensitivity 99%, specificity 86%.

162

EXERCISE C4

In which of the following studies would you suspect that an observed association might be an artifact (or spuriously strong) because of differential validity?

1. A comparison of the incidence of schizophrenia in two countries, based on the diagnoses recorded in clinical files by psychiatrists.
2. A study of the association of retinal disease with diabetes, based on the clinical records of people with and without diabetes.
3. A study of the efficacy of immunization against a specific disease, based on a comparison of the subsequent incidence of the disease in volunteers who were immunized and in people who were not immunized.
4. A study of the efficacy of a new treatment for painful menstruation, in which the proponents of this treatment questioned patients about the persistence of their symptoms, after randomly dividing them into two groups—one whose members received the new treatment (without their knowledge) and one whose members continued their usual treatment.
5. A study of the relationship between exposure to anesthetic gases and a specific immunodeficiency disorder, using a test (for the disorder) with a specificity of 100% but a sensitivity of only 60%.
6. A study of the association of senile dementia with educational level, using simple tests of cognitive functioning (general knowledge and intellectual capacity) to measure senile dementia.
7. A study of the association between fever in early pregnancy and congenital anomalies, in which mothers of deformed and normal babies were questioned about the illnesses they had had during their pregnancy.
8. A study of the effect of smoking on physical fitness, in which smokers were compared with people who had given up smoking.
9. A study of the effectiveness of an intensive educational program on hygienic practices, in which school children who had been exposed to the program were asked whether they washed their hands before eating, and their replies were compared with those of similar children who had not been exposed to this program.
10. A study to determine whether rheumatoid arthritis "runs in families," in which patients with this disease and controls who were free of it were asked whether their parents had arthritis.
11. A study of the association between respiratory disease and disease of the locomotor system (bones, joints and muscles), based on an analysis of the diagnoses recorded in hospital patients.
12. A study of international variations in the prevalence of gallstones, based on the crude findings of all autopsy studies published since 1890 (Brett and Barker, 1976).

U n i t
C5

EFFECTS OF MISCLASSIFICATION

Spurious associations, or spuriously strong ones, could arise in all the studies listed in *Exercise C4*, except in (5), where the only problem is low sensitivity (nondifferential), which would reduce, and could not increase, the strength of any association. In studies (3), (8), and (11), and maybe in (12), however, the problem is not misclassification. In (3), there may be *volunteer bias:* volunteers may differ in many respects from other people, and these differences may be reflected in a different risk of contracting a given disease. In (8), people who give up smoking may differ from continuing smokers in many other ways—for example, in their physical activity—and the effects of these differences may be confounded with the effects of ceasing to smoke. Study (11) provides an example of possible *Berksonian bias*—that is, bias due to selective admission to a study sample. Not all people with respiratory disease, nor all people with locomotor disease are hospitalized; however, people who have both types of disease may be especially likely to be hospitalized. Associations found in a highly selected sample, like hospital patients, may not exist in the general population. In this instance, a study in Ontario demonstrated that the rate of locomotor disease was 25.0% in hospital patients with respiratory disease and 7.6% in hospital patients without respiratory disease—giving a rate ratio of 3.3. There was no such association in the general population, where the corresponding rates were 7.6% and 7.2%, with a rate ratio of 1.1 (Roberts et al., 1978). In (12), we cannot be sure that the methods of determining the presence of gallstones were uniform in all studies; but more obvious reasons for possible spurious differences in prevalence are selection bias (differences in the criteria for doing autopsies) and confounding (age differences).

In studies (1), (2), and (4) there is a possibility of differential validity because of the differences in the methods of measurement or the way they were used. In (1), it is very likely that different diagnostic criteria and techniques are used by psychiatrists in different countries, and these may produce apparent differences in the incidence of schizophrenia. The probability that a person with schizophrenia will receive psychiatric care and be blessed with a psychiatrist's diagnosis also varies from country to country. In (2), diabetics are probably more likely to have retinal examinations than other patients, because of the known hazard of diabetic retinopathy. In a study using clinical records, more retinal disease may therefore be missed in nondiabetics than in diabetics. In (4), there is a possibility that the findings may reflect the unconscious bias of the clinicians, who were proponents of the new treatment and knew which patients had which treatment. The questions they asked, the way they asked them, or the way they interpreted the responses may have differed in the two groups. This possibility of differential validity would not have existed if the appraisal of outcome had been "blind."

In (6), (7), (9), and (10), uniform methods of measurement were used, but their validity may have differed in the groups that were compared. In (6), the validity of the tests of cognitive functioning may well vary with educational status: for example, a low score may be due to lack of education rather than senile dementia. In (7), it is possible that mothers of deformed infants may, because of their concern or feelings of guilt, be especially likely to recall and report minor illnesses that occurred during early pregnancy. In (9), we may suspect that children who have been exposed to intensive brainwashing will tend to give the responses about hand-washing that they think are expected of them. And in (10), we may suspect that people who have a given disease will be especially likely to recall and report the occurrence of the same disease in their family members. In fact, in a study in which people with rheumatoid arthritis were questioned, only 27% reported that their parents were free of arthritis. But when their unaffected siblings were questioned, 50% reported that the same parents were free of arthritis (Schull and Cobb, 1969).

The findings of a study can be taken at their face value only if the study methods are satisfactory. An appraisal of the validity of the measures and the possible effects of misclassification should never be overlooked. If we know what these effects may be, we can avoid unwarranted conclusions, and may be able to gauge the true situation by making allowance for the bias. Formulae are available for estimating the true situation from the observed findings, for both nondifferential (Note C5–1) and differential misclassification (Note C5–2).

Table C5–1. History of Herpetic Blisters in Patients with Lip Cancer and Controls

Herpetic Blisters	Cases	Controls
Yes	60	12
No	76	38

EXERCISE C5

Question C5–1

In a study of the possible relationship of herpes to cancer of the lip, men with cancer of the lip and men with skin cancer elsewhere on the face (controls) were asked about the past occurrence of recurrent blisters on the lips or face. The results (Table C5–1) showed a positive association, with an odds ratio of 2.5 (Lindquist, 1979). Assume that men with lip cancer were more likely to remember and report their blisters. Without doing any calculations, can you say whether the observed association was stronger than the true one?

Question C5–2

A cohort study assessed the prognostic value of exercise electrocardiographic testing in people with no symptoms of coronary disease. The subsequent incidence of coronary events (angina pectoris, myocardial infarction or sudden death) in individuals who initially had abnormal ECG findings was compared with the incidence of these events in those who initially had normal ECG findings (Giagnoni et al., 1983). The results (Table C5–2) showed a positive association, with a rate ratio of 4.5. However, there may have been bias, since the study was not "blind," and the physicians who made the appraisals may have had a greater tendency to diagnose coronary events in people whose previous exercise ECG was abnormal. Assume that this actually happened. Without any calculations, can you say whether the observed association was stronger than the true one?

Table C5–2. Occurrence of Coronary Events in People With and Without Abnormal ECGs

Subsequent Coronary Event	Exercise ECG	
	Abnormal	Normal
Present	21	13
Absent	114	366

NOTES

C5–1. The following formulae can be used to estimate the true situation if there is nondifferential misclassification with respect to one variable, and none with respect to the other. In a cohort study the true absolute difference between rates is the apparent difference (revealed by the survey) divided by $(Se + Sp - 1)$, where Se and Sp are the sensitivity and specificity, expressed as decimal fractions (Fleiss, 1981). In the comparison of Pepi and Quepi (test A data, Tables C3–1 and C3–2), this formula gives a true difference of $(18.38\% - 7.46\%)/(0.8 + 0.98 - 1)$, or 14%; the actual rates were 21% and 7%. If the disease has a low frequency, the true risk ratio can be estimated from the observed risk ratio R, provided that a definitive evaluation can be performed of unexposed people classified as diseased, to determine the proportion C of this group who are truly diseased. The true risk ratio is then approximately $(R + C - 1)/C$ (Green, 1983). In a case-control comparison where exposure to the factor under study has a low prevalence, the true odds ratio can be similarly estimated from the observed odds ratio OR by the formula (OR $+ B - 1)/B$, where B is the proportion of controls classified as exposed who are truly exposed (Kelsey et al., 1986). The algebra of misclassification bias is described by Fleiss (1981, pp. 188–211) and Kleinbaum et al. (1982, chap. 12).

C5–2. The following formulae may be used if there is differential misclassification of one variable (Fleiss, 1981; Kleinbaum et al., 1982). If we use the symbols in Table B11 for the observed findings (after misclassification), the true number of exposed cases (in a case-control study) is $[a - (a + c)(1 - Sp_X)]/(Sp_X + Se_X - 1)$, where Sp_X and Se_X are the specificity and sensitivity (with respect to the measure of exposure) in the cases, expressed as decimal fractions. To obtain the unexposed cases, subtract this number from $(a + c)$. The number of exposed controls is $[b - (b + d)(1 - Sp_Y)]/(Sp_Y + Se_Y - 1)$, where Sp_Y and Se_Y are specificity and sensitivity in the controls. Subtract this from $(b + d)$ to obtain the unexposed controls. In a cohort study the true number with the disease in the exposed group is $[a - (a + b)(1 - Sp_E)]/(Sp_E + Se_E - 1)$, where Sp_E and Se_E are the specificity and sensitivity (for detecting the disease) in those exposed; the true number with the disease in the unexposed group is $[c - (c + d)(1 - Sp_U)]/(Sp_U + Se_U - 1)$, where Sp_U and Se_U are the specificity and sensitivity in those unexposed to the factor under study.

Unit
C6

EFFECTS OF MISCLASSIFICATION
(CONTINUED)

Differential validity can produce spurious associations, spuriously strong ones, or any other kind of distortion. But the correct answer to *Questions C5–1* and *C5–2* is no; it is not possible to guess the effect of differential misclassification. It is possible, however to calculate the true values from the observed results if assumptions are made about the sensitivities and specificities. This computation is easy if there is differential misclassification of only one variable (Note C5–2).

To see how the study described in Question C5–1 might have been affected by misclassification, Sosenko and Gardner (1987) made the assumptions that sensitivity (with respect to prior herpes) was 98% in cases and 92% in controls, and that specificity was 95% in cases and 98% in controls—that is, that the cases had higher rates of both true and false positive responses. Using the first two formulae in Note C5–2, they calculated that the true odds ratio would then be 2.28—only very slightly less than the observed value of 2.50.

But when they made similar assumptions for the study described in Question C5–2, the results were different. They postulated that sensitivity (with respect to coronary events) was 98% in those with abnormal ECGs and 92% in those without, and that the respective specificities were 95% and 98%—that is, that people with prior ECG abnormalities had higher rates of both true and false positive diagnoses of coronary events. Under these conditions, the calculated true rate ratio was 7.0—higher than the observed value of 4.5. The direction of the bias is the opposite of what we might have expected, showing that one cannot guess the effect of differential misclassification. The bias depends on the balance between false positives and false negatives, which is not determined solely by sensitivity and specificity (as we saw in Unit C3).

In both these instances, simple computations demonstrated that (under the stated assumptions) the observed associations were not artifacts caused by differential misclassification. (If you are a martyr for punishment, check the calculations: apply the formulae in Note C5–2 to the data in Tables C5–1 and C5–2; to get the same answers, round off your results.)

When there is misclassification of both the independent and dependent variables, the kind of bias depends on whether the misclassification is differential or not (in the same way as when only one variable is misclassified). If there is no differential misclassification, a true association may be underestimated or obscured, but will not be increased or reversed. However, if there is differential misclassification of one variable or both, bias in *any* direction may be produced. Calculations to determine the true situation are complex if there is misclassification of both variables.

EXERCISE C6

Sensitivity and specificity can be used to gauge validity only in dichotomous (two-category) situations, where we have "yes–no" measures of "yes–no" entities (e.g., disease or no disease), and where a "gold standard" is available. This exercise presents other situations. Methods of appraising validity were reviewed in Unit C2.

Question C6–1

It is proposed to use ten questions about dyspeptic symptoms (belching, burning, nausea, pain, etc.) as a screening test for peptic ulcer, and to test their validity by a comparison with radiological findings. How could specificity and sensitivity be used as measures of validity? If validity is high, can the questions be used to study ethnic differences in the occurrence of peptic ulcer?

Question C6–2

In a survey of a population sample in Auckland, New Zealand, participants were asked their height and weight. People with a Quetelet index (weight in kilograms divided by the square of height in meters) of ≥30 were defined as obese (Stewart et al., 1987). How would you measure the validity of the self-reported measurements and the diagnosis of obesity, using actual measurements as the criteria?

Question C6–3

An epidemiological study of mental health in an Australian university was performed by asking students whether they had experienced any emotional or mental illness during the last year, and if so, whether it was serious, moderate, or minor (McMichael and Hetzel, 1974). How could these self-appraisals be validated?

Question C6–4

One of the variables measured in the Rand Health Insurance Study (a large-scale experiment designed to investigate the effects of different arrangements for financing health care) was "physical health in terms of functioning." A battery of questions about functional limitations was used ("Do you have trouble walking?" "Does your health keep you from working?" "Do you need help with dressing?" etc.). Each response was given a score, and the sum of the scores was used as a measure of physical health (Stewart et al., 1978). How could this measure be validated?

U n i t
C7

OTHER WAYS OF APPRAISING VALIDITY

To appraise the validity of the questions about indigestion (*Question C6–1*), sensitivity and specificity in relation to radiological evidence of peptic ulcer were measured for specific questions, for specific combinations of questions, and for the total number of symptoms reported. For the latter purpose, the range of responses was turned into a dichotomy, using alternative cutting-points: 3 or more, 4 or more, and so forth. Validity was best for a total score of 6 or more; sensitivity was then 80% and specificity 84% (Popiela et al., 1976). However high the validity of such questions, it would be unwise to use them to study ethnic differences, without first measuring their validity in different ethnic groups. Marked ethnic variation has been found in the validity of this kind of question (Epstein, 1969).

Sensitivity and specificity cannot be used for metric-scale variables like weight and height. (What is a metric scale? What kinds of scale of measurement do you know? See Note C7.) The criterion validity of measures of these variables (*Question C6–2*) can be appraised by comparing the findings with "true" ("gold standard") measurements, and using such indices as

1. the correlation between the observed and true measurements. (A correlation coefficient of 1 indicates perfect linear correlation; that is, a higher observed value always means a higher true value.)
2. the size of the discrepancies between the observed and true values (ignoring the direction of the differences), as an indication of the "precision" of the measurements.
3. the difference between the mean values, as an indication of the presence and direction of bias.

In this instance, the comparison showed that self-reported heights and weights had a high degree of accuracy in the population studied

(Stewart et al., 1987). The coefficients of correlation between reported and measured values were .96 for height and .98 for weight. For 75% of participants the absolute discrepancy in height (i.e., ignoring its direction) did not exceed 3.5 cm and the discrepancy in weight did not exceed 2.4 kg. There was slight bias: the reported height tended to be more than the measured height (mean difference, 1.94 cm; 99% confidence interval, 1.78–2.10 cm), and the reported weight was lower than the measured weight (mean difference, 0.58 kg; 99% confidence interval, 0.41–0.75 kg).

The small biases in height and weight acted together to produce a larger bias in the diagnosis of obesity. The prevalence of obesity was 6.2% according to the reported measurements, and 9.3% according to the measured values. The sensitivity of the report-based diagnosis of obesity was 63%, and its specificity was 99.6%.

The self-assessments of mental illness used in the Australian study (*Question C6–3*) were validated in several ways (McMichael and Hetzel, 1974); you may have thought of other possibilities. Criterion validity was tested by a comparison with clinical records; among members of the study sample diagnosed as having an emotional illness during the previous year, the sensitivity of the self-assessment was 73%; the few students who were diagnosed as seriously ill all reported illness. Construct validity was demonstrated by correlations between the self-assessment and attributes that might be expected to go along with mental illness—namely a neuroticism score (the more serious the reported illness, the higher the score) and self-reported psychosomatic disorders. There was no correlation with the student's reported readiness to seek medical help when ill, a fact taken as evidence that the self-assessment of mental illness indicated the occurrence of illness rather than readiness to be labeled "ill." Also, 79% of students who reported mental illness one year reported it again the next year; and the more serious the illness reported the first year, the higher this proportion was. The authors regarded this as predictive validation.

It is not easy to find a "gold standard" for validating the questions used to measure physical health (*Question C6–4*). The investigators satisfied themselves that the questions had face validity (each question appeared to measure what it was supposed to) and content validity (the questions covered the areas included in measures of physical health found in the literature). Construct validity was appraised by seeking (and finding) the expected associations between the score and other questionnaire measures of functioning (physical abilities, role limitations, self-care limitation, performance of physical exercise, etc.), age, and income (Stewart et al., 1978).

The investigators also appraised the extent to which the separate questions "hung together"—how strongly the answers were correlated with each other and with the total score. This kind of *internal consistency* (also called *internal consistency-reliability*) is evidence that the items probably measure much the same thing. Alone, it is no guarantee of validity. But if face and content validity are satisfactory, internal consistency supports the probability that the measure is valid. In this instance, "coefficient alpha" (a measure of internal consistency you are very likely to encounter; possible values, 0–1) was .9; a value of $\geq.7$ is generally regarded as satisfactory.

RELIABILITY

Reliability is defined as

the degree of stability exhibited when a measurement is repeated under identical conditions. Reliability refers to the degree to which a measurement procedure can be replicated. Lack of reliability may arise from divergences between observers or instruments of measurement or instability of the attribute being measured. (Last, 1983)

Reliability is also called *reproducibility* or *repeatability*.

Reliability is no guarantee of validity: people of a certain age may give the same answer whenever they are asked how old they are, even over a period of years, but this may not be their true age. On the other hand, if a measure is unreliable this must detract from its validity. Especially in instances where criterion validity cannot be measured, it may therefore be useful to know how reliable the measure is.

Reliability is usually measured by performing two or more independent measurements and comparing the findings. The object may be to determine whether observers vary in their measurements (interobserver or interrater variation), whether there are differences between measurements made by the same observer at different times (intraobserver or intrarater variation), whether measuring instruments differ, or whether the attribute that is measured is itself labile.

EXERCISE C7

Cataract may be difficult to diagnose, especially in its early stages. A handbook on epidemiology for ophthalmologists states, "One observer may be more apt to diagnose cataracts . . . than another. One man's . . . cataract is not always another's" (Sommer, 1980).

In an imaginary study of the reliability of diagnoses, two ophthalmologists each examined the same 1,000 eyes, without knowing the other ophthalmologist's diagnoses.

Question C7–1

Suppose you are told that each ophthalmologist found 100 eyes with cataract. Does this mean that the diagnoses are reliable? Is there bias?

Question C7–2

Suppose you are told that the *percentage agreement* was 83%—that is, the ophthalmologists agreed with respect to 83% of the eyes they examined. Is this an adequate degree of reliability?

Table C7–1. Presence of Cataract in 1,000 Eyes, According to Two Ophthalmologists

	Dr. Mackay		
Dr. McBee	Absent	Present	Total
Absent	815	85	900
Present	85	15	100
Total	900	100	1,000

Question C7–3

You are now given the findings shown in Table C7–1. Is the reliability of the diagnoses satisfactory? (Can you see how the percentage agreement of 83% was calculated?)

Question C7–4

The full findings are shown in Table C7–2. Were the diagnoses more reliable for early or for advanced cataract?

Table C7–2. Presence and Stage of Cataract in 1,000 Eyes, According to Two Ophthalmologists

	Dr. Mackay			
Dr. McBee	Absent	Early Cataract	Advanced Cataract	Total
Absent	815	85	0	900
Early cataract	85	9	1	95
Advanced cataract	0	0	5	5
Total	900	94	6	1,000

Question C7–5

Using the data in Table C7–1, can you calculate the sensitivity and specificity of the diagnoses?

NOTE

C7. *Scales of measurement.* A *dichotomy* has two mutually exclusive categories (e.g., disease present, disease absent). A *nominal scale* has any number of mutually exclusive categories that do not fall into a natural order (e.g., Easterners, Westerners, Northerners). An *ordinal scale* has mutually exclusive categories that represent relative positions between which a natural order is assumed (e.g., social classes 1, 2, 3, 4, and 5; or no disease and mild, moderate, and severe disease). An *interval scale* is one in which any given difference between two numerical values has the same meaning, whatever the level of the values; the difference between the values reflects the magnitude of the difference in the attribute (e.g., age). The term *ratio scale* is sometimes used for interval scales whose zero values mean absence of the attribute (most interval scales used in epidemiology are ratio scales). Interval and ratio scales may be referred to as *metric.* These scales are *continuous* if an infinite number of values are possible along a continuum—for example, in measurements of height. They are *discrete* if only certain values are possible; for example, a woman's parity cannot be 2.3.

Unit C8

APPRAISAL OF RELIABILITY

The fact that the ophthalmologists detected the same numbers of cases of cataract (*Question C7–1*) does not ensure reliability, since they may not have decided that the same eyes had cataracts. Reliability may be very low. The fact that both ophthalmologists diagnosed the same number of cases does not necessarily mean there is no bias; they may have an equal tendency to overdiagnose or underdiagnose cataract.

The percentage agreement (*Questions C7–2* and *C7–3*) is 83%, since there were 830 agreements in 1,000 eyes (815, no cataract; 15, cataract). This high percentage suggests a high degree of reliability. However, this is misleading: as Table C7–1 shows, the ophthalmologists agreed on the presence of cataract in only 15 eyes, but in 170 others one said there was cataract and the other said there was not.

The percentage agreement is a widely used but obviously unsatisfactory measure of reliability. It does not allow for the fact that chance alone will lead to a large number of agreements; this is illustrated in hypothetical Table C8–1, where there is no association whatsoever between the diagnoses made by two physicians: Dr. Maxcy diagnoses trachoma in 10% of the eyes Dr. MacDee finds diseased, and in 10% of those Dr. MacDee finds free of trachoma. Yet the percentage agreement is 82%!

Table C8–1. Presence of Trachoma According to Two Physicians (No Association)

Dr. MacDee	Dr. Maxcy		Total
	Absent	*Present*	*Total*
Absent	810	90	900
Present	90	10	100
Total	900	100	1,000

A better measure is *kappa* (Note C8–1), which is a measure of agreement "beyond chance." To calculate this for Table C7–1, we first estimate the number of agreements to be expected by chance, on the basis of the totals in the right-hand column and bottom row (the "marginal totals") of Table C7–1. Dr. Maxcy found trachoma in 100/1000 (10%) of the eyes he examined, and if the diagnoses were unrelated, he could therefore be expected to find trachoma in 10% of the 100 cases found by Dr. MacDee, so that there would be 10 agreements on a positive diagnosis. Similarly, there would be agreement on a negative diagnosis in 90% of 900 eyes, or 810 eyes. In all, 820 agreements might be expected by chance (as in Table C8–1). We then subtract these chance agreements from the observed agreements (830), leaving 10 agreements beyond chance. We also subtract the chance agreements (820) from the total number of comparisons (1,000), leaving 180 potential agreements beyond chance. Kappa is then 10/180 = 5.6%; that is, if chance agreements are excluded, the two eye doctors agreed in only 5.6% of instances. In Table C8–1, kappa is 0%.

A kappa value of 75% or more may be taken to represent excellent agreement, and values of 40–74% indicate fair to good agreement. Below 40% indicates poor agreement.

Agreement was closer for advanced than for early cataract (*Question C7–4*): the table shows only one disagreement about the presence of advanced cataract. Kappa can be calculated for this diagnosis only, or for overall agreement (concerning both the presence and the stage of the disease). If you wish, calculate these kappas (solutions in Note C8–2).

In answer to *Question C7–5*, sensitivity and specificity of course cannot be calculated from the data in Table C7–1. We cannot regard either physician as providing us with the "true facts," for use as a criterion in appraising the other physician's diagnoses.

EXERCISE C8

Question C8–1

A medical group in New York City provided a screening program, including chest x-rays, for construction workers who were exposed to asbestos. The x-rays were read by staff radiologists. In addition, separate arrangements were made for the x-rays to be read by specialists in occupational medicine. Table C8–2 presents a comparison of the x-ray interpretations by staff radiologists and specialist readers with respect to the presence of signs typical of asbestosis (Zoloth et al., 1986). The value of kappa is .27. What conclusions can you draw about validity? Can you measure sensitivity and specificity?

Table C8–2. Presence of Typical Signs of
Asbestosis* in 775 X-rays, According to Staff
Radiologists and Specialist Readers

| | Staff Radiologists | | |
Expert Reader	Absent	Present	Total
Absent	660	39	699
Present	54	22	76
Total	714	61	775

*Small opacities (grade 1/0 or higher on the International
  Labor Organization scale) or comments indicative of
  interstitial marking.

Question C8–2

What is the prevalence rate, in these workers, of x-ray signs typical of
asbestosis?

Question C8–3

There have been many studies of concordance with respect to the presence of various clinical signs and symptoms and electrocardiographic,
radiographic, and other findings, based on comparisons between exam-
iners or between repeated examinations by the same observer. How
high do you think kappa generally is, in these studies?

Question C8–4

Suppose that a comparison of repeated examinations yielded a kappa
of .95. What would you conclude about the validity of the measure?

Question C8–5

Suppose that replicate examinations are not feasible; and instead, interobserver variation is studied by comparing the findings of two physicians who examine different groups of patients. What condition or
conditions must be met to make such a study of reliability satisfactory?

Question C8–6

Various statistical measures may be used to summarize the results of
studies of repeated measurements of metric-scale variables. Attention
may be directed to correlation and other coefficients that measure how
closely the measurements are associated, or to the discrepancies

between measurements, with or without consideration of their direction. In the following studies, what statistical measures would be of special interest?

1. A study in which each subject's blood pressure was measured twice, once with a conical cuff and once with a rectangular (standard) cuff. The sequence of the cuffs was changed from subject to subject.
2. Reliability studies of various measures of type A behavior, anger, and hostility, for use in exploring associations with the development of cardiovascular diseases.
3. A study in which the blood pressures of a random sample of Dutch children were reexamined annually.

Question C8–7

The blood pressures of residents of nine homes for the elderly in Nottinghamshire, England, were examined, and people with diastolic pressures of ≥100 mm Hg were randomly divided into two groups, one of which received medication for hypertension, while the other did not. Six months later, the mean diastolic pressure in the control group had decreased by 6.5 mm Hg (Sprackling et al., 1981). How can this change in an untreated group be explained?

NOTES

C8–1. Kappa is explained in detail by Fleiss (1981, chap. 13), who emphasizes the statistical aspects, and Sackett et al. (1985, chap. 2), who emphasize clinical implications. Kappa can be used to compare measurements made by two or more observers or at two or more times, and can be adapted for use with graded categories.

C8–2. According to Table C7–2, the expected number of chance agreements is $(5/1,000) \times 6 = 0.03$ for advanced cataract and the number is $(995/1,000) \times 994 = 989.03$ for the absence of advanced cataract. Total chance agreements $= 0.03 + 989.03 = 989.06$. Observed agreements $= 5$ (advanced cataract present) plus $815 + 85 + 85 + 9 = 994$ (advanced cataract absent); total, 999. Kappa for diagnosis of advanced cataract $= (999 - 989.06)/(1,000 - 989.06) = 91\%$. Kappa for overall agreement is calculated after subtracting $[(900/1,000) \times 900 + (95/1,000) \times 94 + 5/1,000 \times 6]$ from both the numerator $(815 + 9 + 5)$ and the denominator $(1,000)$; its value is 5.6%.

Unit
C9

APPRAISAL OF RELIABILITY
(CONTINUED)

Validity cannot be high if reliability is low. The very low concordance between the two sets of x-ray interpretations (*Question C8–1*) points to the low validity of one or the other or both of the sets of readings. The specialists were more familiar with occupational diseases, and it is probably right to assume that their readings were more valid (face validity). If we take their results as a "gold standard," we can calculate the sensitivity and specificity of the staff radiologists' readings (sensitivity = 22/76 = 29%; specificity = 660/699 = 94%).

In the face of this low concordance, we cannot be sure of the prevalence rate of x-ray signs of asbestosis (*Question C8–2*). A tempting solution is to accept the specialist readers' interpretations—which is what Zoloth et al. (1986) did. The rate is then 76/775 = 9.8 per 100. But there are other possibilities: we can insist on a positive finding by both readers (in which case the rate is 22/775 = 2.8%), or we can be less strict and accept a positive finding by either reader (in which case the rate is 115/775 = 14.8%). If we wanted to compare the prevalence in this group with the rate in other workers, based on readings by other radiologists, we would have a problem.

In answer to *Question C8–3*, most comparisons of clinical examinations, as well as interpretations of x-rays, ECGs, and microscopic specimens yield kappa values in the 40–74% range ("fair to good" agreement).

A high kappa value (*Question C8–4*) means high reliability, but alone it tells us nothing about validity. The findings may be consistent without measuring what they purport to measure.

A reliability study based on a comparison of two physicians' findings in separate groups of patients (*Question C8–5*) can be satisfactory only if there is no selection bias: the two groups must be similar. The allocation of subjects should preferably be random, so that the only differences to be expected are those occurring by chance. If the purpose was to study interphysician reliability with respect to a specific examination procedure, it would be important to know whether they had agreed to use a standard procedure and had in fact adhered to it.

Various statistical measures may be used in studies of repeated measurements of metric-scale variables (Note C9). The choice depends on the objectives of the study. In *Question C8–6*, the aim of study (1) was to see if the conical cuff gave lower blood pressure readings, especially in the obese, and the frequency of differences is therefore of interest: in 74% of subjects the conical cuff gave a lower diastolic reading, and in 18% this difference exceeded 10 mm Hg (Maxwell et al., 1985). In study (2), where "to make a contribution to understanding disease processes, the constructs must not be applicable to one-time, transient states, and their assessment must be consistent over time . . ." (Matthews et al., 1985), the main interest is in coefficients based on test–retest studies with a long time span. The aim of study (3) was to see whether a child's position in relation to the distribution of blood pressures remains the same as he or she grows older, and measures of the predictive value of earlier measurements are of interest: 27% of boys who were in the upper tenth of the distribution when first examined were still there four years later (Hofman et al., 1985).

REGRESSION TOWARD THE MEAN

Whenever there is a "random" element in measurements—whether this is because the characteristic is unstable or its measurement is unreliable—a repeated measurement in the same subject will tend to give a lower value if the initial value was high, and a higher value if the initial value was low. This is called "regression toward the mean." Whatever other suggestions you may have offered for the decrease in the mean blood pressure of untreated people with high blood pressures (*Question C8–7*), you should not have omitted this possible explanation.

This phenomenon may mimic the result of treatment and sometimes presents a problem when one is interpreting the results of trials of therapies and health programs. It may be countered by a comparison with the change seen in an appropriate control group (as in the study cited), or by statistical procedures that measure or compensate for regression to the mean. Sometimes one measurement is used to select the subjects for a trial or follow-up study, and a subsequent one is used as the baseline for measuring change.

TAKING ACCOUNT OF VALIDITY AND
RELIABILITY

A short recap may be useful at this stage, putting what we have done into the framework of the basic procedure for appraising data (as outlined in Unit A16). When we want to interpret data, what do we do about validity and reliability?

First, we should always ensure that we know how the variables were measured. This is part of the process of "determining what the facts are"—the initial step in the basic procedure for appraising data. We can then appraise the face validity of the measures. Before or after inspecting the data, we should review any available evidence of criterion validity (sensitivity and specificity or, for metric-scale variables, correlation coefficients, mean discrepancies from criterion values, etc.). In studies where we are interested in associations, it is important to know whether validity is differential. If evidence of criterion validity is lacking, we should review evidence of predictive, construct, and content validity. Information about reliability and internal consistency–reliability may be important if clear evidence of validity is lacking, or for other reasons, as when regression toward the mean is suspected.

With this information, we can consider the role of validity and reliability when we seek explanations for the findings; specifically, we can give thought to the possibility that rates, means, or other summary statistics may be biased, or that the presence, absence, or strength of observed associations may be artifacts. Consideration of possible explanations may lead us to seek additional information about how the data were obtained and the accuracy of the methods.

We may be able to infer the direction and degree of bias in prevalence or incidence rates, mean values, or other summary measures. If we are interested in associations between variables, we can appraise the possibility that the association is spurious, or spuriously strong or weak; the effects of misclassification are most easily estimated if validity is nondifferential.

In some instances, it may be possible to compensate for the effects of low validity or reliability by appropriate statistical manipulations. In others, the best we can do is to allow for these effects when drawing conclusions from the findings, and to consider them when deciding whether, what, and how additional information should be collected.

SCREENING TESTS

The purpose of a screening test is to identify individuals or groups who have a high probability of having a particular disease or other attribute.

Screening was defined in 1951 by the U.S. Commission on Chronic Illness as, "The presumptive identification of unrecognized disease or defect by the application of tests, examinations or other procedures which can be applied rapidly. Screening tests sort out apparently well persons who probably have a disease from those who probably do not. A screening test is not intended to be diagnostic . . ." Screening is an initial examination only, and positive responders require a second, diagnostic examination. (Last, 1983)

The next two exercises deal with the validity of screening tests and the appraisal of their results.

Sensitivity and specificity are the main measures of the validity of a screening test.

EXERCISE C9

Question C9–1

You will remember that we have two tests for the detection of TV dementia—test A (sensitivity 80%, specificity 98%) and test B (sensitivity 99%, specificity 86%). Which would be a better screening test, and why?

Question C9–2

What other information (besides sensitivity and specificity) would be helpful in appraising the value of a screening test?

NOTE

C9. Indices of the reliability of metric-scale measurements, based on duplicate observations, include the correlation coefficient; the intraclass correlation coefficient; the components of variation according to one-way analysis of variance; regression coefficients; and the mean, frequency distribution, and quantiles of discrepancies.

APPRAISAL OF A SCREENING TEST

The aim of population screening is usually to detect as many cases as possible. Test B can be expected to identify 99% of cases, and test A only 80%. In answer to *Question C9–1*, Test B seems therefore to be a more useful screening test. But we cannot ignore its lower specificity. People with positive results will presumably be submitted to definitive diagnostic examinations, and if test B is used there will be a great deal of unnecessary expense, anxiety, and inconvenience. This may or may not be an important consideration. The cost of diagnostic tests and the availability of the personnel and other resources they require cannot be ignored.

If the purpose of screening is not to detect as many cases as possible, but merely to detect *some* cases—for example, to find subjects for a clinical trial to compare two treatments—test A may be an appropriate one.

There are a number of other measures that may be helpful in appraising the value of a screening test (*Question C9–2*). The *predictive value of a positive result* is probably the most useful. This is the proportion with the disease (or other attribute) among people with a positive test result. It measures the probability that a person with a positive result has the disease, and gives an indication of what cost and effort the screening program will require. Other indices of this effort are the number of positive tests per case identified (which is also the number of definitive diagnostic examinations required per case identified), and the total number of screening tests per case identified. Multiplied by the average costs of the respective investigations, these figures provide an index of the average cost of finding a case. The *predictive value of a negative test,* which is the proportion free of the disease among people with a negative test result, is another measure of validity.

In your answer to Question C9–2, you may rightly have listed additional criteria of the value of a screening test. These include the extent to which there is a need for the test (taking account of the prevalence of undiagnosed cases, the impact of the condition, and the probability that detection will lead to effective action and a substantial impact on health), the side effects of the test (including anxiety caused by false positive results), practicability, acceptability, and the cost both of the test and of the more elaborate diagnostic examinations that are required if the result is positive.

EXERCISE C10

Question C10–1

Table C10–1 (a copy of Table C3–1) shows the results of test A in Pepi. Use these data to calculate the predictive value of a positive test, the predictive value of a negative test, the number of positive tests per case identified, and the total number of tests per case identified.

Question C10–2

Now again calculate these indices for test A, this time using the results in Outer Shepi, where TV transmissions were only recently introduced, and the prevalence of TV dementia is only 1%, not 21% as in Pepi. To do this you may first need to construct a table like Table C10–1, based on your knowledge that the prevalence rate is 1%, the sensitivity is 80%, and the specificity is 98%. (If you have any difficulty, see Note C10.) Compare the results and explain the findings.

Table C10–1. Results of Test A* in Relation to Presence of TV Dementia in Pepi (Prevalence, 21%)

| Test Result | Disease | | Total |
	Absent	Present	
Positive	158	1,680	1,838
Negative	7,742	420	8,162
Total	7,900	2,100	10,000

*Sensitivity 80%, specificity 98%.

NOTE

C10. Each 10,000 people in Outer Shepi include 100 (1%) with TV
       dementia. When test A is used, 80 (80%) of these have positive
       and 20 (20%) have negative results. There are 9,900 people with-
       out TV dementia, of whom 9702 (98%) have negative and 198
       have positive results.

Unit
C11

APPRAISAL OF A SCREENING TEST (CONTINUED)

In answer to *Question C10–1*, the predictive value of a positive test in Pepi was 1,680/1,838, or 91%. The predictive value of a negative test was 7,742/8,162, or 95%. The number of positive tests per case identified (which is the reciprocal of the predictive value of a positive test) was 1,838/1,680, or 1.1; and the total number of tests per case identified was 10,000/1,680, or 6.0.

The sensitivity and specificity of the test were the same in Outer Shepi (*Question C10–2*) as in Pepi. But the other indices differed, as shown by the figures in Table C11–1 (based on a prevalence rate of 1%). The predictive value of a positive test was only 80/278, or 29%. The predictive value of a negative test was 9,702/9,722, or 99.8%. The number of positive tests per case identified was 278/80, or 3.5, and the total number of tests per case identified was 10,000/80, or 125.

Clearly, these indices are determined not only by sensitivity and specificity, but also by the prevalence of the disease or attribute in the population in which the test is used: the lower the prevalence, the lower the

Table C11–1. Results of Test A* in Relation to Presence of TV Dementia in Outer Shepi (Prevalence, 1%)

Test Result	Disease		Total
	Absent	Present	
Positive	198	80	278
Negative	9,702	20	9,722
Total	9,900	100	10,000

*Sensitivity 80%, specificity 98%.

predictive value of a positive test will be. To estimate these indices, we must know—or guess—the prevalence rate.

The value of a screening test can be judged only by considering the results to be expected in the population in which it will be used.

EXERCISE C11

This exercise deals with the appraisal of diagnostic tests. If you are not interested in clinical applications, go straight to Unit C13.

Question C11–1

For what purposes would a diagnostic test with a high sensitivity be useful, even if its specificity is low?

Question C11–2

For what purposes would a diagnostic test with a high specificity be useful, even if its sensitivity is low?

Question C11–3

Go back to Table C10–1, which shows the results of test A in Pepi. On the basis of the prevalence rate, what is the probability that a member of this population (who has not yet been tested) has TV dementia? (This is called the *pretest probability*.) What are the odds in favor of the disease (the *pretest odds*)? If we now do test A and it turns out to be positive, what is the probability that the subject has the disease? If the test is negative, what is the probability that the disease is present? (These are

Table C11–2. Probability of Positive and Negative Results Among People With and Without TV Dementia, When Test A is Used in Pepi

Result	Disease		Likelihood Ratio*
	Present	Absent	
Positive	0.80	0.02	40
Negative	0.20	0.98	0.204
Total	1.00	1.00	

*The ratio of the probability of the given result among people with the disease to the corresponding probability among people free of the disease.

the *posttest probabilities* of the disease.) What are the corresponding odds? (These are the *posttest odds.*)

How useful would test A be in clinical practice in Pepi?

Question C11–4

The facts about test A (sensitivity 80%, specificity 98%) are presented in another way in Table C11–2. Make sure you understand what the figures mean. Then multiply the pretest odds (0.266—is this the result you got in Question C11–3?) by each of the likelihood ratios in turn, and compare the answers with the posttest odds (which you also calculated in Question C11–3). What do you find?

Question C11–5

In this question we use a diagnostic test that yields a range of results. It is a supposititious test for TV dementia, acronymously named the BLIP test. The subject is shown a one-hour video film called "Bird Life in Patagonia," and the time that elapses before his or her eyes close in sleep is measured. The shorter this period of wakefulness (POW) is, the higher the probability of the disease. Table C11–3 is based on the results of a trial in two samples, one with and one without the disease. The results are shown as probabilities. Can you say what you would regard as the normal range? What does "normal" mean?

Table C11–3. Probability of Various Results of BLIP Test Among People With and Without TV Dementia

	Disease		
POW* (minutes)	Present	Absent	Likelihood Ratio†
Under 2	0.20	0.0025	80
2– 4.9	0.30	0.005	60
5– 9.9	0.20	0.01	20
10–14.9	0.15	0.025	6
15–19.9	0.10	0.1	1
20–29.9	0.02	0.2	0.1
30–44.9	0.02	0.35	0.06
45–59.9	0.01	0.3	0.03
60	0	0.0075	0
Total	1.0	1.0	

*POW = period of wakefulness.
†The ratio of the probability of the given result among people with the disease to the corresponding probability among people free of the disease.

Unit
C12

APPRAISAL OF DIAGNOSTIC TESTS

Diagnostic tests are used for at least three purposes: to discover the presence of a disease, to confirm its suspected presence, and to exclude its presence.

A test with a high sensitivity (*Question C11–1*) may obviously be useful as a discovery test, since it will not miss many cases. If its specificity is low, there will be many false positives, but this will not matter much if the additional tests needed to make a firm diagnosis can easily be done. A test with a high sensitivity may also be useful as an exclusion test (however low its specificity): the higher the sensitivity, the more certainly a negative result means absence of the disease.

The higher the specificity of a test (*Question C11–2*), the more useful the test may be as a confirmation test: a specificity of 100% means that a positive result is pathognomonic of the disease. However, a negative result does not mean absence of the disease.

These rough-and-ready rules are not very useful in practice. It is more helpful to see how the test affects our assessment of the likelihood that the disease is present. This is what you did in *Question C11–3*. The likelihood of the disease before test A is done is 21% (because the prevalence rate is 21 per 100). The pretest odds are $2,100/7,900 = 0.266$ to 1; odds can also be calculated from the probability P by the formula $P/(1 - P)$, as we saw in Unit B11; that is, $.21/(1 - .21) = .266$. If the test is positive, the posttest probability becomes $1,680/1,838 = 91\%$, and the posttest odds are 10.6. If the test is negative, the posttest probability is $420/8,162 = 5.1\%$, and the odds are 0.05.

The results of the test have a big influence on our assessment of the likelihood that the disease is present. Test A would therefore be a useful diagnostic tool (it does not appear to be too inconvenient, expensive, or hazardous to use).

As you saw in *Question C11–4*, multiplying the pretest odds by the likelihood ratio provides the posttest odds. If we know the likelihood ratios for the results of a test, it is thus easy to calculate the posttest odds and probabilities; remember that probability = odds/(1 + odds).

To use this procedure for converting the result of the test into a meaningful statement about the certainty of a diagnosis, one requires (a) an estimate of the pretest probability, and (b) information about the likelihood ratios when the test is applied to patients similar to the patient under consideration. The procedure can be used both for tests that have dichotomous results (as was demonstrated in Question C11–4) and for tests that give a range of results. If the test is a dichotomous one, the likelihood ratio for a positive result is the sensitivity divided by the false positive rate.

The procedure can also be used before a test is done, to see how the result can affect the probability of the disease. This may help the clinician to decide whether the test is worth doing (Note C12–1).

As an exercise, suppose that a 55-year-old woman is given a BLIP test (Table C11–3), and that you know that the specific prevalence rate of TV dementia in women of her age is 20%. What is the posttest probability of the disease if she falls asleep in one minute? in six minutes? in 50 minutes? Is the test useful? (For answers, see Note C12–2.)

THE MEANING OF "NORMAL"

The "normal" range of responses to the BLIP test (*Question C11–5*) is not easy to define. "Normal" is used in at least three different ways:

- "What is usual." In this sense, a normal range can be defined in unequivocal terms—for example, "from two standard deviations below the mean to two standard deviations above the mean" or "between the 10th and 90th percentiles." But "abnormal" then only means "unusual."

- "What is desirable"—that is, a range of values that indicate or predict good health. But there may be no sharp dividing line between "healthy" and "unhealthy" findings. In the present instance (Table C11–3), the monotonically decreasing likelihood ratios show that there is a gradient of normality, not a dichotomy; no finding occurs only in disease-free people, and no finding occurs only in people with the disease. Any dividing line must be arbitrary. We can decide, for example, that any result with a likelihood ratio of 1 or less is "normal"; but this "normal" range will include some—and maybe many—people with the disease.

- "What requires no action"—that is, there is no need for further investigations, for surveillance, or for curative or preventive measures. This use of "normal" requires information not only about

associations with health and disease, but also about the likely benefits of intervention.

NOTES

C12–1. For a detailed discussion of the selection and interpretation of
        diagnostic tests, see Sackett et al. (1985, chaps. 3–4) or a series
        of papers by the same authors (Department of Clinical Epi-
        demiology and Biostatistics, McMaster University, 1983).

C12–2. The pretest probability that a 55-year-old woman has TV de-
        mentia is .2. The pretest odds are $.2/(1 - .2) = 0.25$. If the
        subject falls asleep in one minute the likelihood ratio (Table
        C11–3) is 80. The posttest odds are therefore $0.25 \times 80 = 20$,
        and the posttest probability of the disease is $20/(1 + 20) = 95\%$.
        If the POW is six minutes, the posttest odds are $0.25 \times 20 = 5$,
        and the posttest probability is $5/6 = 83\%$. If the POW is 50
        minutes, the posttest probability is 0.7%. The test is obviously
        a useful one.

TEST YOURSELF (C)

To wrap up this section, see if you can do the following (Unit numbers in parentheses):

- List various ways of appraising the validity of a measure (C1).

- Calculate

    sensitivity and specificity of a measure (C1).
    false positive and negative rates (C1).
    predictive values of positive and negative results (C10).
    kappa (C8).

- Explain what is meant by

    criterion validity (C1).
    predictive validity (C1).
    construct validity (C1).
    content validity (C1).
    face validity (C1).
    consensual validity (C1).
    zero preference (C1).
    misclassification bias (C2).
    reliability (C7).
    a screening test (C10).

- Explain the difference between

    differential and nondifferential misclassification (C3).
    interobserver and intraobserver reliability (C7).
    percent agreement and kappa (C7).

- Explain

    how a low sensitivity will affect an estimate of prevalence (C3).
    how a low specificity will affect an estimate of prevalence (C3).

how use of a measure of low validity affects the estimated prevalence of a rare disease (C3).
why the predictive value of a positive test varies with the prevalence
of the disease (C3).

- List

ways of measuring the criterion validity of metric-scale measures
(C7).
various measures of reliability (C8, C9).
different kinds of scale of measurement (C7).

- State how an association between two variables may be affected by

nondifferential misclassification of one variable (C3).
nondifferential misclassification of both variables (C6).
differential misclassification of one variable (C6).
differential misclassification of both variables (C6).

- Appraise a screening test (C10, C11).

- State what factors influence the predictive value of a positive screening test (C11).

- Interpret a kappa value (C8, C9).

- Explain what is meant by

dichotomy (C7).
nominal, ordinal, interval and ratio scales (C7).
metric scale (C7).
continuous and discrete scales (C7).

- Explain (in general terms) what is meant by

Berksonian bias (C5).
internal consistency–reliability (C7).
regression toward the mean (C9).

(The following items refer to diagnostic tests.)

- Compare the importance of sensitivity and specificity in determining the usefulness of a diagnostic test (C12).

- Explain what is meant by

pretest probability and odds (C12).
post-test probability and odds (C12).
likelihood ratio (C12).
a "normal" result (C12).

- Calculate the posttest probability from the pretest probability and a
likelihood ratio (C12).

Making Sense of Associations

"I know what you're thinking about," said Tweedledum: "but it isn't so, nohow."

"Contrariwise," continued Tweedledee, "if it was so, it might be; and if it were so, it would be; but as it isn't, it ain't. That's logic."

(Carroll, 1872)

Unit
D1

INTRODUCTION

Section D deals with the appraisal of associations between variables, using the approach described in Unit A16. By way of a reminder, here is a list of basic questions that may be asked about an association:

- Actual or artifactual? (selection bias? information bias?)

- Strength (rate ratio, odds ratio, rate difference, etc.) and other qualities (direction? monotonic? linear?)

- Nonfortuitous?

- Consistent? (influence of modifying factors?)

- Influence of confounding factors?

- Causal?

We have already done a number of exercises on the detection and examination of associations, the appraisal of selection and information bias, confounding and modifying effects, the use of stratification and standardization to control confounding effects, and other specific aspects.

Topics that will receive special attention in this section include statistical significance, methods of appraising the possibility and likely direction of confounding effects, measures of the strength of associations, synergism, the appraisal of associations in stratified data, and multivariate analysis. The appraisal of causation will be dealt with in more detail in Section E.

EXERCISE D1

Are people with varicose veins especially likely to develop coronary heart disease? This was one of the questions investigated in a prospec-

Table D1. Incidence Rate of Coronary Heart
Disease* (CHD) per 1,000 Person-Years, by
Presence of Varicose Veins at Entry into Study

Varicose Veins	No. of Men	Rate of CHD
None	5,477	2.9
Mild	1,217	4.4
Moderate	731	5.7
Total	7,425	3.4

*Myocardial infarction and deaths from CHD.

tive study of Paris policemen (Note D1). After an initial examination,
7,432 men (French-born, aged 42–53) with no evidence of coronary heart
disease or certain other atherosclerotic diseases were followed up for an
average of 6.6 years, to identify new cases and deaths of coronary heart
disease. The results are shown in Table D1. The rates are person-time
incidence rates.

Question D1–1

Summarize the facts about the association between varicose veins and
coronary heart disease.

Question D1–2

What are the possible explanations for the association between varicose
veins and coronary heart disease? (Ignore Occam's razor.)

Question D1–3

What additional information would you like? (Use Occam's razor.)

NOTE

D1.   The study is by Ducimetière et al. (1981). The exercises use derived
      data, which may not completely conform with the actual findings.

Unit
D2

EXPLANATIONS FOR AN ASSOCIATION

In answer to *Question D1–1*, there is a positive association between the presence of varicose veins and the subsequent incidence of coronary heart disease (CHD). Men with mild varicose veins had a higher rate of CHD than men with no varicose veins, and men with moderate varicose veins had a still higher rate. One way of expressing the strength of this association is to calculate rate ratios, using one group (say, the men without varicose veins) as the *reference category*. The rate ratios are then $4.4/2.9 = 1.5$ for mild varicose veins and $5.7/2.9 = 2.0$ for moderate varicose veins. Ratios of incidence rates are often termed *risk ratios* or *relative risks*.

The possible explanations for the association (*Question D1–2*) are as follows:

1. The association may be an artifact resulting from selection bias, differential misclassification, or other shortcomings in the study methods.
2. The association may be a chance one.
3. The association may reflect the confounding effects of age, social class, fatness or other variables.
4. Varicose veins may be a cause of CHD (rather unlikely).

In seeking additional information (*Question D1–3*), it would be wise to start with information about the methods used in the study. This will give us a better understanding of what the numbers in the table represent, and enable us to appraise the likelihood of selection bias or information bias. We should ask such questions as: How was the study sample chosen? Were there many nonresponders or losses to follow-up? How were varicose veins and CHD measured? Is there information on validity or reliability?

The exercises that follow deal with possible information bias, statistical significance, confounding, and the uses of the study. We will assume that there is no reason to suspect selection bias.

EXERCISE D2

The report on the study states that

during the examination, the clinician visually inspected and palpated the legs of each subject and noted any venous enlargement or tortuosity. The severity of the varicosities when present were coded as mild or moderate . . . [There were] significant differences in the observations of individual clinicians. Among the 12 physicians who [each] examined at least 200 patients . . . the observed prevalence varied from 14% (of which 5% were moderate) to 40% (15% moderate). [The men] were followed up by annual examinations or in the case of retirement by mailed questionnaires, and new cases of atherosclerotic diseases and deaths were identified. . . All events were confirmed by a medical committee from documents available . . . [indicating] appearance of new Q waves on the electrocardiogram . . . or clinical symptoms with electrical changes. Enzymatic data were evaluated when available.

Question D2–1

Can you reach a conclusion about the validity of the diagnoses of varicose veins and CHD?

Question D2–2

How may possible misclassification affect the association between varicose veins and CHD?

Question D2–3

How may possible misclassification of cases affect the association between CHD and other variables?

Unit

D3

EFFECTS OF MISCLASSIFICATION

In answer to *Question D2–1*, we cannot be certain that the differences in the findings of the 12 physicians occurred only because of interobserver variation in the diagnosis of varicose veins, since there may have been real differences in prevalence among the groups they examined. But it is probably correct to conclude that reliability was low, particularly in the absence of information about any efforts to standardize the examination methods or diagnostic criteria. The investigators themselves inferred that the diagnosis of varicose veins was "partially subjective" and "far from satisfactory."

If we conclude that reliability was not high, we must also conclude that validity was not high. The term used by the investigators was "uncertainty of diagnostic accuracy." As the presence of varicose veins was measured at the outset of the study, misclassification was probably nondifferential; that is, sensitivity and specificity were probably similar in men who subsequently developed CHD and men who did not. If this is so, the effect would be to reduce the strength of the association between varicose veins and CHD. We cannot, however, be absolutely sure that misclassification was nondifferential: possibly the diagnosis was less valid, for example, in fat subjects, who may also have been more likely to develop CHD.

The diagnoses of CHD cannot be completely valid; cases may well have been missed, especially among pensioners (who were not examined). There is no reason, however, to suspect that the validity of the diagnosis was related to the presence of varicose veins; information was obtained about all subjects annually, and the same methods and criteria were used for men with and without varicose veins. We may conclude that this misclassification, too, probably weakened the association between CHD and varicose veins. The true association is thus probably stronger than the observed one.

In answer to *Question D2–3*, the validity of the diagnoses of CHD probably differed in nonpensioners (who were examined) and pensioners (who were not), resulting in differential misclassification. This might strengthen, attenuate, or reverse the association between CHD and age or any other variable closely linked with retirement.

STATISTICAL SIGNIFICANCE

We test the statistical significance of an association to enable us to decide whether to regard the finding as nonfortuitous. The test provides a P value, which tells us the probability that, if no association actually exists, chance processes alone would produce an association as strong as, or stronger than, the one actually observed (see Note D3).

A critical value ("alpha") of 0.05 is often used for appraising significance. That is, a P value of under 1 in 20 is often regarded as justification for regarding an association as nonfortuitous. Lower critical values of P—for example, .01 or .001—may be used.

In the present example, the value of P was .0042; that is, the likelihood that chance processes alone would produce the observed association between varicose veins and CHD was 42 in 10,000, or 1 in 238. The association was highly significant.

EXERCISE D3

Question D3-1

Compare the make-believe data in Table D3–1 with the data in Table D1. In Table D3–1 the sample size is half that in Table D1, but the incidence rates are identical. Which table shows a stronger association? Which set of data will yield a higher P value? Which set of data will yield more precise estimates of the rate ratios (i.e., narrower confidence intervals)?

Table D3–1. Incidence Rate of Coronary Heart Disease (CHD) per 1,000 Person-Years, by Presence of Varicose Veins at Entry into Study: Imaginary Data

Varicose Veins	No. of Men	Rate of CHD
None	2,738	2.9
Mild	608	4.4
Moderate	365	5.7

Question D3–2

Are the following statements true or false?

1. When we detect an association that is of interest, we should always test its statistical significance.
2. A test of statistical significance will tell us whether an association is present.
3. A test of statistical significance will tell us whether an association is strong.
4. A test of statistical significance will tell us whether an association is causal.
5. If an association is statistically significant, it is not a chance association.
6. If an association is not statistically significant, it is a chance association.

Question D3–3

If you had to choose between a significance test and the confidence interval of a measure of association, which would you prefer?

Question D3–4

A well-designed trial in which a new treatment and a conventional treatment were compared in similar groups of patients shows that the new treatment is more effective. The P level is .045, according to a one-tailed significance test. Do you know what a one-tailed test is? What hypothesis was tested in this trial? How would you appraise the finding of the trial?

Question D3–5

Before returning to Paris, we take a brief look at a study in Cambridge, England, where Davies et al. (1986) compared the mothers of boys with undescended testes with the mothers of normal boys born on the same day in the same hospital, in order to test the hypothesis that undescended testis is caused by an excess of maternal estrogen in pregnancy. The specific hypothesis was that the mothers of boys with undescended testes would have had a higher prevalence, during pregnancy, of nausea, vomiting, and hypertension (believed to be associated with a high estrogen level). The findings are shown in Table D3–2. Assume that these are the only results of the study. Would you regard the difference with respect to threatened abortion as a finding not attributable to chance?

Table D3–2. Comparison of Pregnancies of Mothers Whose Boys Had Undescended Testes and Mothers of Normal Boys

Variable	Odds Ratio	P
Mean age at conception	—	NS*
Mean length of gestation	—	NS
Mean birth weight	—	NS
Birth weight <2,500 g	—	NS
Threatened abortion	4.9	.04
Breech presentation	0.5	NS
Nausea	1.3	NS
Consultation for nausea	1.1	NS
Antiemetics prescribed	1.4	NS
Vomiting	1.1	NS
Consultation for vomiting	1.1	NS
Hypertension	1.3	NS
Proteinuria	0.5	NS
Any of the above seven	1.1	NS
Any x-rays	0.8	NS
Any ultrasound	1.0	NS
Cigarette smoking (≥1/day)	1.4	NS
Alcohol (≥1 unit/day)	0.8	NS
Iron preparation taken	0.8	NS
Hypnotics	0.2	NS
Analgesics	1.8	NS

*NS: not significant ($P \geq .05$).

NOTE

D3. At the risk of oversimplification, most significance tests can be said to calculate the probability (P) that an association that is as strong as (or stronger than) the one that was observed will occur in a random sample (of the size actually used) drawn from a wider population in which this association does not exist (i.e., in which the null hypothesis holds true). The P value is the probability of concluding that there is a real association when actually there is none. Significance testing may be concerned not only with random sampling variation, but also with random measurement error and other "chance" processes. The test "can't do its job unless the word 'chance' has been given a precise definition . . . Unless there is a clearly defined chance model, a test of significance makes no sense" (from Freedman et al., 1978, who explain "chance models" at length). Refer to a statistics textbook for a full explanation of statistical significance.

STATISTICAL SIGNIFICANCE
(CONTINUED)

In answer to *Question D3–1*, the incidence rates are the same in both tables. This means that the associations are equally strong. But the sample size is smaller in Table D3–1. Therefore the data in Table D3–1 will yield a higher P value: that is, there is a higher probability that chance processes alone would produce the association seen in this sample. The data in Table D1 will provide more precise estimates of the rate ratios.

All the statements in *Question D3–2* are false:

1. We may sometimes be interested in an association without caring whether it occurred by chance or not. If the immunization rate is lower in one neighborhood than in another, this may require special action, whatever the reason for the difference; statistical significance is irrelevant.
2. A significance test cannot tell us whether there is an association. What it does is to help us decide whether to regard an observed association as nonfortuitous.
3. One of the factors determining statistical significance is sample size. Even a trivial association may be statistically significant if the sample is large enough.
4. Statistical significance does not tell us whether an association is causal. A statistically significant association may be an artifact or a consequence of confounding.
5. A verdict of significance does not prove that the association is not a chance one; it tells us only that the association is unlikely to be due to "chance" processes alone (see Note D3), so that we can have some degree of confidence in regarding it as nonfortuitous.
6. A "nonsignificant" result does not prove that the association is a chance one. It tells us only that "chance" processes might easily produce such an association. The verdict is "not proven." (But a

"nonsignificant" result in a very large sample indicates that there is probably no *strong* nonfortuitous association.)

There is no simple correct answer to *Question D3-3*; in some circumstances a significance test is more appropriate than the confidence interval of a measure of association (Fleiss, 1986a). In general, however, confidence intervals are more informative, since they

provide estimates of the gamut of true relations consistent with a given set of observations. As such they may allow reconciliation of apparently divergent results, and they generally (since confidence intervals are almost always wider than one would wish) introduce an appropriate note of caution into the interpretation of 'clear' findings. (Walker, 1986)

There is currently a debate about the value of significance tests, summarized as follows by a proponent:

Some epidemiologists believe that significance tests are dead, and in some journals they've succeeded in burying tests and p-values. Investigators who are comfortable using them should be reassured that, nevertheless, significance tests are alive and well. (Fleiss, 1986a)

A *one-tailed (one-sided) significance test* tests for the presence of a difference in a specified direction, unlike the "ordinary" (two-tailed) test used in most epidemiological studies, which ignores the direction of the difference. The hypothesis tested in the trial described in *Question D3-4* was that the new treatment was better than the conventional one (the null hypothesis being that it was not better). A two-tailed test would have tested the hypothesis that the two treatments differed in their effectiveness (the null hypothesis being that there was no difference, in either direction).

One-tailed tests are quite valid, and their results can be taken at their face value, provided the test has not been misused. On this condition, we can compare the P value with whatever critical level (say, .05) we choose to use, and decide whether to regard the superiority of the new treatment as nonfortuitous.

There may be a temptation to use one-tailed tests inappropriately, because the one-tailed P value is generally half the two-tailed value: in this trial, the two-tailed P value would have been .09 ("not significant"). In the planning stage of a study, temptation may arise because one-tailed tests require smaller sample sizes. Statisticians agree that the decision to use a one-tailed test must be made before the data are examined (no data-snooping!). Such a test should obviously be used only if there is interest in a difference in a specific direction. An extreme, but "safe" (i.e., conservative) view is that "one should decide to use a one-sided test only if it is quite certain that departures in one particular direction will always be ascribed to chance, and therefore regarded as nonsignificant, however large they are. This situation rarely arises in practice" (Armitage and Berry, 1987). If the original intention was to use a one-tailed test but when the data became available a switch was made to a two-tailed test because of a surprising difference in the unexpected direction, Cochran (1983) suggests that the P value be multiplied by 1.5.

Significance tests have "built-in" errors. If a critical level of .05 is used, chance processes will produce a verdict of "statistically significant" in about five of every 100 tests performed, even if no real associations exist (Note D4). In *Question D3–5*, where 21 differences were tested and one of them was found to be (just) significant, it is difficult to be confident that this difference was not a "statistically significant" fluke. To play safe, we could lower the critical level—for example, if 21 tests are done, by dividing .05 by 21, and demanding a P value of $<.0024$; alternatively (which comes to the same thing), we could multiply each P value by 21 before comparing it with our critical level of .05. In some circumstances, special tests may be used for multiple comparisons.

EXERCISE D4

We have decided that the association between varicose veins and CHD is probably a real one (underestimated by our data), and can be regarded as nonfortuitous. We now consider possible confounding.

Table D4 shows the prevalence of varicose veins in police of different ranks.

Question D4–1

Summarize the facts shown in Table D4. Use rate ratios.

Question D4–2

May the association between varicose veins and CHD be confounded by rank?

Table D4. Prevalence (%) of Varicose Veins by Rank

Varicose Veins	Officers (N = 1,270)	Subofficers (N = 1,895)	Policemen (N = 4,260)
None	78.6	73.1	72.6
Mild	13.6	17.2	16.9
Moderate	7.8	9.7	10.5
Total	100.0	100.0	100.0

Question D4–3

The association between rank and varicose veins is highly significant: P = .000013. How does this finding affect the probability that rank may confound the association between varicose veins and CHD?

Question D4–4

If there were no association between rank and varicose veins, could rank confound the association between varicose veins and CHD?

Question D4–5

If rank is a confounder, in what direction will it bias the results?

Question D4–6

How can we determine whether rank is actually a confounder?

Question D4–7

Can you suggest other possible confounders of the CHD–varicose veins connection?

NOTE

D4. Spurious "statistically significant" results (indicating that there is a real association when actually there is none) are called "type I" errors. A type II error is the erroneous failure to find a true association. The *power* of a test is its capacity to avoid type II errors.

Unit
D5

CONFOUNDING EFFECTS

In answer to *Question D4–1*, there is an inverse relationship between rank and varicose veins. The main difference is between officers and other ranks; both mild and moderate varicose veins are slightly less prevalent in officers than in other ranks. The differences between subofficers and policemen are small. Table D5–1 shows rate ratios. In a table of this sort, the reference category, with which the other groups are compared, has a rate ratio of 1.0.

The conditions necessary for confounding were considered in Units A10, A11 and A14: the association between an independent and dependent variable can be confounded by a third variable that influences the dependent variable and is associated with the independent variable (without being an intermediate link in the chain of causation connecting the other two variables). In answer to *Question D4–2*, therefore, confounding by rank is a possibility; to meet the conditions completely, rank must also affect the incidence of CHD. However, a confounding effect of any importance is possible only if the associations between the confounder and the other variables are strong ones. As Table D5–1 shows, the association between rank and varicose veins is weak. Rank can have a substantial confounding effect only if the association between rank and CHD is very strong indeed.

Table D5–1. Association Between Varicose Veins and Rank: Rate Ratios

Varicose Veins	Officers*	Subofficers	Policemen
Mild	1.0	1.3	1.2
Moderate	1.0	1.2	1.3
Total	1.0	1.3	1.3

*Reference category.

The confounding effect is determined by the presence, direction and strength of the associations between the potential confounder and the other variables. The statistical significance of these associations (*Question D4–3*) is irrelevant. Weak associations—even if statistically highly significant—are unlikely to produce an important confounding effect, whereas strong associations that are not statistically significant (usually because the sample is small) may produce a substantial confounding effect. (Despite this, significance testing may have a role as a strategy for deciding which potential confounders to control; see Note D5.)

A variable can confound the association between two other variables only if it is associated with both of them. The simple answer to *Question D4–4*, then, is no: if rank is not associated with both varicose veins and CHD, it cannot confound the association between varicose veins and CHD.

This forms the basis for a strategy frequently used when considering possible confounders: we know the conditions that must be met if confounding is to occur, and can see whether they are met. If they are definitely not met, we can decide to disregard the possibility of confounding.

This *exclusion test* is useful, but unfortunately not foolproof. Confounding may occur even when the crude data do not demonstrate associations between the suspected confounder and the other variables, since conditional associations (see Unit A9) may be present; that is, an association with the dependent variable may exist when the independent variable is held constant in the analysis, or vice versa. An association between rank and CHD, for example, might exist in men without varicose veins, and this association might easily be missed if we looked only at the data as a whole, ignoring the presence of varicose veins. These conditional associations may satisfy the requirements for confounding (Kleinbaum et al., 1982, chap. 13). What this means, in effect, is that an exclusion test based on the easily observed "crude" associations may be misleading; not only may the crude data fail to reveal an existing conditional association between the suspected confounder and the dependent variable (if the suspected confounder is also a modifier), it may also obscure a conditional association between the suspected confounder and the independent variable (for a fictional example, see Kahn and Sempos 1989, p. 86). In these exercises, we will generally ignore this complication, remembering only that the exclusion test, as usually applied, is not foolproof. This is a calculated risk that many epidemiologists take in real life.

The direction of a confounding effect can be predicted by a simple and useful although not always reliable *Direction Rule*. If the associations of C (the confounder) with A and B are both in the same direction (i.e., if both are positive or both are inverse), confounding will tend to produce a positive association between A and B. On the other hand, if the associations of C with A and B are in opposite directions (one positive and one inverse), confounding will tend to produce an inverse association between A and B. (This rule may be misleading if C is also a modifier, such that the direction of the association between A and B differs in the categories of C: the effect will depend on the relative size of these categories; paradoxical situations may occur.)

In this instance (*Question D4–5*), the direction of the possible confounding effect of rank cannot be predicted, as we have no information on the direction of the association between rank and CHD.

To determine whether rank is actually a confounder (*Question D4–6*), we can compare the crude relative risks—that is, the risk ratios based on the crude rates (Table D5–1)—with the relative risks seen when rank is controlled by stratification, standardization, or some other procedure. In the next exercise, we will see rates standardized for rank.

The candidates for inclusion in a list of possible confounders (*Question D4–7*) are variables that are known or suspected to be causally related to the dependent variable, and that may be associated with (but not affected by) the independent variable as well; consideration should always be given to the "universal variables" (see Unit A11). Your list probably includes age, smoking, blood pressure, obesity, diabetes, and other known risk factors for coronary heart disease.

EXERCISE D5

Question D5–1

The incidence rates of CHD were standardized for rank, using the indirect method. The rates in the total study sample were used as the standard. The results are shown in Table D5–2, together with the crude rates. According to these figures, was the association between varicose veins and CHD confounded by rank?

Table D5–2. Incidence of CHD by Presence of Varicose Veins

Varicose Veins	Crude Rate*	Standardized for Rank	
		SMR	Rate*
Absent	2.9	0.86	2.9
Present	4.9	1.37	4.7

*Mean annual rate per 1,000.

Question D5-2

Are the following statements true or false?

1. A variable can confound the association between two other variables only if it is associated with both of them.
2. Confounding often produces very strong associations.
3. If no association is detected between the variables that interest us, there is no point in considering possible confounding effects.
4. If the association between two variables becomes weaker or disappears when a third variable is controlled, this shows that the third variable is a confounder.
5. A confounding effect is always completely controlled by stratification.
6. A confounding effect is always completely controlled by standardization.

Question D5-3

You may remember that in a previous exercise (B12), we found that fractures of the femur were more common in Oxford than in Epiville, and considered the possibility that age might be a confounder. Older people had a higher incidence of fractures, and people in Oxford were older than in Epiville. Use the Direction Rule to predict how controlling for age will affect the association between fractures and place of residence.

Question D5-4

Is there any way of appraising the possible confounding effect of a variable that was not measured in the study under consideration?

NOTE

D5. Experts disagree on the role of significance testing in the identification of possible confounders. The general view is that statistical significance is irrelevant. As pointed out by Fleiss (1986a, 1986b), however, significance testing provides explicit rules and hence a reproducible method for use in appraising the relative importance of potential confounders and deciding which to control.

Unit
D6

CONFOUNDING EFFECTS (CONTINUED)

A change in the strength of an association when a suspected confounder is controlled is suggestive of confounding. To answer *Question D5–1*, we must know the strength of the association according to both the crude and standardized results. The crude relative risk was 4.9/2.9, that is, 1.7, and the standardized relative risk was 1.37/0.86 or 4.7/2.9, that is, 1.6. There was thus a very slight—and hence unimportant—confounding effect.

The answers to the "true–false" questions (*D5–2*) are:

1. True. However, the associations with the other variables may not be obvious; they may be conditional ones.
2. False. Even if the confounder is strongly associated with the other variables, "the spurious effect is only a relatively weak echo" (Note D6).
3. False. The apparent absence of an association may be due to confounding.
4. False. The third variable may be a confounder, but it may also be an intervening cause that mediates the causal relationship between the two variables.
5. False. Stratification controls the confounding effect completely only if the categories are homogeneous. If we were controlling for systolic blood pressure, and used broad categories such as "<140," "140–159," and ≥160 mm Hg, there would still be much variation *within* the strata: blood pressure would not be altogether "held constant," and some of its confounding effect might remain.
6. False. In the same way, the use of broad categories may also impair the value of standardization.

To use the Direction Rule (*Question D5–3*), we must be able to designate associations as positive or negative. This may require the choice of reference categories (the choice is arbitrary, and does not affect the conclusions). In this instance, let us choose "Epiville" as the reference category for place of residence. The facts, then, are that age is negatively associated with the independent variable (residence in Epiville) and positively associated with the dependent variable (incidence of fractures). As these associations are in opposite directions, we can predict that if age is a confounder it will probably tend to produce a negative association between residence in Epiville and fractures of the femur. If the confounding effect is controlled, the association will therefore become "more positive." Because the crude incidence rates showed a negative association between residence in Epiville and fractures, we can expect that if age is controlled the negative association will become weaker or disappear, or even change to a positive one—as it actually did when we controlled for age by stratification (Table B14–1) or standardization (Table B14–2).

In answer to *Question D5–4*, it is sometimes possible to make inferences about a confounding effect even if the suspected confounder was not measured. This requires knowledge (from other studies) of the strength and direction of the suspected confounder's associations with other variables. It is then possible to apply the "exclusion test" and the Direction Rule, and even to estimate the magnitude of the possible confounding effect (Note D6).

EXERCISE D6

In this exercise we glance at multivariate analysis. (We will return to this topic later.)

A multivariate analysis was used in the study of Paris police, to control simultaneously for the possible confounding effects of six variables known or suspected to be associated with CHD. These were age, number of cigarettes smoked per day, systolic blood pressure, serum cholesterol, the presence of diabetes, and Quetelet's body mass index. The adjusted relative risks of CHD when these variables were controlled (i.e., held constant) are shown in Table D6, together with the relative risks based on the crude data. The association between varicose veins and CHD remained statistically significant ($P = .0053$) when these six variables were controlled.

Question D6–1

According to Table D6, can the association between varicose veins and CHD be attributed to the confounding effects of the six variables controlled in this analysis?

Table D6. Relative Risk of CHD
by Presence of Varicose Veins

Varicose Veins	Crude*	Adjusted†
None	1.00	1.00
Mild	1.52	1.34
Moderate	1.97	1.78

*Based on rates in Table D1.
†Controlling for six variables (see text).

Question D6–2

The following explanation was provided for the method of multivariate analysis used in this study. (Don't worry if you don't understand it.)

Multivariate analysis of the relationship between annual incidence rates and different variables was performed by an exponential model with covariates which allowed for unequal follow-up durations (Lellouch, J. and Rokotovao, R., 1976). During follow up, the hazard rate for illness is assumed to be constant (r) for each subject. This assumption is equivalent to stating that the probability that the subject will get the illness before the instant t is $1 - \exp(-rt)$, the classical exponential survival model. The individual hazard rate, r, is chosen as an exponential function of the covariates $x_i \ldots x_k$:

$$r = r_0 \exp(b_i x_i \cdots + b_k x_k)$$

Writing the likelihood of observations for cases and noncases and maximising this quantity by an iterative technique gives an estimate of r_0 and the b_j's as well as their asymptotic standard error, allowing a test of the significance of the b_j's by a t test.

Just for argument's sake, pretend you don't understand this explanation. Do you feel that, despite this, you can safely use the results?

NOTE

D6. See Bross (1966 and 1967), who explains how to find whether a possible confounder's associations with two other variables are strong enough to account for the observed association between these other variables.

MULTIVARIATE ANALYSIS

The use of multivariate analysis to control six possible confounders (Table D6) reduces the strength of the association between varicose veins and CHD, but the association remains apparent. The answer to *Question D6–1*, therefore, is that the association can be only partly explained by the confounding effects of these factors.

Question D6–2 poses a real dilemma. We have seen how even a simple statistical manipulation like standardization may, under some circumstances, yield misleading results (Units B14 and B15). How much more likely is it that a complicated procedure—especially one that we do not understand—may mislead us.

We cannot avoid this dilemma. Multivariate analysis provides a shortcut way of handling the effects of a number of variables at the same time, and of looking at complicated interrelationships. With ready access to computers and ready-made computer programs, such analyses are easy to do and increasingly popular. But this does not make their results easier to appraise. Must we just take them on trust?

Ideally, we should understand the procedures well enough to know when they are appropriate, and how to relate to the findings. But what if we don't, and can't find a friendly statistician to ask? There are many forms of multivariate analysis: multiple linear regression, analysis of variance and covariance, discriminant analysis, log-linear analysis, logit analysis, multiple logistic regression, and others. Each uses its own mathematical model (Note D7–1) and is based on its own set of assumptions, which are not always clearly spelled out, and may or may not be justified.

A basic general understanding of the main multivariate methods is not difficult to acquire (see Note D7–2). But if we lack this and cannot obtain help, we should not ourselves use a multivariate procedure; and if we come across one in a published paper, we should see whether the investigators present a plausible case for the validity of the method: are the assumptions explained and justified, and has the model as a whole been tested to see how well it fits the observed facts? Failing this, the best we can do may be to consider the qualifications and stature of the investigators and the reputation of the journal, and decide whether these inspire us with confidence. (Maybe this is a cop-out, but there may be no alternative.)

In any case, it is prudent to regard the results of any multivariate analysis as providing only an *approximate* picture of the truth. A mathematical model rarely fits the facts perfectly. It is probably wise not to take the findings too literally; associations may be somewhat weaker or stronger than they appear, adjustment for confounding effects may be incomplete, and levels of statistical significance may be misleading. Clear-cut findings are probably correct, but borderline ones—associations that are weak or of marginal statistical significance—should be taken with a pinch of salt.

EXERCISE D7

In this exercise, we review possible explanations for the association between varicose veins and CHD, and consider the possible uses of the findings.

Question D7–1

This study has shown an association between varicose veins and CHD which (because of misclassification) is probably stronger than it appears.

1. In the light of what you now know, is it possible that the association is a chance finding?
2. Is it possible that the association is a consequence of confounding?
3. May the association be explained by an effect of CHD on the occurrence of varicose veins?
4. May the association be explained by an effect of varicose veins on the occurrence of CHD?
5. Is it possible that varicose veins and CHD are associated because they share a common cause or causes?

Question D7–2

Summarize the additional information that Table D7 provides about the varicose veins–CHD association. Can you suggest an explanation for the new findings?

Making Sense of Associations

Table D7. Occurrence of CHD by Presence of Varicose Veins and Rank (Numbers of Cases and Mean Annual Rates per 1,000)

	Rank					
	Officers		Subofficers		Policemen	
Varicose Veins	Cases	Rate*	Cases	Rate*	Cases	Rate*
Absent	21	3.3	28	3.1	54	2.9
Present	5	3.1	11	3.4	44	5.9
P		NS*		NS		.0005

*NS = not significant ($p \geq .05$).

Question D7–3

The title of the paper on which these exercises were based asks "Varicose veins: a risk factor for atherosclerotic disease?" What is your answer to this question?

Question D7–4

Brandishing the results shown in Table D7, the health officer of the Paris police force excitedly announces that he intends to institute a program using varicose veins as a risk marker. In order to reduce the incidence of CHD, all rank-and-file policemen with varicose veins will be identified and subjected to intensive health surveillance and risk factor intervention, including advice on diet and smoking, and treatment of blood pressure where necessary. Do you have any reservations about his decision? What criteria would you use for appraising the value of a risk marker (i.e., an indicator of increased risk)?

Question D7–5

What are the possible other uses of what we have learned about the association between varicose veins and CHD in Paris policemen?

NOTES

D7–1. *"Mathematical model.* A representation of a system, process or relationship in mathematical form in which equations are used to simulate the behaviour of the system or process under study"—*A Dictionary of Epidemiology* (Last, 1983).

D7–2. For a brief general explanation of multivariate analysis, see Kahn and Sempos (1989, chap. 6). In their view, "epidemiologists require a general understanding of some multivariate methods, but most need statistical assistance in carrying out the specific analyses required by specific studies."

U n i t
D8

EXPLANATIONS FOR THE FINDINGS

In answer to *Question D7–1:*

1. Yes, the association may be a chance finding. The probability that it is due to chance is .0053 (according to the multivariate analysis), or 1 in 189.
2. Yes, the association may be a consequence of confounding by factors that we have not yet examined, or maybe thought of.
3. No, the association cannot be due to an effect of CHD on the risk of incurring varicose veins—an impossibility if we accept the investigators' assurance that the men were free of CHD at the outset of the study. An effect cannot precede its cause.
4. Yes, the association may be explained by an effect of varicose veins on the occurrence of CHD. The "dose–response" relationship shown in Table D1—that is, the monotonic increase in CHD incidence when men with no varicose veins, mild varicose veins, and moderate varicose veins were compared—is consistent with a causal explanation. The only argument against this explanation is that it is difficult to suggest a plausible etiological mechanism. This low biological plausibility may lead us to regard a causal explanation as improbable, but we may be wrong: maybe the explanation is correct, and current biological knowledge is defective.
5. Yes, it is possible that varicose veins and CHD have a common cause (or causes), even if we cannot identify it. A common cause may have a confounding effect (Fig. A14–2). Finding a variable that confounds the association between varicose veins and CHD because of its effect on both these disorders would add to our understanding of etiology; a confounder is not always just a "nuisance variable."

In answer to *Question D7–2,* stratification of the data (Table D7) shows that the association between varicose veins and CHD is modified by

220

rank. There is no noteworthy association in officers (relative risk = 3.1/3.3 = 0.9) or suboffa cers (relative risk = 1.1); however, in rank-and-file policemen the relative risk is 2.0, and this is statistically highly significant. In other words, the presence of varicose veins is a risk marker for CHD, but only in rank-and-file policemen.

To explain why the association between varicose veins and CHD is restricted to rank-and-file policemen, we must consider how these men differ from police of higher ranks—in the nature of their work, the conditions they are exposed to, their life-style, or the characteristics or experiences that led to their being rank-and-file policemen and not officers or suboffa cers. We need to identify some factor whose presence is a condition for the processes (which we do not yet understand) that link varicose veins and CHD. The factor we are seeking must, of course, be one that is associated with the incidence of CHD (see Unit A13). It need not, on the other hand, be associated with the independent variable (varicose veins); this is a requirement for a confounding effect, but not for a modifying effect.

No explanation for the effect modification was suggested by the investigators. You may have been more successful. If so, check that the factor you have named meets the above condition. Your suspected factor may, for example, be excessive standing. It is not enough to know that (as the investigators tell us) the average Paris policeman spends a large amount of time standing relatively motionless; we must also know, or at least believe it plausible, that prolonged standing is associated with CHD. If these conditions are met, we can proceed to seek facts that will test the hypothesis that excessive standing accounts for the findings seen in Table D7. (To do this, we will need data on the amount of standing.) Note that the possible association between excessive standing and varicose veins (found in other studies) is not relevant to the hypothesis that excessive standing modifies the association between varicose veins and CHD.

RISK FACTORS AND RISK MARKERS

"Yes," "no," and "don't know" are all acceptable answers to *Question D7–3*, depending mainly on how "risk factor" is defined. There is unfortunately no agreed definition. To cite the *Dictionary of Epidemiology* (Last, 1983):

Risk factor. This term is used by different authors with at least three different meanings.

1. An attribute or exposure that is associated with an increased probability of a specified outcome, such as the occurrence of a disease. Not necessarily a causal factor. A risk marker.

2. An attribute or exposure that increases the probability of occurrence of disease or other specified outcome. A determinant.
3. A determinant that can be modified by intervention, thereby reducing the probability of occurrence of disease or other specified outcomes. To avoid confusion, may be referred to as a "modifiable risk factor."

If we use definition 1, the answer to the question is "yes." If we use one of the other definitions, our answer may be "no" (not proved by the study) or "don't know" (not disproved).

In the interests of clarity, it is probably best to use the term "risk factor" only if we know that the factor is causal—that is, that it increases the risk (definition 2) and does not merely *point to* an increased risk (definition 1). If the factor points to—but does not necessarily bring about—an increased risk, it is advisable to call it a risk marker. These are the terms we will use in these exercises. If we thought that varicose veins were a cause of CHD and that treating them would reduce the incidence of CHD, we could use the term "modifiable risk factor" (definition 3).

APPRAISING A RISK MARKER

A risk marker should be appraised in the same way as a screening test (Units C10 and C11). The only difference between them is that screening tests identify people with a high probability of *having* a disease, whereas risk markers identify people with a high probability of *developing* the disease. Before deciding to use varicose veins as a risk marker in his program (*Question D7-4*), the police health officer should review statistical indices such as sensitivity and predictive value, and compare them with the corresponding indices for alternative risk markers—as well, of course, as having satisfactory evidence for the effectiveness of preventive intervention.

The sensitivity of varicose veins as a predictor of CHD in rank-and-file policemen was 45%. (Do you know where this figure comes from? If not, see Note D8-1). The risk marker would have identified under half of those who incurred CHD by the end of the study. If cases in all ranks are taken into account, we see from Table D7 that only 44/163, or 27%, of cases would have been identified in the program. The health officer should certainly take these facts into consideration. Even if the proposed intervention can completely prevent CHD (which is unlikely), the program will prevent only part of the cases. Maybe the health officer should consider the provision of preventive care to the whole police force (irrespective of individual risk), or seek a more sensitive risk marker.

The predictive value of a risk marker (equivalent to that of a screening test) is the risk associated with the marker. The health officer knows that in rank-and-file policemen this risk is 5.9 per 1,000 per year (Table D7), or about 3.5% in six years, and has presumably decided that this provides sufficient justification for his program.

Additional factors to be taken into account in appraising the value of a risk marker in a program of this sort include the risk marker's prevalence. If this is very high, so that the high-risk group requiring special attention is very large, it may be more effective and efficient to give extra care to the total population. (Do you know the difference between effectiveness and efficiency? If not, see Note D8–2.) In this instance, the prevalence rate of varicose veins in rank-and-file policemen is 27% (Table D4). Also, the use of the risk marker must be practicable in terms of cost, resources, acceptability, and convenience. Obviously, there must also be good reason to believe that the detection of vulnerability will lead to an appreciable reduction of risk, and the expected benefit must outweigh any harm that may be done by labeling apparently healthy people as being "at risk" and involving them in surveillance and preventive activities.

USES OF THE FINDINGS

In considering the possible uses of knowledge about the association of varicose veins with CHD in Paris police (*Question D7–5*), we should take account of the various categories of users (Unit A17).

First, for users whose chief interest is in the health care of Paris police, the results point to a way of identifying men with an especially high risk of CHD, who may merit special surveillance and preventive care. This may be applied not only in a special program, but in the clinical care of individual policemen. Second, the results may possibly serve the same purpose for those who want to identify high-risk individuals or groups in other populations. And third, for users whose basic interest is in "research," the association may provide clues that will lead, in the long run, to a better understanding of etiological processes and methods of prevention. This is probably the most important potential contribution of the study. Why does the association exist? Do varicose veins and coronary heart disease have common etiological factors, such as dietary factors or decreased blood fibrinolytic activity (Ducimetière et al., 1981) or hitherto unsuspected causes? In particular, why is the association strongest in rank-and-file policemen? What clues to etiology does this provide? *Unexplained effect modification—like any other unexplained or unexpected finding—should always be regarded as a possible clue to etiology.*

We now bid adieu to the Paris gendarmérie.

EXERCISE D8

Question D8–1

Using the terms "risk factor" and "risk marker" in the way recommended above, are the following statements true or false?

1. Every risk marker is a risk factor.
2. A factor cannot be both a risk marker and a risk factor.
3. Every risk factor is useful as a risk marker.
4. Every factor that brings about a change in the probability of a disease is a risk factor.
5. There are risk factors whose effects are irreversible; removing the risk factor does not reduce the risk.

Question D8–2

A large-scale follow-up study of army veterans, initiated in the United States in 1954, demonstrated strong relationships between smoking and mortality (Kahn, 1966). The findings in Table D8 show that in the veterans aged 65–74 (as in other age groups) cigarette smoking was an indicator of an increased risk of dying.

According to these data, what is the approximate risk of dying within the next five years, for a 68-year-old man in each of the three smoking categories?

Question D8–3

For geniuses only. A study of a large sample of seven-year-old boys showed that 4.77% had been diagnosed as having inguinal hernia, and 8.1% of the boys with such diagnoses had low birth weights (<5 lb). A representative sample of seven-year-old boys without hernias was investigated, and in this control group the proportion with low birth

Table D8. Annual Probability of Death* for Veterans Aged 65–74 Years by Smoking Category

Smoking Category	Annual Probability of Death (%)	Relative Risk
Never smoked (or occasional only)	2.4	1.0
Ex-cigarette-smokers (who stopped for reasons other than "doctor's orders")	3.1	1.3
Current cigarette smokers	4.0	1.7

*Equivalent to the annual cumulative mortality rate.

weights was 2.1%. Can you estimate the risk of having an inguinal hernia diagnosed by the age of seven, for a live-born boy who weighs <5 lb at birth and survives to the age of seven? (See Note D8–3.)

NOTES

D8–1.   The *sensitivity of a risk marker* is the proportion of incident cases in whom the risk marker was previously present. Table D7 tells us that 98 cases of CHD occurred in rank-and-file policemen during the period of the study. Of these, 44 had varicose veins at the outset. In these circumstances, sensitivity was thus 44/98 = 45%.

D8–2.   *Effectiveness* refers to the extent to which desirable effects are achieved. *Efficiency* refers to the balance between these effects and the expenditure (in time, effort, money, and other resources) required to achieve them.

D8–3.   Data from Depue (1984); modified slightly.

U n i t
D9

RISK FACTORS AND RISK MARKERS
(CONTINUED)

The following are the answers to the "true–false" questions in *Question D8–1*.

1. False. Varicose veins may point to an increased risk of CHD, without being responsible for the increased risk.
2. False. Hypertension, for example, points to an increased risk of CHD, and is also a reason for the increased risk.
3. False. Considerations such as low sensitivity, low predictive value, and the cost or inconvenience of examinations to determine the presence of a given risk factor may render it of little practical value as a marker.
4. False. A factor that affects the probability of occurrence of a disease is, of course, a risk factor only if it *increases* the probability of the disease: "risk" is generally used to refer to the probability of an unfavorable outcome. If the factor *reduces* the probability of the disease, it is a *protective* or *preventive* factor.
5. True. Hypertension, for example, is unquestionably a risk factor for myocardial infarction, but there is little evidence that treating it has an appreciable effect on the risk of myocardial infarction, although the risk of strokes, congestive heart failure, and other complications is much reduced.

In answer to *Question D8–2*, we can make a rough estimate of the risk of dying within five years by multiplying the annual probability of death by five. This gives a risk of 12% for the "never smoked" group, 15.5% for ex-smokers, and 20% for cigarette smokers (see Note D9–1).

Question D8–3 (skip this paragraph if you didn't try the question) is difficult; you probably were not able to do it if you skipped the exercise on diagnostic tests (C11). The risk that is required is the "exposure-specific" risk, for individuals exposed to a specific factor (a low birth weight). This is analogous to the predictive value of a positive test—that is, the disease probability associated with a positive test result (a low birth weight), or the posttest probability (see Unit C12)—and it can be computed in the same way. Calculate the likelihood ratio (8.1/2.1 = 3.86), and then multiply the pretest odds in favor of a hernia diagnosis— that is, $0.0477/(1 - 0.0477) = 0.050$—by the likelihood ratio (3.86), to obtain the posttest odds of 0.193. The posttest probability—which is what we require—is $0.193/(1 + 0.193)$, or 16.2%. You may have reached this answer in a different way.

MEASURES OF THE STRENGTH OF AN ASSOCIATION

A wide variety of indices may be used to measure the strength of associations between variables. They include absolute differences (e.g., between rates, proportions, or means), ratios (e.g., risk ratios and other rate ratios, the odds ratio, and other measures of relative differences), and other statistical indices (e.g., correlation and regression coefficients). (See Note D9–2.)

The choice of a measure of strength depends, inter alia, on the scales of measurement of the variables (Note C7), the purpose of the study (are we more interested in absolute or relative differences?—see Unit A3), and the kind of study.

The next two exercises test your ability to interpret and use some of these measures.

The *relative risk* or *risk ratio* is the ratio of two incidence rates (or, more strictly, of two cumulative incidence rates). An odds ratio is sometimes referred to as the *estimated relative risk,* since if the risk is low the odds ratio and risk ratio are very close to each other (Note B11–1).

EXERCISE D9

Question D9–1

The incidence rate of disease A is twice as high in vegetarians as in nonvegetarians. The incidence rate of disease B is 0.2 times as high in vegetarians as in nonvegetarians. Which disease is more strongly associated with eating habits?

Question D9–2

A large follow-up survey showed that mortality from cancer of the lips, tongue, and mouth was 4.1 times as high in cigar smokers as in people who had never, or only occasionally, smoked (Kahn, 1966). Does this show that cigar smoking is a modifying factor?

Question D9—3

Is this association (relative risk = 4.1) likely to be due solely to confounding?

Question D9—4

Assuming you had no other information, could you conclude from this association that preventive activities with respect to these cancers should center on efforts to reduce the smoking of cigars?

Question D9—5

What does a relative risk of 1 mean?

Question D9—6

If we conduct a follow-up study and obtain a relative risk by comparing the incidence of a disease in a cohort (group) of smokers and a cohort of nonsmokers, will this tell us what the relative risk is in the total population?

Question D9—7

If we compare the previous smoking habits of people who have a certain disease (cases) and people who do not (controls), will the results tell us the relative risk? Can the results of such a study be generalized to the population as a whole?

Question D9—8

One of the findings of a 19-year follow-up study of 5,135 male Japanese physicians (Kono et al., 1986), in which the relationship between drinking habits and mortality was investigated, was that the age-adjusted death rate from coronary heart disease per 10,000 person-years was 26.3 in nondrinkers and 16.2 in occasional (less than daily) drinkers. The difference between the rates was 10.1 deaths per 10,000 person-years, and the ratio of the rates was 1.6 (or 0.6). Is the difference or the ratio a better measure of the strength of the association?

Table D9. Association Between Occasional Drinking and Mortality from Coronary Heart Disease: Relative Risks Adjusted for Age and Smoking Habits

Drinking Habits	Relative Risk (with 95% Confidence Interval)
Nondrinker	1.0
Occasional drinker	0.6 (0.4–0.9)
Daily drinker	
<2 go of *sake*	0.7 (0.5–1.1)
≥2 go of *sake*	0.7 (0.4–1.1)
Ex-drinker	1.5 (1.0–2.4)

Question D9–9

More findings from the study of Japanese physicians are shown in Table D9. Are any of the associations shown in the table statistically significant? What do you think may explain the finding in ex-drinkers?

Question D9–10

The response rate in the above study was low. Only 51% of the physicians in the region participated. The authors discuss the possibility that this may have biased the associations between drinking and mortality. What kind of bias are they referring to?

Question D9–11

If a risk ratio is statistically significant, does this mean it is significantly different from 0, from 1, or from some other value? If a rate difference is statistically significant, does this mean it is significantly different from 0, from 1, or from some other value? If an odds ratio is statistically significant, does this mean it is significantly different from 0, from 1, or from some other value?

NOTES

D9–1. Better estimates of the five-year risk, using the formulae in Note B5–4, are 11.5% (never smoked), 14.6% (ex-smokers) and 18.5% (current smokers). For the "never smoked" group, for example, the person-time rate is $0.024/[1 - (0.024/2)] = 0.0243$, and the five-year cumulative rate is $(0.0243 \times 5)/[(0.0243 \times 5/2) + 1] = 11.5\%$.

D9–2. The concept that differences as well as ratios and other indices can serve as measures of the strength of an association is a useful one, although not consistent with a narrow statistical definition of "strength," which requires "free" (nondimensional) measures.

Unit
D10

MEASURES OF STRENGTH

In *Question D9–1*, disease B exhibits a stronger association with eating habits than disease A. The risk of disease A is only twice as high in one group as in the other, whereas the risk of disease B is five times as high in one group as in the other. Whether the ratio of two rates is 0.2 or 5 depends only on which rate we decide to divide by which; this decision does not affect the strength of the association.

A relative risk of 4.1 (*Question D9–2*) tells us that cigar smoking is strongly associated with the disease, but a single relative risk can tell us nothing about effect modification. Effect modification is detected by comparing the associations found in different groups or different circumstances. If we found that the relative risk was 5 in older men and 2 in younger men (and if this difference was statistically significant, not an artifact, and not caused by confounding), we would conclude that age modified the association between cigar smoking and the disease—or, as a corollary, that cigar smoking modified the association between age and the disease (Unit A13).

A relative risk as high as 4.1 (*Question D9–3*) is unlikely to be due solely to confounding, except in unusual circumstances. The stronger an association is, the more likely it is to be a causal one.

Decisions about the institution of preventive activities (*Question D9–4*) do not depend solely on the strength of an association. Other considerations would come into play even if cigar smoking was to be used only as a risk marker, as we saw when we considered a proposed preventive program based on the presence of varicose veins (Unit D8). In this instance, we are considering preventive activities that center on the reduction of cigar smoking. Such activities presuppose that cigar smoking is causal and that its reduction will have an important impact on the incidence of mouth cancers in the population. More evidence is required.

A relative risk of 1 (*Question D9–5*) means that there is no association: the rates under comparison are identical.

A comparative study of groups of smokers and nonsmokers (*Question D9–6*) will tell us the relative risk in the total population only if the groups are representative samples of all smokers and nonsmokers, respectively, in the population.

A case-control study can provide an odds ratio and a rate ratio—in this instance (*Question D9–7*) the ratio of smoking rates—that can serve as measures of the association. But a case-control study does not tell us the incidence rates in smokers and nonsmokers, and therefore cannot itself provide a relative risk. If the risk is low, however, the odds ratio will be a good estimate of the relative risk. Also, if ancillary information is available, such as the incidence of the disease in the total population, risks—and hence risk ratios—can be derived from case-control studies (we had an example in Question D8–3). Application of the findings to the total population is of course warranted only if the samples of cases and controls are representative of cases and noncases, respectively, in the population.

The choice of an absolute or relative difference as a measure of association (*Question D9–8*) depends on the use we want to make of the finding. If we wish to study processes of causation, the rate ratio will serve our purpose well. If we think that occasional drinking saves lives, and want to know how many lives it saves, we should use the absolute difference.

In answer to *Question D9–9*, if the 95% confidence interval of a rate ratio lies wholly above 1 or wholly below 1, it is generally safe to conclude that P is under .05. The association with occasional drinking is thus statistically significant, and the association with being an ex-drinker *may* be statistically significant: the unrounded value of the lower confidence limit may be below 1 (e.g., 0.951) or above 1 (e.g., 1.049). The investigators' comment on the high CHD rate in ex-drinkers is: "It is possible that ex-drinkers may have drunk heavily before they abstained, but it seems more likely that ex-drinkers stopped drinking because of their illnesses" (Kono et al., 1986).

The possibility of biased associations (*Question D9–10*) in this study does not arise from the low participation rate itself, but from the possibility that participation rates may differ in people with different drinking habits and also in people with different probabilities of dying, and that the interplay of these selection factors may produce associations in the sample that differ from those outside the sample and in the population as a whole. This kind of selection bias (which we encountered in Unit C5) is called *Berksonian bias*.

In answer to *Question D9–11*, statistical significance means a significant difference from 1 in the case of risk and odds ratios, and a significant difference from zero in the case of a rate difference.

EXERCISE D10

In this exercise we look at some other measures of the strength of an association.

Question D10–1

Table D10–1 shows the correlation of diastolic blood pressure with age and weight in a random population sample in the West Indies (Khaw and Rose, 1982).
     Are the correlations strong?

Question D10–2

What modifying effects are shown in Table D10–1?

Question D10–3

Can you tell whether the association with weight in the older age group is confounded by age?

Question D10–4

Do you know a simple way to see whether the association with weight in the younger age group is confounded by age?

Question D10–5

The association between malignant melanoma and geographical latitude was examined, using the age-standardized mortality rates from melanoma in 1950–1967 in the states of the United States and the provinces of Canada, and the latitude of the largest city in each state or province (Elwood et al., 1974). Are the results (Table D10–2) consistent with the hypothesis that exposure to sunlight plays a part in the etiology

Table D10-1. Association of Diastolic Pressure
With Age and Weight in Two Age Groups:
Correlation Coefficients

Age Group (yr)	Correlation With Age	Correlation With Weight
30–44	0.24*	0.36*
≥45	0.00	0.24*

*$P < .01$.

Table D10–2. Relationship of Melanoma Mortality
to Latitude

	Correlation Coefficient	Regression Coefficient of Mortality on Latitude (Deaths per Million)*
Male	−0.79	−0.056 (0.044–0.068)
Female	−0.72	−0.034 (0.026–0.042)

*95% confidence intervals shown in parentheses.

of malignant melanoma (as it does in other skin cancers?) Do you know
how to calculate what proportion of the variation in melanoma mortality
can be explained by the association with latitude?

Question D10–6

What do the regression coefficients in Table D10–2 tell us? Does sex
have a statistically significant modifying effect?

Question D10–7

In a follow-up study of a population sample in Wales, it was found that
between 1957 and 1966 the mean height of a sample of men aged 25–34
(in 1957) declined by 2.24 cm, whereas the mean height of men aged 55–
64 declined by 3.13 cm (Cole, 1974). The difference between these differences (0.89 cm) was highly significant ($P<.001$). What association is
measured by the difference between the differences?

Question D10–8

In this Welsh study, there was apparently an error in the measurement
of height in 1966, when the measuring pole was fitted to the wall in the
wrong place—about 2.5 cm too high—so that the measured heights

Table D10–3. Purchase of Raw Milk by Cases
and Matched Controls

	Purchased		Not Purchased		Total	
	No.	%	No.	%	No.	%
Cases	51	67	25	33	76	100
Controls	29	38	47	62	76	100

Table D10–4. Purchase of Raw Milk by Cases
and Matched Controls

Controls	Cases		Total
	Purchased	Not Purchased	
Purchased	19	10	29
Not purchased	32	15	47
Total	51	25	76

were lower than the true values. How would this error affect the difference between the differences in the two age groups?

Question D10–9

During an investigation of an outbreak of gastroenteritis in a rural community, 76 patients and 76 controls (individually matched for age, sex, and street) were questioned about their food purchases and consumption (Tillett, 1986). Data on the purchase of raw (unpasteurized) milk are shown in two different ways in Tables D10–3 and D10–4. Make sure you understand the tables.

What was the reason for using matching? Which table makes fuller use of the information? Do you know how to calculate an odds ratio from these data? Do you know what significance tests you could use?

Unit
D11

MEASURES OF STRENGTH (CONTINUED)

A *correlation coefficient* (r) measures the linear relationship between two variables. A coefficient of 1 means that a higher value of one variable is always associated with a higher value of the other, and a coefficient of -1 means that a higher value of one is always associated with a lower value of the other. The correlation coefficient does not indicate *how much* each variable changes when the other changes; this is what a regression coefficient tells.

As a rough rule of thumb, an r of $>.8$ (or $<-.8$) can be regarded as a strong correlation, $.5 - .8$ as moderate, and $.2 - .5$ as weak. It is often helpful to calculate r^2, which expresses the proportion of the variance of each variable that is "explained" by its linear relationship with the other. The answer to *Question D10–1* is clearly "no"; the correlations shown in the table are not strong.

In answer to *Question D10–2*, the correlations of blood pressure with both age and weight appear to be modified by age, since the coefficients differ in the two age groups. The correlations with age are significantly different from each other, but we do not know whether the differences between the correlations with weight are larger than might easily occur by chance: the P values refer to differences from zero, not to the differences between the coefficients.

The exclusion test for possible confounding (Unit D5) indicates that the correlation between blood pressure and weight in the older age group (*Question D10–3*) cannot be confounded by age (because age is not correlated with blood pressure in this group).

A simple way to see whether the association with weight in the younger age group is confounded by age (*Question D10–4*) is to compute a *partial correlation coefficient* that controls for linear relationships with age. This is easy to calculate if we also know the correlation between age and weight.

In *Question D10–5* the correlations between melanoma mortality and

236

latitude are fairly strong, and are negative. The higher the latitude (i.e., the further from the equator and the less the exposure to sunlight), the lower the mortality. The findings are thus consistent with the hypothesis that sunlight is a cause of this disease. The square of the correlation coefficient tells us what proportion of the variation (variance) of one variable can be explained by the linear correlation with the other; for males this is $(-.79)^2$, or 62%; for females it is 52%.

A *regression coefficient* tells us the mean change in one variable when there is a change of one unit in the other. The answer to *Question D10–6* is that an increase of one degree in latitude is associated, on average, with a decrease in melanoma mortality of .056 per million (in males) and .034 per million (in females). The statistical model is the linear regression equation $y = a + bx$, in which y is the melanoma mortality rate, x is the latitude, a (the *intercept*) is the value of y when x is zero, and b is the regression coefficient of the mortality rate on latitude. If melanoma mortality rates are plotted against latitude on a graph, the correlation coefficient measures how close the points are to a straight line, and the regression coefficient b measures the slope of this line.

The regression coefficients are different in the two sexes (Table D10–2), and there is no overlap between their confidence intervals, clearly showing that sex has a statistically significant modifying effect on the regression coefficients.

In answer to *Question D10–7*, the difference between the differences observed between 1957 and 1966 in the two age groups is an index of the association between age and the change in height. The systematic error in measurement (*Question D10–8*) does not bias this association. The error can be corrected by adding 2.50 cm to all 1966 heights; the mean changes are then +0.26 cm (25–34 years) and −0.63 cm (55–64 years), and the difference between the differences is still 0.89 cm.

MATCHED SAMPLES

When a matching procedure is used in the selection of samples that are to be compared, the purpose is to prevent confounding. If these samples (cases and controls, in *Question D10–9*) are similar with respect to certain variables, these variables cannot have a confounding effect.

The samples may be selected by choosing individuals who are similar in defined respects (individual matching), or just by ensuring that the groups as a whole are similar in certain respects (group matching). When individual matching is used, the findings are best tabulated as in Table D10–4, where each entry represents a *pair* of observations: it indicates the findings for each member of the pair (both members consumed raw milk, neither did, etc.). This table makes fuller use of the information than does a table like Table D10–3, which shows the data as if the two samples were unrelated. The observations in a table like Table D10–4 need not relate to cases and controls. They may, for example, relate to matched pairs whose one member was exposed and the other not exposed to a suspected risk factor, or to paired observations (e.g., before and after treatment) in the same subjects. We used this sort of table when we compared the diagnoses of two ophthalmologists who examined the same eyes (Table C7–1).

In such studies the odds ratio is the ratio of the two numbers of pairs with discrepant findings. In Table D10–4, the discrepant pairs are those whose one member purchased raw milk whereas the other did not. There were 32 such pairs in which it was the case who bought raw milk, and 10 in which it was the control. The odds ratio is 32/10, that is, 3.2, or 10/32, that is, 0.31. The appropriate significance test, which uses the same two numbers, is a McNemar test or an exact binomial probability test.

EXERCISE D11

This exercise deals with synergism.

Table D11–1 shows death rates from suicide in the United States in 1984 (National Center For Health Statistics, 1986), by race and sex. It also shows rate differences and rate ratios, as two measures of the strength of the associations with race and sex.

Question D11–1

Does Table D11–1 show effect modification?

Table D11–1. Death Rates from Suicide, United States (Age-Standardized Rates per 100,000), with Rate Differences and Rate Ratios

	Rate		Difference	Ratio
	Black	White	(black − white)	(black : white)
Male	11.2	19.7	−8.5	0.57
Female	2.3	5.6	−3.3	0.41
Difference (male − female)	+8.9	+14.1		
Ratio (male : female)	4.9	3.5		

Table D11–2. Effects of Race and Sex
on Death Rate from Suicide:
Rate Differences

	Black	White
Male	+8.9	+17.4
Female	0*	+3.3

*Reference category.

Question D11–2

Table D11–2 shows the strength of the same associations by comparing each mortality rate with the rate in black females (the group with the lowest rate). It shows the rate differences. Is there evidence of a synergistic effect on the death rate from suicide? That is, is the effect of being both male and white greater than the combined separate effects of being male and being white?

Question D11–3

Table D11–3 again shows the strength of the associations, this time in terms of rate ratios. Is there evidence of a synergistic effect in this table?

Question D11–4

Table D11–4 shows lung cancer death rates by smoking habits and occupational exposure to asbestos. It is based on a large study in the United States (Hammond et al., 1979). Do smoking and exposure to asbestos have a synergistic effect on the risk of the disease? (You will find it helpful if you first construct tables like Tables D11–2 and D11–3, showing the strength of the associations with the incidence rate.)

Table D11–3. Effects of Race and Sex
on Death Rate from Suicide:
Rate Ratios

	Black	White
Male	4.9	8.6
Female	1.0*	2.4

*Reference category.

Table D11−4. Age-Standardized
Death Rates (per 100,000 Man Years)
from Lung Cancer, by History of
Cigarette Smoking and Occupational
Exposure to Asbestos Dust

	Exposure to Asbestos	
Cigarette Smoking	*No*	*Yes*
No	11.3	58.4
Yes	122.6	601.6

Question D11−5

Why is synergism based on rate ratios worth detecting?

Question D11−6

Why is synergism based on rate differences worth detecting?

U n i t
D12

SYNERGISM

Table D11–1 shows that the strength of the association between the death rate from suicide and race differs in men and women (whether use is made of rate differences or rate ratios), and the strength of the association between the death rate and sex differs in blacks and whites. Thus in answer to *Question D11–1*, there is clear evidence of effect modification: there is interaction between race and sex in their effects on the death rate from suicide.

Synergism refers to *positive interaction*—a situation where the joint effect of two or more factors is greater than their combined separate effects. (Sometimes the use of the term is confined to situations where the factors act together in a biological or mechanistic sense.) *Question D11–2* refers to the absolute differences connected with race and sex. The separate effect of being male is to increase the death rate (in comparison with the rate of black females) by 8.9 per 100,000 (Table D11–2). The separate effect of being white is to increase the rate (again in comparison with the rate of black females) by 3.3 per 100,000. A combination of these factors may therefore be expected to raise the rate to a value that is higher than the rate in black females by (8.9 + 3.3), or 12.2 per 100,000. In fact, the rate was higher by 17.4 per 100,000. The findings therefore indicate a synergistic effect.

This conclusion is based on an *additive* model, wherein effects are measured as rate differences, and combined by adding them to one another.

In *Question D11–3* we use a *multiplicative* model: effects are measured as ratios, and must be combined by multiplying them by one another. Table D11–3 shows that being male multiplies the rate (of black females) by 4.9, and being white multiplies the rate by 2.4. The predicted combined effect is to multiply the rate by (4.9 × 2.4), or 11.8. In fact, the rate in white males was only 8.6 times the rate in black females. Using this model, there is no synergism.

Table D12–1. Effects of Smoking and
Exposure to Asbestos on Lung Cancer
Deaths: Rate Difference

Cigarette Smoking	Exposure to Asbestos	
	No	Yes
No	0.0*	+47.1
Yes	+111.3	+590.3

*Reference category.

The data on smoking and asbestos (*Question D11–4*) yield a similar conclusion. When rate differences are examined (Table D12–1), the joint effect of these factors on lung cancer deaths is an increase of 590.3 per 100,000 person-years, which is greater than the combined separate effects (47.1 + 111.3 = 158.4). But when rate ratios are examined (Table D12–2), the joint effect is a 53.2-fold increase, which is less than the combined separate effects (5.2 × 10.8 = 56.2). There is synergism only if an additive model is used.

The occurrence of multiplicative synergism (*Question D11–5*) has etiological implications, and may provide useful clues to causative processes. Additive synergism (*Question D11–6*) is meaningful if we are interested in the absolute magnitude of a public health problem or an individual's risk. In the instance of asbestos and smoking, the findings provide no clue to etiological processes, but the fact that asbestos workers who smoke have especially high lung cancer death rates has obvious practical implications.

The fact that we found effect modification with respect to one measure of an association (the rate difference) but not with respect to another (the rate ratio) should not surprise us. *Whenever we examine modifying effects— or, for that matter, confounding effects—we do so in relation to a specific*

Table D12–2. Effects of Smoking and
Exposure to Asbestos on Lung Cancer
Deaths: Rate Ratios

Cigarette Smoking	Exposure to Asbestos	
	No	Yes
No	1.0*	5.2
Yes	10.8	53.2

*Reference category.

measure of association, that we have chosen as a suitable one for our purposes. If we use a different measure, we may come to different conclusions.

EXERCISE D12

This exercise introduces a procedure commonly used in the appraisal of associations, based on stratification.

The association of oral contraceptives with myocardial infarction was investigated in a case-control study in 155 hospitals in the United States (Note D12). The cases were women admitted to a coronary-care unit for a first episode of definite myocardial infarction, and the controls were women who had never had a myocardial infarction. The women, who were aged 25–49 and premenopausal, were asked whether they had used oral contraceptives in the previous month. The crude findings are shown in Table D12–3, and the findings stratified by age appear in Table D12–4.

Question D12–1

Is the association between oral-contraceptive use and MI confounded by age?

Question D12–2

Is the association between oral-contraceptive use and MI modified by age?

Question D12–3

Can you suggest a simple way of using the data in Table D12–4 to obtain a single odds ratio that circumvents possible confounding by age?

Table D12–3. Use of Oral Contraceptive ("Pill") by Women with Myocardial Infarction (MI) and Controls (Ctl)

Pill	MI	Ctl
Yes	29	135
No	205	1,607

Odds ratio: 1.7 (95% confidence interval, 1.1–2.8). *P* (by chi-square test) = .011.

Table D12-4. Use of Oral Contraceptive ("Pill") by Women with
Myocardial Infarction (MI) and Controls (Ctl), by Age

Pill	25–29 yr		30–34 yr		35–39 yr		40–44 yr		45–49 yr	
	MI	Ctl	MI	Ctl	MI	Ctl	MI	Ctl	MI	Ctl
Yes	4	62	9	33	4	26	6	9	6	5
No	2	224	12	390	33	330	65	362	93	301
Odds ratio	7.2		8.9		1.5		3.7		3.9	

NOTE

D12. This exercise is based on data from Shapiro et al. (1979), using the
Cornfield–Gart procedure (Fleiss, 1981) for confidence intervals
and heterogeneity tests. The same example is treated in more
detail by Schlesselman (1982).

Unit
D13

APPRAISING STRATIFIED DATA

The discrepancy between the findings based on crude and age-stratified data is clear evidence of confounding by age (*Question D12–1*). The odds ratio that expresses the strength of the association between "the pill" and myocardial infarction is 1.7 in the sample as a whole, but much higher than this in all but one of the age strata.

There is also evidence that the association is modified by age (*Question D12–2*), since the odds ratios in the various age strata differ. The differences may, however, be due to sampling variation (Note B3–2). We can, if we wish, do a significance test to determine the probability that heterogeneity of this degree might occur by chance (see Note D13–1). If we do so, we will find that $P = .17$; that is, there is no significant heterogeneity.

The odds ratios in the separate age strata are not confounded by age, since the strata have such narrow age spans (five years) that there cannot be much age variation within them. Therefore, if (in answer to *Question D12–3*) we can combine the stratum-specific odds ratios to obtain some sort of average, this too will be an odds ratio that is not affected by age confounding. The method most often used for this purpose is the Mantel–Haenszel procedure (Note D13–1), which in this instance provides a value of 4.0—much higher than the crude odds ratio of 1.68. This value, 4.0, is a *point estimate* of the common odds ratio; the confidence interval is 2.4–6.7. Unlike standardization, this and similar procedures do not require the use of a standard reference population. The Mantel–Haenszel chi-square test, which is often used to test the significance of an association when effects connected with suspected confounders are controlled, yielded a P of less than one in a million.

A procedure that pools the stratum-specific findings in this way provides an odds ratio that controls for possible confounding by the stratifying variable. This may be regarded as the common "underlying" odds ratio, in instances where the absence of significant variation between the findings in the various strata makes this an acceptable concept. Where appropriate, the Mantel–Haenszel procedure can also provide a point estimate of the common rate ratio.

The data may be stratified by two or more variables. Each of the five age strata in Table D12–4, for example, may be divided into three cigarette-smoking categories, producing 15 two-by-two tables, and the Mantel-Haenszel procedure can be applied to these. When this is done, the common odds ratio is 3.3. (What does this tell us? For answer, see Note D13–2.)

The data can also be rearranged so as to study a different independent variable. For example, we could stratify the same data by age and the use of oral contraceptives, and then use the Mantel–Haenszel procedure to examine the association between smoking and myocardial infarction (controlling for the other variables).

MAKING SENSE OF A MULTIVARIATE ANALYSIS

The last three exercises in Section D are devoted to multivariate analysis. Multiple linear regression analysis and multiple logistic regression analysis will be used as illustrations.

As was stressed in Unit D7, a basic general understanding of multivariate procedures (see Note D7–2) is an essential condition for their intelligent use. The following brief notes are no substitute for this, but serve only as reminders of some salient features. If at present you know nothing at all about these procedures, you should probably leave these exercises until you do (go to Unit D17).

Multivariate analysis looks at a number of variables at the same time (generally in relation to a single dependent variable), using a mathematical model to represent the processes being studied. The model may be additive or multiplicative (using these terms as they were defined in Unit D12).

Multivariate analysis has two main purposes in epidemiology:

- For appraising the strength and significance of the relationships of a number of variables (separately or jointly) with the dependent variable, paying attention both to the variables' "main effects" and to their interactions (modifying effects). The relationship of each independent variable with the dependent variable can be examined while controlling for effects connected with other variables, by holding the other variables constant in the analysis. Multivariate analysis is a way of controlling for confounding.

- For making predictions of risk, based on the effects of multiple factors.

Multiple linear regression analysis, which generally has a metric-scale dependent variable, is based on an additive model:

$$y = a + b_1 x_1 + \cdots + b_i x_i$$

where y is the predicted value of the dependent variable, and each b is the coefficient (estimated from the data) by which the value of the corresponding independent (predictor) variable x is multiplied; a (the intercept) is another constant estimated from the data).

Multiple logistic regression uses a model that is multiplicative with respect to odds (it is additive with respect to log odds; adding the logarithms of numbers is the same as multiplying the numbers). The variable of interest is generally a disease or other "yes–no" characteristic. The model is expressed in terms of the log odds of the disease (i.e., the natural logarithm of the predicted odds in favor of the disease):

$$\text{Log odds of disease} = a + b_1 x_1 + \cdots + b_i x_i$$

In this formula, each x is the value of a specific independent variable. The variable may be a metric-scale one. If it is dichotomous, the values 0 for "absent" and 1 for "present" are commonly used. If the variable has more than two categories, one is generally designated as a reference category, and the others become "dummy variables." For example, if there are three categories of cigarette-smoking ("none," "moderate," and "heavy"), two of these would appear as variables in the model—probably "moderate" and "heavy"—each of them being scored (say) 0 for "not in this category" or 1 for "in this category."

The probability of the disease can be estimated by the formula

$$\text{Probability of disease} = 1/\{1 + \exp[-(\text{Log odds of disease})]\}$$

The regression coefficient b expresses the strength of the association with the dependent variable when the other variables in the model are held constant. In a multiple linear regression analysis, it is similar to the simple regression coefficient we encountered in Unit D12. It "indicates an average change in y for a unit change in x_i after their linear association with all other x variables has been removed from both y and x" (Kahn and Sempos, 1989). In a multiple logistic analysis, the coefficient b is the natural log of the odds ratio; the exponential ("antilog") of b is the odds ratio for the variable's association with the disease, adjusted for effects connected with other variables; this odds ratio indicates the change in the disease odds when there is a change of one unit (e.g., from 0 to 1) in the independent variable.

The analysis generally provides P values and standard errors or confidence intervals for the b coefficients. The P values indicate whether the coefficients are significantly different from zero—that is, whether the relevant association with the dependent variable (controlling for effects connected with other variables) is statistically significant.

A multivariate analysis may include additional terms that express interactions of specified variables.

There may be information on the validity of the model as a whole. A multiple regression coefficient R, for example, expresses the degree to which predictions based on a multiple regression analysis model fit the observed facts; its square R^2 expresses the proportion of the variation (variance) of the dependent variable that is explained by the total set of independent variables. A multiple logistic analysis generally provides at least one chi-square test of the model, the interpretation of its result depending on what kind of test it is (see Note D13–3); but if the test result throws doubt on the model's validity, the value of any findings based on the model is open to question. Also, as we will see in the coming exercises, simple comparisons can be used to see how well the values predicted by a model conform with observed data (Kahn and Sempos, 1989). Validity is most convincing if the model was developed and tested in one sample (or part of a sample) and then retested in another.

By using models that include smaller or larger sets of variables and interactions, and comparing their R^2 values or likelihood-ratio statistics, it is possible to see whether specific variables or interactions contribute appreciably to the validity of the model.

Once the a and b coefficients are available, the effects of a specific constellation of factors can be estimated by inserting the appropriate values of each x in the formula and calculating y or the log odds or probability of the disease.

EXERCISE D13

Table D13 shows some results of a multiple logistic regression analysis of the same study of oral contraceptives and myocardial infarction (MI) that we looked at in the last exercise. The analysis was done with a microcomputer program (McGee, 1986).

Question D13–1

Explain in words the meaning of the figure 8.47 in this table; do you know how this figure was obtained?

Question D13–2

Which is more strongly associated with myocardial infarction: age or taking oral contraceptives?

Table D13. Associations with Myocardial Infarction: Multiple Logistic
Regression Analysis*

Variable	Coeff.	S.E.	P	Odds Ratio (with 95% Confidence Interval)
Oral contraceptive				
(0 = no, 1 = yes)	1.188	0.260	.032	3.28 (1.97–5.47)
Age (years)	0.152	0.014	.0010	1.16 (1.13–1.20)
1–24 cigarettes/day				
(0 = no, 1 = yes)	1.125	0.209	.020	3.08 (2.04–4.64)
≥25 cigarettes/day				
(0 = no, 1 = yes)	2.137	0.208	.0013	8.47 (5.64–12.74)
Constant	−9.283	0.629		

*Likelihood ratio statistic (4 degrees of freedom): 272.8.

Question D13–3

Do the results in the table tell us whether the association between the
pill and MI is confounded by smoking? If not, what extra information do
you need? (Can you guess what the likelihood ratio statistic tells us? See
Note D13–4.)

Question D13–4

Do the results in the table tell us whether the association between the
pill and MI is modified by smoking—that is, whether this association is
the same in nonsmokers and women who smoke various numbers of
cigarettes per day? If not, what extra information do you need?

Question D13–5

According to the results in the table, what (controlling for effects connected with age) is the ratio of the odds in favor of MI among women
who use oral contraceptives and smoke ≥25 cigarettes a day, to the
corresponding odds among women who do neither?

NOTES

D13–1.   Methods for estimating a common odds ratio, rate ratio, or rate
difference from stratified data include the Mantel–Haenszel,
precision-based, and maximum-likelihood procedures. The measure computed by these methods is variously called the common, underlying, overall, summary, pooled, or uniform measure. In this book the term "Mantel–Haenszel" refers not only
to the original Mantel–Haenszel procedure for odds ratios, but
to similar procedures now used for rate ratios and rate dif-

ferences; an extension of the Mantel–Haenszel procedure may be used when the dependent and/or independent variable has more than two (ordered) categories (Mantel, 1963; Rothman, 1986, 346–348). All these methods for estimating a common measure, as well as methods for testing the heterogeneity of the findings in the various strata, are described by Rothman (1986, chap. 12); methods using the odds ratio are explained by Fleiss (1981, chap. 10); formulae are summarized by Kleinbaum et al. (1982, pp. 359–361).

D13–2.   A Mantel–Haenszel odds ratio of 3.3 when the data are stratified by age and smoking habits tells us how strong the pill–MI association is when age and smoking are controlled; it also tells us that this association was to some extent confounded by smoking, since the value is now lower than it was when only age was controlled (4.0).

D13–3.   The chi-square statistic for a multiple logistic regression analysis may test how well predictions based on the model fit the observed data. The goodness-of-fit chi-square test provided by the SPSS logistic regression program is an example. A low P value (say $<.05$) indicates a poor fit; the higher the P value is, the more confidence we can have in the model's validity. The same interpretation is given to a chi-square statistic that appraises how well the findings estimated from the logistic coefficients fit with the observed findings. The "-2 log likelihood" chi-square provided by the SPSS program is an example. On the other hand, a chi-square statistic may be used that tests whether the independent variables, considered jointly, are associated with the dependent variable; in this instance, a *low* P value points to the model's validity. The "model chi-square" provided by the SPSS program is an example. The contribution of specific variables or interactions to the model's validity can be appraised by doing the analysis with and without them, and comparing the chi-square values. The difference between the chi-square values— sometimes called the partial chi-square—tests the significance of the effect of these added variables or interactions (using the difference between the degrees of freedom in the two analyses).

D13–4.   A likelihood-ratio statistic is a kind of chi-square statistic. As explained in Note D13–3, different chi-squares are used for testing multiple logistic models. In this instance, chi-square $=$ 272.9 with 4 degrees of freedom, so that $P <.000001$. If this were a goodness-of-fit test, it would indicate a very poor fit. It is actually a test of the association between the pill, age and smoking (considered together), and myocardial infarction, and the null hypothesis (of no association) can be rejected.

Unit
D14

MULTIPLE LOGISTIC REGRESSION

In answer to *Question D13–1*, the odds ratio of 8.47 is the odds ratio when women who smoke ≥25 cigarettes a day are compared with women who smoke none (i.e., the ratio of the odds in favor of MI among women who smoke ≥25 cigarettes day to the odds in favor of MI among women who smoke none), with the other variables (age and oral contraceptives) held constant. Alternatively, it is the ratio of the odds in favor of smoking ≥25 cigarettes (rather than none) among women with MI, to the odds in favor of smoking ≥25 cigarettes among women without MI (you will remember from Unit B11 that the disease odds ratio and exposure odds ratio are identical). The figure was obtained by taking the exponential (antilog) of the coefficient 2.137; $e^{2.137}$ is 8.47.

The coefficient and odds ratio for age express the effect of a one-year difference in age when the other variables in the analysis remain unchanged. A comparison of these values with those for oral contraceptives, as requested in *Question D13–2*, is meaningful only if a specific age difference is stated. For a 20-year difference, for example, the coefficient 0.152 may be multiplied by 20 to obtain 3.04. This is the natural log of 20.9, so the appropriate odds ratio for comparison with that for oral contraceptives (3.28) would be 20.9. The P values can of course not be used to measure the strength of the associations.

The odds ratios in the table are adjusted for effects connected with smoking. The only way to tell whether the association between the pill and MI is confounded by smoking (*Question D13–3*) is to compare the findings with those when smoking is *not* controlled in the analysis. We could do another analysis, excluding smoking from the list of variables. This hardly seems worth doing, as we have already controlled for possible confounding.

The table tells us nothing about modifying effects (*Question D13–4*). We can examine the modifying effect of smoking on the association between the pill and MI by repeating the analysis after adding a term or

251

terms that express the interaction of smoking and the pill. We can then
see how this changes the findings (we will do this in the next exercise),
and can appraise the strength and significance of the interaction effect.
Alternatively, we could conduct separate analyses in nonsmokers and
moderate and heavy smokers, using only oral contraceptives and age as
independent variables, and compare the strength of the associations
shown in the three analyses.

The multiple logistic model is a multiplicative one, in the sense that
we obtain the odds ratio for a combination of two factors (*Question D13–
5*) by multiplying their separate odds ratios. The odds ratio for use of the
pill is 3.28, and the odds ratio for smoking ≥25 cigarettes a day is 8.47.
The odds ratio for both factors together is therefore 3.28 × 8.47, or 27.8.

EXERCISE D14

Question D14–1

Different logistic regression models, that included different sets of variables, yielded different odds ratios for the association between oral contraceptives and MI, as shown in Table D14–1. How do you account for
this? Compare the figures in the table with the corresponding Mantel–
Haenszel odds ratios (Unit D13).

Table D14–1. Odds Ratios Expressing Association
Between Oral-Contraceptive Use and Myocardial
Infarction in Three Logistic Regression Models

Variables Included in Model	Odds Ratio
Oral contraceptive	1.68
Oral contraceptive, age	3.81
Oral contraceptive, age, cigarettes	3.28

Question D14–2

When contraceptive–cigarette interaction is included in the logistic
model used in Table D13 (i.e., in addition to contraceptives, age, and
cigarettes), the overall validity of the model (as appraised by likelihood-
ratio chi-square statistics) does not change significantly, and the coefficients for the interaction terms are not statistically significant. The odds
ratios for the pill–MI association are different, however, from those
based on the no-interaction ("main effect") model. Odds ratios based on
the two models are shown in Tables D14–2 and D14–3. In their summary of their results, the investigators say that the combined effect of oral
contraceptives and smoking

Table D14–2. Age-Adjusted Odds
Ratios Expressing Association Between
Use of Oral Contraceptives and MI,
by Contraceptive Use and Smoking
Habits: No-Interaction Model

	Oral Contraceptives	
Cigarettes/Day	*No*	*Yes*
None	1.0	3.6
1–24	3.3	10.1
≥25	8.5	27.8

was appreciably larger than could be accounted for by the separate effects of
cigarettes and oral contraceptives, and this suggests a considerable accentuation
by cigarette smoking of the effect of oral contraceptive use on myocardial infarction (Shapiro et al., 1979).

Do the results of the multiple logistic analyses support this conclusion?

Question D14–3

The relationships of social class and educational level with obesity were
examined in an imaginary population. Social class and education, which
were treated as dichotomies ("low" and "high") were strongly correlated; 90% of the people in the "low" category of one were also in the
"low" category of the other, and 90% of those in the "high" category c

Table D14–3. Age-Adjusted Odds
Ratios Expressing Association Between
Use of Oral Contraceptives and MI,
by Contraceptive Use and Smoking
Habits: Interaction Model

	Oral Contraceptives	
Cigarettes/Day	*No*	*Yes*
None	1.0	3.6
1–24	3.1	3.7
≥25	8.0	40.3*

*Calculated by multiplying the odds ratios for
   contraceptives (3.6), ≥25 cigarettes (8.0),
   and their interaction (1.4).

Table D14—4. Odds Ratios for Relationships of Low Social Class and Low Educational Level with Obesity in Four Logistic Regression Models: Imaginary Data

	Odds Ratio	
Variables Included in Model	Social Class	Education
Social class	0.30	—
Education	—	0.30
Social class, education	0.50	0.50
Social class, education, social class–education interaction	0.50	0.50

one were also in the "high" category of the other. The results of logistic regression analyses are shown in Table D14–4. How can the differences be explained?

Question D14—4

For the purpose of this question, assume that Table D13 was based on a ten-year follow-up study of the incidence of myocardial infarction in a representative population sample, so that it can be used as a basis for predictions of incidence (it cannot actually be so used). Do you know how to calculate the risk of having an infarction in the next ten years, for a 30-year-old woman who uses oral contraceptives and smokes 30 cigarettes a day? How could we appraise the validity of the model as a predictor of risk?

Unit
D15

MULTIPLE LOGISTIC REGRESSION
(CONTINUED)

Different logistic models may provide different odds ratios for the same association (*Question D14–1*) because the odds ratios express the strength of the association after controlling for effects connected with other variables in the model. The results thus vary, depending on what other variables are included. The odds ratios in Table D14–1 are very close to the Mantel–Haenszel odds ratios, which were 4.0 (controlling for age only) and 3.3 (controlling for age and smoking).

Similarly, the addition of interaction terms may appreciably change the results, as Tables D14–2 and D14–3 show. It is probably wise to treat the results of any multiple logistic analysis with reserve if the possible importance of interactions (effect modification) has not been investigated. If interaction is unimportant, the results of a main-effect analysis will fit the data accurately and the meaning of the odds ratios will be straightforward. However, if there is important interaction and it is ignored, the results may be misleading (Note D15–1).

Question D14–2 is not easy to answer. The fuller model, including interactions, shows a definite synergistic effect. However, the interaction term was not statistically significant, so that we cannot be confident that this is not a chance finding. In a detailed discussion of this study, Schlesselman (1982) suggests that the interpretation based on the no-interaction model is preferable, because the analysis using the interaction model (Table D14–3) indicates that oral contraceptives increase the risk of MI markedly in nonsmokers and heavy smokers but not in moderate smokers, which is "biologically implausible"; there may be uncontrolled confounding factors.

In Table D14–4, we again see that the strength of an association in a logistic regression model may change when the model is changed. The specific answer to *Question D14–3* is that the inclusion of highly correlated independent variables in a single model may have a marked effect on the findings (this is referred to as *multicollinearity*). The associations

Table D15–1. Fit of Multiple Logistic Risk Function to Data: Comparison of Predicted and Observed Incidence of Diabetes

Risk (Quartile)	Cases of Diabetes	
	Number Expected	Number Observed
1	72.1	70
2	31.3	28
3	19.5	23
4	10.5	10

Source: Data from Kahn et al. (1971).

with both social class and education became weaker (odds ratios closer to 1) when the other variable was included.

To use multiple logistic regression for predicting the probability of a disease, we must substitute the appropriate values in the equation. In this instance (*Question 14–4*) the log odds (the natural logarithm of the odds) in favor of myocardial infarction is

$$-9.283 + (1.188 \times 1) + (0.152 \times 30) + (1.125 \times 0) + (2.137 \times 1)$$

or -1.398. The risk of the disease is $1/[1 + \exp(1.398)]$, or $1/(1 + 4.047)$—that is, 0.198 or 19.8%.

The model's validity as a predictor of risk—that is, the degree to which the model conforms with observed facts—can be tested in the sample from which the coefficients were derived or (more convincingly) in other samples. One method is illustrated in Table D15–1 (from Kahn and Sempos, 1989). Each individual's probability of developing the disease was calculated from the model, the individuals were divided into quartiles according to their level of risk, and the predicted number of cases in each group was calculated (by adding together the probabilities of the members of the group) and then compared with the observed number. Does Table D15–1 show a good fit with the data? (For answer, see Note D15–2.) If we have them, we can of course also use the chi-square results described in Note D13–3.

EXERCISE D15

Multiple linear regression, with its simple additive model, is easier to use and understand than multiple logistic regression. We will take a single example. The indices used in this example are the regression coefficient b (see formula in Unit D13) and the proportion of total variation (variance) explained by a variable or set of variables.

Data from the National Study of Health and Growth in England and

Scotland were analyzed to appraise the relationship between parents' smoking and children's growth. Children, aged 5–11 years, in a stratified random sample were examined, and their parents were asked to fill in self-administered questionnaires. Information was available for 5,903 children out of 8,120 (Rona et al., 1985).

Question D15–1

The dependent variable in the analysis was the difference between the child's height and the mean height of children of the same age, sex, and country (England or Scotland), divided by the standard deviation for that group. It was denoted the standard deviation score. Why was this score, rather than the height itself, used as the dependent variable?

Question D15–2

The following independent variables were initially included in the multiple regression model. Why were variables c to i included?

a. Smoking at home: the sum of cigarettes currently smoked at home in a day, by the father and the mother; this was used as a measure of passive smoking by the child.
b. Smoking in pregnancy: the number of cigarettes smoked a day during the pregnancy with the given child.
c. Birth weight.
d. Father's height.
e. Mother's height.
f. Number of older siblings.
g. Social class (based on father's occupation).
h. Duration of pregnancy.
i. Household crowding index (number of persons per room).

Question D15–3

A multiple regression analysis that included a similar set of factors yielded a multiple correlation coefficient (R) of .56 (Rona et al., 1978). What does this tell us about the validity of the model?

Question D15–4

The proportion of the total variation in the child's height that was explained by parents' smoking, according to two different regression models, is shown in Table D15–2. What does the discrepancy between the figures in the first two columns and the third column tell us?

Table D15–2. Proportion of Variation in Height Explained by Parents' Current Smoking at Home, Mother's Smoking in Pregnancy, and Both These Factors Combined

| | Proportion Explained by: | | |
Variables Included in Model	Smoking at Home	Smoking in Pregnancy	Smoking at Home and in Pregnancy
Smoking at home, smoking in pregnancy	1.34%	0.67%	1.41%
Smoking at home, smoking in pregnancy, birth weight, father's and mother's height, number of older siblings, crowding index	0.23%	0.14%	0.26%

Question D15–5

What does the discrepancy between the figures in the two rows of Table D15–2 tell us? Can we always conclude that such discrepancies are due to confounding effects?

Question D15–6

Social class and duration of pregnancy were omitted from the analyses summarized in Table D15–2, on the grounds that "they did not explain a significant amount of variation in height." "Significant" may refer either to statistical significance, or to a "meaningful," "substantial," or "appreciable" effect. Which would be a more valid reason for omitting these variables?

Question D15–7

Regression coefficients expressing the relationship of parents' smoking to their children's height, based on four different linear regression models, are shown in Table D15–3. Explain what the coefficients tell us. ("What are the facts?")

Question D15–8

Can we conclude that smoking in pregnancy does not affect the child's height?

Table D15–3. Relationship of Parents' Smoking (Number of Cigarettes per Day) to Child's Height (Standard Deviation Score): Linear Regression Coefficients

Variables Included in Model	Smoking at Home		Smoking in Pregnancy	
	Coeffic.	P	Coeffic.	P
Smoking at home	−0.0099	<.001		
Smoking in pregnancy			−0.0122	<.001
Smoking at home, smoking in pregnancy	−0.0086	<.001	−0.0045	NS
Smoking at home, smoking in pregnancy, birth weight, father's and mother's height, number of older siblings, crowding index	−0.0034	<.01	−0.0028	NS

Question D15–9

What explanations can you suggest for the association between passive smoking and child's height?

Question D15–10

What use or uses does this study serve?

NOTES

D15–1. For a detailed discussion of the impact of effect modification on the results of multiple logistic regression analysis, with examples, see Lee (1986).

D15–2. Yes (by visual inspection). This may be confirmed by a goodness-of-fit test (see Note F2–1). An appropriate test (Lemeshow and Hosmer, 1982; described simply by Schlesselman, 1982, p. 264) yields a high P value (.58), indicating that there is no significant difference between the observed and predicted distributions.

Unit
D16

MULTIPLE LINEAR REGRESSION

In Unit A15, we discussed the control of confounding by use of a dependent variable that incorporates, and neutralizes the effect of, the confounder. The illustrations included the use of the IQ, which is a test score expressed as a percentage of the average score of children of the same age in order to neutralize the effect of age. In *Question D15–1*, the replacement of height by its discrepancy from the mean height of children of the same age, sex, and country similarly obviates possible confounding by age, sex, and country. Dividing this discrepancy by the standard deviation to obtain a standard deviation score (often called a *z score*) takes this a step further, by controlling for the spread as well as the central tendency of the distribution: the same discrepancy may have different meanings in narrow and wide distributions. (This method also has other statistical advantages.)

Regression analysis is sometimes used as a way of "purging" unwanted influences from a variable for this purpose. If we have a valid regression model for predicting blood pressure from age, sex, and other biological attributes, for example, we can calculate each subject's expected blood pressure and determine the discrepancy between the actual and predicted values. This discrepancy (the *"residual,"* or "what is left after the model is fit") is a measure that is not influenced by these biological attributes; using it as a dependent variable in other analyses will therefore control for confounding by these attributes.

Residuals may also be used to see how well a multiple regression model fits the observed facts. For example, Table D16 (from Kahn and Sempos, 1989) presents a simple test of a model that used age and weight to predict systolic blood pressure. (Would you conclude that the fit was good? See Note D16.)

The independent variables in the model used for parents' smoking and children's height (*Question D15–2*) were included because it was thought they might have a confounding effect on the association be-

260

Table D16. Agreement Between Observed and
Predicted Blood Pressure (mm Hg)

Age (yr)	Weight (lb)	Mean Residual (Observed BP Minus Predicted* BP)
<53	<172	−0.3
<53	≥173	−4.6
≥53	<172	−4.0
≥53	≥173	+3.8

*Predicted from age and weight.

tween smoking and height. In each instance there was reason to believe there might be a relationship with smoking, height, or both.

The square of the multiple correlation coefficient is the proportion of the variation of the dependent variable that is "explained" by the total set of independent variables. In *Question D15–3*, the square of .56 is .31, or 31%. This is higher than the explained proportion in most epidemiological studies.

The discrepancy between the proportions of variation explained by the smoking factors when considered separately and together (*Question D15–4*) obviously points to an overlap between their effects. We can compute from the figures in the top line that when nonsmoking variables are not taken into consideration (1.41 − 0.67)%, or 0.74%, of the variation is attributable only to smoking at home and (1.41 − 1.34)%, or 0.07%, only to smoking in pregnancy; the remaining (1.41 − 0.74 − 0.07)%, or 0.60%, is a shared effect. When other variables are included, the proportions are 0.12% (smoking at home), 0.03% (smoking in pregnancy), and 0.11% (shared). This overlap means that the number of cigarettes currently smoked at home and the number smoked during pregnancy are correlated; the correlation coefficient (for smoking by mothers) was in fact .64. We cannot determine which part of the overlap is attributable to current smoking, and which to smoking during pregnancy. This is another example of multicollinearity (Unit D15).

The reduction in the proportion of variation explained by an independent variable when other factors are included in a model (*Question D15–5*) may mean that the other factors (or some of them) are confounders, or it may mean that the other factors (or some of them) are intermediate causes. The statistical constellations in the two instances are the same (Unit A14). In this analysis there is one factor that may be an intermediate cause. This is birth weight: smoking in pregnancy is known to reduce the mean birth weight, and small size at birth may be one of the factors leading to low stature.

Absence of a statistically significant association (*Question D15–6*) does not prevent a variable from being a confounder. Strong associations can produce important confounding effects whatever their statistical significance. However, since there are no explicit criteria for deciding whether an association is sufficiently strong to produce confounding, opinions are divided about the use of significance tests for the purpose of deciding which potential confounders to control (Note D5).

A multiple linear regression coefficient indicates the average change in the dependent variable when there is a change of one unit in the relevant independent variable, with no change in the other variables in the model. The figure -0.0099 (*Question D15–7*) means that every additional cigarette currently smoked in the home, by mother or father, is associated with an average decrease in height of 0.0099 standard deviations. This is true if other variables are held constant. When smoking in pregnancy is added to the model, the specific ("unique") effect connected with smoking in the home (i.e., excluding the area of overlap) becomes slightly smaller, and it becomes still smaller (height decreases by only 0.0034 standard deviations for every cigarette) when other variables are added to the model and adjustment is made for their effects. But the association with smoking in the home remains statistically significant. Smoking a cigarette in pregnancy has a stronger effect than currently smoking one in the home, when other factors are held constant. But when the latter are taken into account, the effect is smaller and not statistically significant.

We cannot, however, conclude that smoking in pregnancy does not affect the child's height (*Question D15–8*). First, absence of statistical significance does not mean that an association is necessarily a chance finding. Second, one of the variables whose control weakened the association was birth weight, and (as pointed out above) small size at birth may be a link in a causal chain connecting smoking in pregnancy with low stature in childhood. Holding an intermediate cause constant weakens the statistical association between cause and effect. Such a finding supports a causal explanation; but we do not have data to enable us to separate the effects of controlling for birth weight and for other (confounding) variables. Third, as we have seen, there is a correlation between current smoking and smoking in pregnancy, and an overlap between their effects. The coefficients for smoking in pregnancy when current smoking is controlled express the effect that is "unique" to smoking in pregnancy, and may underestimate the true total effect of smoking in pregnancy. Our conclusion must be that the results do not tell us whether smoking in pregnancy affects height in childhood.

The association between passive smoking and the child's height (*Question D15–9*) is statistically significant, and remains apparent when variables expressive of genetic and other biologic attributes and social circumstances are held constant in the analysis. But adjustment for these factors may be incomplete: controlling for social class, number of older siblings, and household crowding may not hold socioeconomic factors completely constant. This is the first of the competing explanations considered by the investigators. Second, there may be an indirect causal association, mediated by other changes attributable to smoking, such as changes in family food consumption resulting from the effects of smoking on appetite or the family budget, or an increase of respiratory diseases in children exposed to the smoke. And third, tobacco smoke may have components that have a more direct effect on growth. You may have thought of other explanations—for example, the possibility of Berksonian bias, particularly since information was available for only 5,903/8,120, or 73%, of the study sample.

In answer to *Question D15–10*, this study may serve at least two purposes. First, an endeavor to identify the associated or intermediate reasons for the association may lead to new insights into factors affecting growth. Second, the results may serve pragmatic purposes. The effect of smoking on the child's height may or may not be thought important: assuming that the association is causal, parents who between them daily smoke 50 cigarettes in the home reduce their children's height by an average of (50×0.0034), or 0.17 standard deviations, which is approximately a centimeter. But even if this specific effect is regarded as unimportant, the study's additional evidence of the hazards of passive smoking may, if properly used, help to reduce the prevalence of smoking.

NOTE

D16.   Table D16 shows that the mean residuals differ in different subgroups of the study sample. This would not happen if the model had a perfect fit with the observed facts. But we might well decide that the mean discrepancies are so small that they do not matter.

U n i t
D17

TEST YOURSELF (D)

Check that you can do the following:

- Judge whether the possibility of confounding can be excluded (D4).

- Predict the probable direction of a confounding effect (D4).

- Detect synergism (D12).

- Calculate

  the sensitivity of a risk marker (Note D8–1).
  the predictive value of a risk marker (D8).
  an odds ratio from paired data (D11).
  an odds ratio from a logistic regression coefficient (D14).
  risk from multiple logistic regression coefficients (D15).

- Explain

  when statistical significance should be tested (D4).
  the various meanings of "risk factor" (D8).
  when to use a rate difference and when to use a rate ratio (D10).
  the difference between additive and multiplicative models (D12).

- Explain what is meant by

  a reference category (D5, D6).
  a risk ratio (D8).
  a relative risk (D8).
  a risk marker (D8).
  a statistically significant risk ratio or odds ratio (D10).
  a statistically significant rate difference (D10).
  a z score (D16).
  an intercept (D11).
  a statistically significant correlation coefficient (D11).

- Infer statistical significance from a confidence interval (D10).

- Appraise a risk marker (D8).

- Make sense of

  a P value (D4).
  a correlation coefficient (D11).
  a simple regression coefficient (D11).
  a multiple regression coefficient (D13, D16).
  a logistic regression coefficient (D13, D14).

- Explain (in general terms) what is meant by

  a conditional association (D4).
  a dose–response relationship (D8).
  synergism (D12).
  the Mantel–Haenszel procedure (D13).
  multiple logistic regression (D13).
  multiple linear regression (D13).
  residuals (D16).

SECTION
E

Causes and Effects

"Don't let us quarrel," the White Queen said in an anxious tone. "What is the cause of lightning?"

"The cause of lightning," Alice said very decidedly, for she felt quite certain about this, "is the thunder— oh, no!" she hastily corrected herself. "I meant the other way."

"It's too late to correct it," said the Red Queen: "when you've once said a thing, that fixes it, and you must take the consequences."

(Carroll, 1865)

Unit
E1

INTRODUCTION

This final set of exercises deals with three main topics—the kinds of epidemiological study used to investigate causal processes, criteria for the appraisal of causal associations, and ways of measuring the impact of causal factors.

KINDS OF STUDY

Epidemiological studies of causal processes can be broadly divided into *experiments* (in which the researcher decides which subjects or groups will be exposed to, or deprived of, the factor whose effect is under study) and *analytical surveys* (where surveys are defined as nonexperimental or "observational" studies). There is also a gray zone of *quasi-experiments*, which do not meet all the requirements of a well-designed experiment. We need not here concern ourselves with *descriptive surveys*, which aim to describe a situation rather than explain it; we have had examples in previous exercises, such as the studies of fractures of the femur in Oxford (Exercise B8) and suicide death rates in the United States (Exercise D11).

Analytic surveys can be classified in different ways (Note E1). The main types are:

- *Cross-sectional studies* (sometimes called *"prevalence studies"*). These are studies of total populations or population groups (or representative samples of them), in which information is collected about the present and (sometimes) the past characteristics, behavior, or experience of individuals. Examples in previous exercises are the studies of correlations with blood pressure in a population sample in the West Indies (Exercise D10) and of children's height and parents' smoking in England and Scotland (Exercise D15).

- *Case-control studies*, which compare cases and controls with respect to their present or past characteristics, behavior, or experience. Examples are the studies of cancer of the lip and previous herpes (Exercise C5), gastroenteritis and food consumption (Exercise D10), and myocardial infarction and the use of oral contraceptives (Exercise D12).

- *Cohort studies,* in which a total population group, a sample, or samples of people with known differences in their exposure to a supposed causal factor are followed up to determine the subsequent development of a disease or other outcome ("follow-up" or "prospective" studies). Examples are the studies of electrocardiographic abnormalities (Exercise C5), varicose veins (Exercise D1), and drinking (Exercise D9) in relation to subsequent coronary heart disease, and the study of smoking and mortality (Exercise D8).

- *Group-based studies,* which compare groups (e.g., countries) and not individuals; these are sometimes called "ecologic" studies, or "studies of groups of groups" (Friedman, 1980). The study of the relationship between melanoma mortality rates and latitude (Exercise D10) is an example.

Each kind of study has its own special features, which affect the use of its results. These relate especially to the use of measures of association, sources of bias (artifactual findings), confounding, and the study's external validity.

We start with a cross-sectional study.

EXERCISE E1

The association between caffeine consumption and indigestion, palpitation, and other symptoms was investigated in a cross-sectional survey of 4,558 Australians (Shirlow and Mathers, 1985). The subjects were volunteers aged 20–70 years collected "off the street" by a voluntary screening clinic, and by a mobile unit that visited places of employment. Questions were asked about the usual intake of coffee, tea, cola drinks, chocolate, and medications, the kind of coffee drunk, and the strength of the

Table E1–1. Mean Daily Caffeine Intake (mg) by Frequency of Indigestion (Men)

Indigestion	No.	Caffeine Intake
Never/rare	1,370	233
Sometimes/frequent	754	251
P		<.001

Table E1–2. Prevalence Rates of Indigestion in Low, Medium, and High Caffeine Consumption Groups, with Rate Ratios (Men)

Caffeine Consumption	Rate %	Rate Ratio
Low (0–150 mg/day)*	33.2	1.0
Medium (151–250 mg/day)	33.0	0.99
High (>250 mg/day)	39.3	1.18

*Reference group.

tea or coffee. Caffeine consumption was calculated, using standard figures for the caffeine content in different sources. The frequency of symptoms was reported as "never or rarely," "sometimes" (1–3 times a month), or "frequently" (once a week or more). Selected findings in men are shown in Tables E1–1 and E1–2 (the findings in women were similar).

Question E1–1

Two different approaches to the examination of associations are used in Tables E1–1 and E1–2. Do you know what these approaches are called? Summarize the facts shown in the tables. Are the rate ratios in Table E1–2 risk ratios?

Question E1–2

Table E1–2 shows rate ratios, and Table E1–3 shows odds ratios calculated from the same raw data. Which are preferable?

Question E1–3

May the respondents' or interviewers' awareness that symptoms were present have influenced the association with caffeine consumption?

Table E1–3. Association Between Indigestion and Caffeine Consumption: Odds Ratios

Caffeine Consumption	Odds Ratio
Low (0–150 mg/day)*	1.0
Medium (151–250 mg/day)	0.99
High (>250 mg/day)	1.30

*Reference group.

Table E1–4. Relationships of Caffeine
Consumption to Prevalence of Symptoms
(Men): Odds Ratios Based on Multiple
Logistic Regression

Symptom	Odds Ratio*	P
Indigestion	1.1	NS
Palpitation	1.3	<.01
Headache	1.4	<.0001
Tremor	1.2	<.05
Insomnia	1.3	<.0001

*The odds ratios indicate the change in the odds
   when daily caffeine consumption increases by
   200 mg.

Question E1–4

The data were submitted to multiple logistic regression analyses in
which indigestion and other symptoms were dependent variables. The
independent variables were caffeine consumption, age, Quetelet index,
smoking, and alcohol consumption. Odds ratios derived from the results are shown in Table E1–4. Summarize the findings. Can you conclude that caffeine consumption produced these symptoms?

Question E1–5

Would you have any hesitation in applying the results of this study to
Australian adults in general?

NOTE

E1.   The different kinds of study and their pros and cons are explained
      in all epidemiological textbooks. For more detailed classifications,
      see Abramson (1990, chap 2) or Kleinbaum et al. (1982, chap. 5).
      There are many hybrid designs.

APPRAISING THE RESULTS OF A
CROSS-SECTIONAL STUDY

A *retrospective* or *prospective* approach may be used when examining a postulated causal association (*Question E1–1*). Table E1–1 uses a retrospective
approach: the subjects are classified according to the supposed outcome
(indigestion), and we see whether the groups differ in their exposure to
the supposed cause (caffeine); we move from the postulated outcome to
the postulated cause. In Table E1–2, we start at the other end: the subjects
are classified according to their exposure, and we see whether they differ
in the frequency of the outcome. This is a prospective approach. Both approaches are feasible in a cross-sectional study, in contrast to a case-control study (which is characterized by a retrospective approach) or a cohort
study or experiment (where the approach is prospective). The terms "retrospective" and "prospective" may unfortunately be used with other
connotations, which can cause confusion (Note E2).

Both tables show positive associations between caffeine intake and
indigestion; the association is statistically significant. The prevalence
rate of indigestion is similar in the low and medium caffeine consumption groups, and higher in the high-caffeine group.

If we use the usual definition of risk (Note A6), the rate ratios in Table
E1–2 are not risk ratios; they are not ratios of incidence rates. A cross-
sectional study cannot provide a direct measure of risk.

There is no compelling reason to prefer either rate ratios or odds ratios
(*Question E1–2*). Both are good measures of the strength of an association.

In answer to *Question E1–3*, respondents who thought their symptoms were caused by coffee drinking might tend to report a higher
consumption; and interviewers inclined to this view might try harder to
get full information about caffeine consumption. The investigators say,
however, that "the questionnaire . . . did not indicate to the subject
that an association was expected . . . The possibility of such a bias was

lessened by the questions forming part of a general health screening examination aimed primarily towards the identification of cardio-vascular risk factors" (Shirlow and Mathers, 1985).

The subjects' awareness of their symptoms may have influenced the association in another way: it may have led them to drink less coffee. (But the authors report that only 2.6% of the subjects said they avoided coffee because of palpitation.)

These possibilities of effects arising from the fact that the postulated outcome occurs before the study is done also apply to case-control studies.

In answer to *Question E1–4*, all the symptoms except indigestion showed statistically significant, if weak, associations with caffeine consumption when possible confounders were controlled. The authors report that the association with indigestion was accounted for by strong correlations with adiposity (Quetelet index), and disappeared when adiposity was controlled in the analysis. We have no grounds for concluding that caffeine consumption produces indigestion. The findings are consistent with the hypothesis that it produces the other symptoms; but there may be unidentified confounders. The investigators concluded "that this study presents *suggestive* evidence that habitual caffeine consumption causes palpitations, tremor, headaches, and sleep disturbances" (Shirlow and Mathers, 1985).

The main reservation about the external validity of the study (*Question E1–5*) is the possibility of Berksonian bias. The associations observed in this volunteer sample may be different from those in the community at large. This might happen, for example, if people who drank a lot of coffee, and those with symptoms, were especially prone to volunteer.

A frequent problem in cross-sectional studies is that it may be difficult to know which came first, the supposed cause or the supposed outcome.

EXERCISE E2

Exercises D12 to D14 were based on a case-control study that showed a strong association between the use of oral contraceptives and myocardial infarction. The study was done in 155 hospitals in a region of the United States. The cases consisted of all premenopausal women aged 25–49 who were admitted to a coronary-care unit during a two-year period for a first episode of definite myocardial infarction (by WHO diagnostic criteria). Five potential controls were interviewed for each case of definite or possible myocardial infarction admitted. The controls were premenopausal women who had never had a myocardial infarction and were admitted to the surgical, orthopedic, or medical service of the same or a nearby hospital for conditions judged to be unrelated to oral-contraceptive use or cigarette smoking; controls who turned out not to meet these criteria were disqualified. The women in both groups were asked (inter alia) whether they had used oral contraceptives in the last month. Permission for the interview was refused by the patient or physician in 6% of cases and 6% of controls (Shapiro et al., 1979).

Question E2–1

Can a case-control study (like this one) measure

- risk?

- relative risk?

- a risk difference?

- a rate ratio?

Question E2–2

An obvious problem with case-control studies is that the samples of cases and controls may not be closely comparable, and the differences between them may confound the associations with the disease. What, therefore, do you think should be one of the first steps in the analysis?

Question E2–3

In a case-control study, the occurrence of the postulated effect (in this instance, myocardial infarction) precedes the collection of information about the postulated cause (oral contraceptives). How may this produce bias?

Question E2–4

As we have seen, the results of this study are consistent with the hypothesis that oral contraceptives increase the risk of myocardial infarction. Are they consistent with a completely different hypothesis—that oral contraceptives protect the lives of women who have an infarction?

Question E2–5

Under what circumstances can the odds ratio found in a case-control study be regarded as an estimate of the relative risk in a target population?

NOTE

E2.   The terms "retrospective" and "prospective" are often used to indicate whether a study is based on already available data. To avoid confusion, Feinstein (1977) has suggested use of the term *"retrolective"* for a study based on previously recorded data, and *"prolective"* for one in which data collection is planned in advance. These terms use the Latin root of the word "collect."

U n i t
E3

APPRAISING THE RESULTS OF A CASE-CONTROL STUDY

A case-control study cannot generally provide a direct measure of risk (*Question E2–1*): the number of cases in the study is determined by the investigator, not by the incidence of the disease. Thus the study cannot yield a direct measure of relative risk, or a risk difference. A case-control study can, of course, provide a rate ratio that is not a risk ratio—in this instance, the ratio of the rate of contraceptive use in cases to that in controls.

In certain circumstances, and if ancillary information is available, the risk associated with a specific factor *can* be estimated; we had an example in Question D8–3. Risk can be estimated in a *nested case-control study*, in which new cases of a disease are identified during a follow-up study of a cohort and are then compared with controls drawn from the same cohort.

An obvious early step in the analysis of data from a case-control study (*Question E2–2*) must be a comparison of the characteristics of the two samples. In this study, the cases and controls were found to be similar in ethnic group, religion, marital status, parity, and education, but they differed in geographical area (Boston, New York, or Philadelphia), cigarette smoking, obesity, and a history of diabetes, hypertension, lipid abnormality, angina pectoris, and preeclamptic toxemia. The latter variables were controlled by including them in a multiple logistic regression model; the adjusted odds ratio for the association between oral contraceptives and myocardial infarction was then 4.1.

In answer to *Question E2–3*, in a case-control study (as in a cross-sectional study), the fact that information about the "cause" is collected after the "effect" has occurred may produce bias in various ways. Those listed by Sackett (1979) in a catalog of biases are "rumination bias" (cases may ruminate about causes for their illnesses and thus report different prior exposures than controls), "obseqiousness bias" (subjects may alter their responses to fit what they think the investigator wants), "exposure suspicion bias" (a knowledge of the subject's disease status may influence the intensity and outcome of a search for exposure to the putative cause), and "recall bias" (caused by repeatedly asking cases about specific exposures, but asking controls only once). In this study, the investigators could not rule out the possibility of information bias, since the nurses who did the interviewing and many of the patients were aware of the hypothesis.

If a postulated causal factor (in this instance, oral-contraceptive use) affects the chance of inclusion as a case or control in the study, this will produce selection bias. This study did not include women who died immediately after having an infarction, before admission to hospital. If oral contraceptives protect infarction patients from death (*Question E2–4*), the lucky women who stayed alive and entered the study would include a high proportion of users of the pill—producing the observed association. The results are therefore consistent with the hypothesis that oral contraceptives keep infarction patients alive. (The investigators refute this interpretation by citing studies of patients with fatal infarction.)

The odds ratio can be regarded as a direct estimate of the relative risk in a target population (*Question E2–5*) if (a) the outcome condition is rare; and (b) there is no selection bias—that is, the cases are representative of cases in the target population and the controls are representative of noncases. The latter conditions are seldom met.

EXERCISE E3

Our example of a cohort study is a follow-up study conducted in a rural district of southern India, in which the association between tobacco-chewing and mortality was investigated (Gupta et al., 1984). In that part of the world, tobacco is chewed in the form of "pan"—that is, with betel leaf, areca nut, and slaked lime. A random sample of villagers aged 15 years and over—about 5,000 males and 5,000 females—were questioned about their tobacco habits. Deaths were ascertained through follow-up surveys conducted three years later, and then annually until ten years had passed.

Table E3 shows the results in females, 41% of whom chewed tobacco; tobacco smokers (1%) are excluded. Rates were age-standardized by the direct method, using specific rates for ten-year age intervals and the world standard population (Note B14–3).

Question E3–1

Person-time mortality rates were calculated, not cumulative mortality rates. Can you guess why? Does this study provide measures of risk?

Table E3. Mortality Rates per 1,000 Person-Years and Relative Risks, by Tobacco-Chewing Habit (Females)

	Crude		Age-Standardized	
	Rate	Relative Risk	Rate	Relative Risk
Tobacco chewers	12.8	3.4	8.3	1.3*
Nonchewers	3.8	1.0	6.2	1.0

*$P<.05$.

Question E3–2

What is the explanation for the difference between the crude and age-standardized relative risks?

Question E3–3

May the statistically significant association shown by the age-standardized data be a spurious one caused by confounding?

Question E3–4

Do you want to know anything about losses to follow-up? If so, why and what?

Question E3–5

Can you conclude that tobacco-chewing increased the risk of dying?

Question E3–6

In men, the age-standardized relative risk of mortality in tobacco chewers was 1.2. Does this alter your reply to Question E3–5?

Question E3–7

Can the results of this study be applied to the population from which the sample was drawn?

Unit
E4

APPRAISING THE RESULTS OF A COHORT STUDY

In answer to *Question E3–1*, some people were lost to follow-up before the end of the ten years of the study, so that direct measurement of cumulative mortality rates was not possible. By using person-time denominators it was possible to utilize all the available information about each subject, until loss of contact. Cumulative mortality rates can, of course, be estimated from the person-time rates (Note B5–4). With rates as low as those reported, the person-time and cumulative mortality rates would be almost identical. Both can be used as measures of risk. One of the advantages of a cohort study, with its prospective approach, is that it provides measures of risk.

The difference between the crude and age-standardized relative risks (*Question E3–2*) shows that there is confounding by age. (Can you say whether tobacco chewers were older or younger than nonchewers? See Note E4 for answer.) If the chewers and nonchewers were very different in age, some degree of confounding may remain even after age standardization (*Question E3–3*), since there may be substantial age differences between chewers and nonchewers *within* the broad (ten-year) age groups used for standardization. There may also be other confounders. The only other variable mentioned by the authors is socioeconomic status, which was not measured because of practical difficulties and because it was estimated that 90–95% of the population were in the lower socioeconomic strata. (But if the other 5–10% did not chew tobacco and had a low death rate, this could account for part of the association seen in Table E3.) We thus cannot exclude the possibility that the association is, at least in part, spurious.

Information about losses to follow-up (*Question E3–4*) is important in any cohort study. If people whose traces are lost have a different risk from those whose fate is known, the observed risk will be biased; and if this bias is different in the groups under comparison, the relative risk will be biased. We should therefore seek information about losses to follow-up and their reasons. The report tells us that most losses were due to leaving the district, probably because of marriage. Since nubile women tend to be healthy, these losses probably produced an upward bias of the death rate. Losses were more frequent in nonchewers, whose mean follow-up period was shorter (7.7 years) than that of chewers (8.8 years). This suggests that bias due to losses would tend to reduce rather than produce a difference in mortality.

It is difficult to be confident that tobacco-chewing increased the risk of dying (*Question E3–5*), as confounding can easily produce a weak association such as the one seen in this study, and it is not certain that age and other possible confounders were adequately controlled. If similar results were obtained in another sample or study, this would support the inference that the association was causal, and not due to chance, bias, or confounding. But the similar relative risk found in men in this study (*Question E3–6*) may mean only that the same confounding factors were operative in both sexes.

The results of the study, which was based on a random sample, can obviously be applied to the population from which the sample was drawn (*Question E3–7*). The results of any cohort study can be applied to a target population if the exposed and unexposed individuals in the sample (i.e., those exposed or not exposed to the suspected cause) are representative of the exposed and unexposed, respectively, in the population.

EXERCISE E4

As an example of a group-based ("ecologic") survey, we will use a study of correlations between the infant mortality rate and other national statistics in 18 developed countries—the U.S., Canada, Australia, New Zealand, and 14 European countries—in 1970 (Cochrane et al., 1978). These countries were chosen because they met criteria based on population size, the gross national product (GNP) per caput, and the availability of data.

Multiple regression analysis showed that 97% of the variation (variance) of infant mortality was explained by seven variables: the GNP per head, population density, the percentage of health expenditure covered by public expenditure, the number of doctors per 10,000 population, the annual cigarette consumption per head, the annual alcohol consumption per head, and the annual consumption of sugar per head. Other variables—the numbers of nurses, pediatricians, midwives, hospital beds, protein and fat consumption, and education—made little additional contribution.

Question E4-1

There was a negative correlation ($r = -.46$) between infant mortality and the GNP per head; that is, richer countries had lower infant mortality rates. This correlation was statistically significant. The GNP per head alone explained 21% of the variation of infant mortality. According to the multiple regression analysis the infant mortality rate decreased by 16%, on average, for a rise of one standard deviation in the GNP per caput, when the other six factors in the analysis were held constant. How would you explain the association between infant mortality and the GNP per head?

Question E4-2

There was a positive association ($r = .67$) between infant mortality and the number of doctors per 10,000 population; that is, countries with a higher prevalence of doctors had higher infant mortality rates. This correlation was statistically significant. The number of doctors alone explained 45% of the variation of infant mortality. According to the multiple regression analysis the infant mortality rate increased by 17%, on average, for a rise of one standard deviation in the number of doctors per 10,000 population when the other factors in the analysis were held constant. An analysis of data for 1960 revealed similar results, suggesting that the findings "cannot too easily be dismissed as a chance curiosity." How would you explain the association between infant mortality and the number of doctors per 10,000 population?

NOTE

E4.   Confounding by age produced spurious strengthening of the association, and mortality obviously has a positive association with age. According to the Direction Rule (Unit D5), therefore, tobacco-chewing, too, was probably positively associated with age.

Unit
E5

APPRAISING THE RESULTS OF A GROUP-BASED STUDY

There are two kinds of explanation for the negative correlation between infant mortality and the GNP per head (*Question E4–1*). Richer countries may have lower rates because they are richer (better hospital facilities, better food, better sanitation, etc.), or the correlation may be due to confounding factors that are correlates but not necessarily consequences of wealth, such as differences in knowledge, attitudes, and practices with respect to infant care.

Similarly, the positive correlation with the prevalence of doctors (*Question E4–2*) may be causal or due to confounding. As an iatrogenic explanation is implausible, confounding seems likely. But by what? The investigators were not able to find an explanation: "we must admit defeat and leave it to others to extricate doctors from their unhappy position" (Cochrane et al., 1978).

Two main problems beset the appraisal of group-based studies. The first is the influence of confounding factors which, especially in studies based only on official statistics, may be difficult to investigate. The second is the "ecological fallacy" of concluding that an association found at a group basis also exists at the individual level. (There is more malaria in poor countries than in rich ones; but this does not necessarily mean that poor people are at higher risk than rich people in the same country.)

EXERCISE E5

This exercise deals with three studies of the effects of health care procedures.

Question E5–1

The first is a clinical trial of the effect of acupuncture (Godfrey and Morgan, 1978). The subjects were patients with chronic, dull, moderate pain at any site, attending outpatient clinics in a Toronto hospital; 57% volunteered for the study in response to a public announcement, and 43% were referred by physicians. The most frequent diagnoses were osteoarthritis (24%), degenerative disk disease (20%), and lumbosacral strain (8%). Patients found to have inflammatory conditions were excluded. The subjects were randomly allocated to two groups: one whose members received acupuncture (i.e., needling at the sites where, according to acupuncture theory, this was most likely to relieve their pain) and a control group who received sham acupuncture (needling at the sites least likely to reduce their pain). The study was double-blind: the acupuncturist (a Chinese expert) did not know whether he was administering true or sham acupuncture, nor did the subject. The patients used a six-point scale to measure the level of pain. Table E5–1 shows the results after five treatments.

Do the results prove that acupuncture does not work—that is, that "appropriate" acupuncture does not relieve pain better than sham acupuncture? If not, why not? What extra information would you like?

Question E5–2

If there had been 8,400 subjects in each group and the P value was the same (.21), would this affect your appraisal of the results?

Question E5–3

If the trial had showed a clearly beneficial effect, could the results be applied to everyone with pain?

Question E5–4

What kinds of bias are reduced by "blinding" experimental subjects or observers?

Table E5–1. Reduction of Pain After Five Treatments: Double-Blind Randomized Trial of Acupuncture

	Acupuncture	*Controls*
Number of subjects	84	84
Number with reduction of pain	53	45
Success rate (%)	63	54
$P = .21$.		

Table E5-2. Deaths From All Causes Other Than Breast
Cancer: Ten-Year Follow-up After Entry to Study

	Death Rate*
Members of study group who were screened	54.9
Control group	64.8

*Deaths per 10,000 person-years.

Question E5-5

The effect of breast cancer screening on mortality from breast cancer was
examined in a randomized trial (Shapiro et al., 1982). Women aged
40–64 who were members of the Health Insurance Plan of New York
were randomly allocated to two groups: a "study group," whose members were offered four annual screening examinations (clinical examination and mammography); and a control group, who continued to receive
their usual medical care. There were about 31,000 women in each group.
The groups were very similar with respect to a wide range of demographic and other characteristics.

Mortality rates from causes other than breast cancer are shown in
Table E5-2. How can the findings be explained?

Question E5-6

Table E5-3 shows the numbers of breast cancer deaths in the nine years
following entry to the study (Shapiro, 1977). (Since the denominators in
the two groups are almost identical, we can use numbers instead of
rates.) What would you conclude from these results? You may assume
that the differences are not fortuitous.

Table E5-3. Deaths from Breast Cancer: Nine-Year Follow-up After Entry
to Study

Age (yr) at Diagnosis	Number of Deaths		Ratio
	Study Group	Control Group	
40–49	30	27	1.1
50–59	42	67	0.6
≥60	19	34	0.6
Total	91	128	0.7

Table E5—4. Mortality from Cardiovascular Disease in Treated and Control Groups: Rates per 1,000 Person-Years

Type of Analysis	Group		Ratio
	Treatment	Placebo	
"Intention to treat"	34	47	0.72
"On randomized treatment"	30	48	0.63

Question E5—7

A multicenter randomized trial was conducted to determine the value of treatment for mild hypertension in the elderly (Amery et al., 1985). The trial was double-blind, the subject's allocation to the treatment or control (placebo) group remaining undisclosed until the end, unless an event occurred—such as a severe increase in blood pressure—that necessitated "breaking the code." The mortality rates in the treatment and placebo groups are shown in Table E5—4, using two different methods of analysis. The "intention to treat" analysis is based on deaths during the whole follow-up period, in the subjects originally allocated to each group—whether they persisted with their allotted treatment or not. The "on randomized treatment" analysis is confined to the findings while the subjects were in the double-blind part of the study, on their allocated treatment. Which form of analysis is better?

Unit
E6

APPRAISING THE RESULTS OF AN EXPERIMENT

The trial of acupuncture did not demonstrate a statistically significant effect. The slight benefit observed could easily be a chance finding. The absence of statistical significance does not, however, mean that the benefit *was* a chance finding; we have no way of telling. The study does not prove that acupuncture works, but (in answer to *Question E5–1*) neither does it prove that it does not.

Randomization (random allocation into treatment groups, based on tossing a coin, using random numbers, etc.) minimizes the likelihood of confounding, but it cannot completely prevent it. Substantial differences may occur between the groups, just by chance, and these may exaggerate or weaken the apparent effects of treatment. Information on the characteristics of the groups (age distribution, diagnoses, sites of pain, etc.) would satisfy us that confounding was unlikely. We should also have information on withdrawals from the study, for the same reasons as in a nonexperimental cohort study.

In answer to *Question E5–2*, a statistically nonsignificant result based on large numbers—that is, where the power of the test (Note D4) is high—may be taken as evidence that no real effect of any importance exists.

Clinical trials are never conducted on random samples; the requirement that subjects must give their informed consent is enough to ensure this, let alone the trials's specific eligibility criteria. The results can be generalized only to a reference population that the subjects are believed to represent. In this instance (*Question E5–3*), the subjects were certainly not representative of all people with pain. We do not know just what the selective factors were. At best, we might decide that the results can be applied to the sort of hospital outpatient with chronic pain who is likely to request acupuncture or be referred by a physician for acupuncture.

The use of blind methods (*Question E5–4*) reduces the chance that the subjects' reactions or reports, or their readiness to remain in the study, will be influenced by their knowing what treatment they are having. Keeping clinicians and other observers in the dark prevents them from communicating this knowledge to the subjects and from handling the experimental groups differently, and it keeps their own findings unbiased.

Randomization ensures that the subjects in a trial are divided into groups that have only chance differences. But if after randomization we remove people who refuse to participate or are withdrawn from the study (because the treatment is inappropriate, etc.), the groups may no longer be comparable. This is illustrated in *Question E5–5*, where the reason for the difference in mortality is that members of the study group who refused the offer of screening were omitted. The fuller facts (Table E6–1) show that the study and control groups did not differ in their mortality from causes other than breast cancer.

In answer to *Question E5–6*, the table shows fewer breast cancer deaths among women allocated to the study group. As this difference cannot easily be attributed to bias or confounding, the results indicate that screening decreases mortality from breast cancer. This benefit is not apparent below the age of 50.

The stratification by age in Table E5–3 represents one of the procedures commonly used in the analysis of trials (Note E6). Prognostic factors that are associated with the outcome are identified. It is then possible, by appropriate analyses, to examine their modifying and possible confounding effects. The term *post-stratification* may be used to distinguish this method from stratified allocation to treatment and control groups (i.e., stratification of the potential subjects according to supposed prognostic factors, followed by random allocation of the members of each stratum, so as to obtain matched treatment and control groups).

Excluding randomized subjects of a therapeutic trial from the analysis may lead to bias, and the correct answer to *Question E5–7* is that an *"intention-to-treat" analysis,* comparing the outcomes in all the subjects

Table E6–1. Deaths from All Causes
Other Than Breast Cancer: Five-Year
Follow-up After Entry to Study

	Death Rate*
Study group	
Screened	42
Refused	86
Total	57
Control group	58

*Deaths per 10,000 person-years.

originally allocated to each group (including those who did not have or who stopped having the specified treatment) is preferable. This stringent approach may sometimes, however, underestimate the efficacy of the treatment. This probably happened in this study, where a proportion of the subjects in the treatment group stopped treatment, and a proportion of those in the placebo group received antihypertensive treatment: 15% of the subjects in the placebo group (but only 1% of those in the treatment group) were removed from the double-blind part of the study because of a severe increase in blood pressure.

EXERCISE E6

This exercise deals with another two studies of health care.

Question E6–1

An "early stimulation" program for promoting children's development (by encouraging mothers to speak and play with their infants) was instituted and tested at two maternal and child health (MCH) clinics operated by a university department in two neighborhoods of Jerusalem. It was decided not to allocate mothers to the program randomly, partly for practical and ethical reasons, and partly because dissemination to other mothers living in the same neighborhoods and using the same clinics (i.e., "contamination" of controls) was inevitable.

It was therefore proposed to appraise effectiveness by comparing the development of infants served by these clinics with that of infants served by two clinics in neighborhoods where there was no such program. This plan was abandoned when it was found that, mainly because of poor attendance, it would not be possible to measure the status of the control children. Instead, a "before–after" design was chosen, comparing the development of two birth cohorts of infants served by the intervention clinics—those born after implementation of the program and those born before. At two years of age, the mean developmental quotient (DQ) turned out to be higher in children born after implementation of the program (Palti, 1983).

If the first study plan had been practicable, would this have been a good experiment? (And if not, why not?) After the change of design, was this a good experiment? If the two designs had been combined (so as to compare the "before–after" differences in the intervention and control communities), would this have made a good experiment?

Question E6–2

What precaution would be needed when appraising the results?

Question E6–3

Some years later, another evaluative study was done, by comparing the IQs of two groups of five-year-old children who were attending nursery schools in the neighborhoods in which the experimental clinics were situated: children who as infants had received care in these clinics, and control children who had received care at other MCH clinics (Palti et al., 1986). The controls were individually matched by ethnic group, mother's education, and birth rank. The groups were found to be similar with respect to mother's age, mother's work outside the home, father's education, social class, number of years in nursery school, number of languages spoken in the home, and other variables. Would you call this an experiment?

Question E6–4

Selected results are shown in Table E6–2. Summarize the findings. What would you conclude?

Question E6–5

The effect of obstetric care on the outcome of pregnancy was appraised in a hospital in Oxford by comparing fetal deaths ascribed to asphyxia or trauma with randomly selected live-born control infants (Niswander et al., 1984). By use of the clinical records, "blind" assessments were made of the quality of care in pregnancy, and of the complexity of the pregnancy and labor (poor obstetric history, intrauterine growth retardation, abnormalities of fetal heart rate, preterm delivery, etc.). Selected results are shown in Table E6–3.

What conclusion can you reach about the effect of the quality of antenatal care on the outcome of pregnancy?

Table E6–2. Mean IQ of Five-year-old Children Exposed to Early Stimulation Program and Matched Controls, by Mother's Education

Mother's Education	Mean IQ		Difference	P
	Exposed	Control		
5–8 years	106.3	92.0	14.3	.021
9–12 years	111.7	104.6	7.1	.012
>12 years	121.9	121.6	0.3	NS
Total	114.4	108.6	5.8	.003

Table E6–3. Relationship of Fetal Deaths Ascribed to Asphyxia or Trauma
to Quality of Care in Pregnancy

Quality of Care	Fetal Deaths	Controls	Odds Ratio (With 95% Confidence Interval)	P	Adjusted Odds Ratio*
Suboptimal	8	17	3.7 (1.6–8.6)	<.01	3.4
Satisfactory	45	355			

*Controlling for complexity of the pregnancy and labor (by use of the Mantel–Haenszel procedure).

Question E6–6

The above study was obviously not an experiment. An experiment to study the effect of suboptimal antenatal care would have serious ethical objections. Was it a quasi-experiment or a survey? If a survey, what kind? A cross-sectional, case-control, or cohort study?

NOTE

E6. The design, conduct, and analysis of trials are explained in many textbooks. For a simple but thorough exposition, see Peto et al. (1976, 1977). Design and analysis are dealt with in detail by Fleiss (1986c).

Unit
E7

APPRAISING THE RESULTS OF A
QUASI-EXPERIMENT

Quasi-experiments, which do not fully satisfy the criteria of a sound experiment, are usually performed because a better design is not feasible (Note E7–1).

All three of the studies described in *Question E6–1* are quasi-experiments. In the first—the comparison of children served by intervention and control clinics—there was no randomization of clinics (because the investigators were able to implement the program only in their own clinics). Also, the design took no account of the possibility that children living in the different neighborhoods might have differed in their development before the program was started: there were "after" measurements but no "before" measurements. In addition, it can be claimed that there were too few sampling units. In effect, two clusters of children (in different neighborhoods) were compared with two others. If children in different neighborhoods differ much in their development, a good experiment would require a fair number of clusters—certainly more than two—in each group.

The second design—a "before–after" comparison based on the findings in different birth cohorts in the neighborhoods where the program was implemented—makes no allowance for the possibility that a change might have occurred even without the program. Observations in control neighborhoods over the same period might have demonstrated a similar change. To mitigate the problem of a possible "secular trend" (a change with time), the investigators actually used a *time series* instead of a simple "before–after" comparison. They included two birth cohorts born before the program was started, and showed that there was no evidence of a change before the program was instituted (Palti, 1983).

A combination of these two designs—that is, a comparison of "before–after" changes in intervention and control communities—

would remedy some of these drawbacks. But here, too, there is no randomization.

The main precaution to be taken when appraising the results of a quasi-experiment (*Question E6–2*) is that the same careful attention to the possibility of confounding is needed as in an analytic survey.

The design described in *Question E6–3* is also quasi-experimental. It is again a comparison of children served by different clinics, this time using matching to control selected confounders, but still with no randomization or "before" measurements.

The main findings (*Question E6–4*) were that children in the exposed group had a significantly higher mean IQ, that this difference was apparent only in the children of mothers with 12 or fewer years of education, and that there was a positive association between maternal education and the child's IQ (in both the exposed and control groups).

Since some possible confounders were controlled by matching, and others could be disregarded because of the results of the "exclusion test," the findings suggest that the program was probably effective. This interpretation is supported by the interaction with maternal education, since if early stimulation works it might be expected to work best with the disadvantaged children of less educated mothers. The findings conform with this expectation. The program appears to reduce the gap in development between the children of less educated and better educated mothers.

The results of the study in Oxford (*Question E6–5*) suggest that suboptimal antenatal care is a cause of fetal death. The association was strong and statistically significant, it was based on appraisals that were apparently unbiased (because they were "blind"), and it was only slightly attributable to the confounding effect of the complexity of the pregnancy or labor. There is, however, a reservation: the control of confounding may not be as good as it appears. The appraisals of complexity may not have provided sufficient control of prognostic factors. The investigators admit that "failure to achieve adequate control of confounding factors . . . may have led us to overestimate some of the risks associated with suboptimal care. In future studies we shall try to match cases and controls more closely by the clinical problems for which the quality of care is to be assessed" (Niswander et al., 1984).

In answer to *Question E6–6*, this is of course a case-control study. Case-control studies in which the case is a person with a condition that may be due to poor care are becoming increasingly popular as a way of evaluating health care procedures and programs.

EXERCISE E7

In this exercise we appraise causal associations in three studies.

Question E7–1

A study of all infants born in Michigan from 1950 to 1964 showed a strong positive association between birth rank and the rate of Down's syndrome (Note E7–2). There was a threefold variation in rates. Do the findings in Table E7–1 indicate that birth-rank influences the risk of the disease?

Question E7–2

An English study of over 2,500 patients who were treated for hypertension showed that 6% died during four years of follow-up (Bulpitt et al., 1979). Patients were entered into the study at presentation to a hospital hypertension clinic (86%) or when seen in general practice with hypertension (14%). The cumulative mortality rate after four years was 12% for smokers and 5% for nonsmokers. This difference was statistically significant ($P<.001$).

Can you think of any reason to suggest that the difference may be an artifact?

Question E7–3

The investigators compared the characteristics of the hypertensive patients who subsequently died and those who stayed alive. Weight, serum cholesterol, pulse rate, and a history of angina pectoris were not associated with mortality, and could be exonerated from suspicion as confounders. Characteristics that were related to mortality were included, together with smoking, in multiple regression and multiple logistic regression models. The multivariate analyses (in which mortality was the dependent variable) showed significant associations with smoking, age, systolic blood pressure level, and plasma urea; doubtfully significant associations with retinal hemorrhages, proteinuria, and a histo-

Table E7–1. Down's Syndrome in Michigan by Birth Rank: Rates, Relative Risks, and SMRs

Birth Rank	Rate per 100,000 Live Births	Relative Risk	SMR*
1	56.3	1.0	1.0
2	67.6	1.2	1.0
3	83.3	1.5	1.1
4	115.5	2.1	1.0
≥5	167.1	3.0	1.1

*Maternal age controlled by indirect standardization, using the "birth rank 1" group as the standard.

ry of myocardial infarction; and no significant associations with diastolic blood pressure before treatment, serum uric acid, and other variables.

The multiple logistic analysis showed that, controlling for other variables, the odds ratio for the association between smoking and death was 3.6 ($P<.001$). Can we conclude that smoking increased the risk of dying in this group of treated hypertensive patients?

Question E7–4

If we conclude that the patients who smoked had a higher risk of dying because of their smoking, can we infer that their risk would have been reduced if they had stopped smoking?

Question E7–5

The next two questions are based on a study of the association between the use of artificial sweeteners and weight change, in which women who said they added sweeteners (mainly saccharin) to beverages or food were compared with women who said they did not (Stellman and Garfinkel, 1986). The dependent variable was weight change during a one-year period.

The information was obtained from a single questionnaire, which included questions about the use of sweeteners, current weight, and weight one year previously. The difference between these two weights was the dependent variable. The questionnaire was administered during the baseline investigation of subjects enrolled in a prospective mortality study in the United States, in which over a million people were enlisted.

"Rather than attempt to adjust for a multitude of factors," this analysis was confined to 78,694 white women aged 50–69 with at least a high school education, with no history of diabetes, heart disease, or cancer,

Table E7–2. Percentage of Women Who Lost Weight During a One-year Period, by Use of Sweeteners and Relative Weight* at Start

| Relative Weight | Percentage Who Lost Weight | | Ratio | P |
	Sweeteners Used for ≥10 Years	Sweeteners Never Used		
Very low	11.9	12.0	0.99	NS
Low	14.9	16.0	0.93	NS
Average	18.5	19.2	0.96	NS
High	22.2	23.8	0.93	NS
Very high	28.2	25.6	1.10	NS

*Quetelet index (quintiles).

Table E7–3. Percentage of Women Who Gained Weight During a One-year Period, by Use of Sweeteners and Relative Weight* at Start

Relative Weight	Percentage Who Gained Weight		Ratio	P
	Sweeteners Used for ≥10 Years	Sweeteners Never Used		
Very low	32.3	29.6	1.09	<.001
Low	39.0	33.5	1.16	<.001
Average	41.5	35.0	1.19	<.001
High	41.5	32.4	1.28	<.001
Very high	31.9	26.3	1.21	<.001

*Quetelet index (quintiles).

who said there had been no major change in their diet in the past ten years and that they had not changed their smoking status for at least two years. To simplify the analysis only two groups were compared: women who said they had used sweeteners for ten or more years, and women who said they had never used them.

How would you classify this study? Cross-sectional? Case-control? Cohort?

Question E7–6

There were no differences between users and nonusers of sweeteners with respect to the mean number of times per week they reported eating beef, pork, liver, ham, smoked meats, franks or sausages, carrots, squash, citrus fruits or juices, cereal or oatmeal, ice cream, and chocolates. Users ate green leafy vegetables, tomatoes, cabbage, chicken, and fish more frequently than nonusers; and ate butter, white bread, and potatoes less frequently. Information on quantities was not available.

The percentages who reported losing and gaining weight during the previous year are shown in Tables E7–2 and E7–3. The results are stratified by relative weight at the start of the year. The percentages are age-standardized by the direct method, using five-year age intervals.

Do the findings show that artificial sweeteners cause a gain in weight? What other explanations may there be?

NOTES

E7–1. Quasi-experimental designs and their strengths and weaknesses are described by Campbell and Stanley (1966), Campbell (1969), and Cook and Campbell (1979).

E7–2. Stark and Mantel (1966). For a detailed explanation of standardization, using this example, see Fleiss (1981, chap. 14).

Unit
E8

ARTIFACT, CONFOUNDING OR CAUSE?

When an association is found, a causal explanation can be seriously considered only if the association cannot readily be explained as an artifact or a consequence of confounding.

In answer to *Question E7–1*, the association between birth rank and Down's syndrome virtually disappears when maternal age is controlled by indirect standardization. The findings thus provide no support for the hypothesis that birth-rank influences the risk of the disease. The strong association shown by the crude data can be attributed to the confounding effect of maternal age. Confounding does not usually produce strong associations. But it can, as these findings show.

The cohort study of hypertensive patients (*Question E7–2*) showed a higher four-year mortality for smokers than for nonsmokers. The difference may, however, be due to lead time bias (Unit B10), since the starting-point for follow-up was the beginning of treatment—in most cases, the first attendance at a hypertension clinic. It is possible that the smokers were people who tended to take less care of themselves, and began to get treatment for their hypertension at a later stage in the natural history of the disease than did nonsmokers. Their mortality may have been higher because their disease was more advanced.

The results of the subsequent analysis (*Question E7–3*) suggest that the association was not an artifact caused by lead-time bias, since the variables controlled in the multivariate analyses include some that are indicative of the stage of the disease at the outset (the initial blood pressure level and the presence of cardiac, renal, and eye complications of hypertension at entry into the study). The results also show that the association was not caused by the confounding effects of the other variables examined. It is probably safe to infer that smoking increased the risk of dying.

It does not follow, however, that giving up smoking would necessarily have lessened the risk of dying (*Question E7–4*), since some etiological factors have irreversible effects that remain after the factor is removed. We would require other evidence, based on observational or experimental comparisons of the mortality of hypertensives who cease and continue to smoke.

The study of artificial sweeteners (*Question E7–5*) is best classified as a cross-sectional study in which information was obtained about past as well as present characteristics. A prospective approach was used in the analysis. It is not a typical cohort study—although a cohort study can be based on historical data (a *historical prospective study*)—because the information about the use of sweeteners was not collected before the occurrence of the outcome. The study has the potential biases of a cross-sectional study.

A causal relationship between sweeteners and weight gain (*Question E7–6*) is not inconceivable. The mechanism might be pharmacological or psychological—for example, a tendency to regard the addition of sweeteners as a substitute for caloric restriction. However, we should consider other explanations. First, the data concerning weight change (calculated from reported weights) may be biased. It can be claimed that "since changes in weight between two points in time are used . . . any bias due to systematic under-estimation by individuals will tend to be minimized" (Stellman and Garfinkel, 1986). But the validity of the information may be different in users and nonusers. Women who are "weight-conscious"—and therefore take sweeteners and avoid butter, white bread, and potatoes—may, because of this awareness, be especially likely to report that they are gaining weight. Second, there may be confounding by some factor not controlled by the procedures used (these were: limiting the study to a homogeneous group of subjects, stratifying for relative weight, and standardizing for age). One possible confounder is weight change prior to the year under consideration. Women who had previously been gaining weight (and were therefore using sweeteners) may have tended to continue their weight gain during the year of the study, producing the association that was found. Weight gain may have *preceded* the use of sweeteners.

You may have thought of other explanations.

EXERCISE E8

An association cannot be regarded as causal if it can be completely explained by confounding—that is, if it disappears when other variables (that cannot be regarded as intermediate causes) are held constant. We have encountered many ways of dealing with confounding in these exercises. How many can you list?

Unit
E9

COPING WITH CONFOUNDING

Confounding may be handled in various ways. The following methods have been mentioned or used in previous pages.

1. Confounding may be reduced or prevented by the manner of selecting the study sample or samples:
   - individual and group matching (Unit D11).
   - restriction of the study to a homogeneous group (Question E7–5).
   - random allocation to experimental groups (Unit E6).
   - stratified allocation to experimental groups (Unit E6).
2. In the analysis, confounders may be held constant by stratifying the data and then using the stratum-specific findings (Unit A11). Post-stratification may be used when analyzing the results of a trial (Unit E6).
3. Other methods that may be used in the analysis include
   - direct standardization (Unit B14).
   - indirect standardization (Unit B13).
   - Mantel–Haenszel and similar procedures based on stratified data (Unit D13).
   - multivariate analysis (Unit D7)—for example, multiple regression analysis (Units D13, D16) and multiple logistic regression analysis (Units D13–D15).
   - current life table analysis (Note B9–3).
   - partial correlation coefficients (Unit D11).
4. Use is sometimes made of dependent variables that incorporate, and thus neutralize the effect of, the confounder(s) (Unit A15). These include "residuals" based on regression analysis (Unit D16).
5. Confounding is sometimes handled by ratiocination, based on the (non-foolproof) logic of the exclusion test (Unit D5), the Direction Rule (Unit D5), and estimates of the magnitude of the possible confounding effect (Note D6).

DELVING INTO CAUSES

We cannot "prove" a causal relationship. The best we can hope for is that new facts will consistently conform with what we would expect to find if the association were causal. The key to the study of causation is the development of hypotheses that can be subjected to empirical testing (Units A6, A15, A16). Clues, ideas, and new specific hypotheses often arise during the analysis, in the form of inferences that emerge when associations are elaborated and variables are refined. Hypotheses may be tested in the framework of a single study, by subjecting the available data to additional analyses, or may need new data.

In the long run, judgments about causal relationships are based on evidence that comes from many studies, including nonepidemiological ones (Note E9–1). Studies may be reviewed and appraised in an informal way, or their results may be subjected to an integrated statistical analysis (*meta-analysis;* see Section F).

A great deal has been written about methods and criteria for the appraisal of causality (Note E9–2).

EXERCISE E9

What would persuade you that one variable is causally related to another? List as many criteria as you can.

NOTES

E9–1.   For examples of the way that etiological knowledge has evolved from the complementary contributions of population studies, clinical observations, and laboratory experiments, see Morris (1975, pp. 250–261).

E9–2.   Methods of deciding whether an association is causal are discussed in all epidemiology textbooks. For a fuller discussion, see Susser (1973, pp. 140–162) or Susser (1986). For a set of rules (Evans's criteria) for use in deciding whether a factor is a cause of a disease, see Lilienfeld and Lilienfeld (1980, pp. 317–318). See Note A6–1.

Unit
E10

EVIDENCE FOR A CAUSAL RELATIONSHIP

A well-designed experiment can provide better evidence for a causal relationship than a survey can, and the evidence is strongest if the findings are replicated in other experiments.

Whatever kind of study the evidence comes from, there are four basic conditions that must be met before a causal relationship between two variables can be seriously contemplated. These prerequisites are that

- The variables are associated with one another.

- The association cannot readily be explained as an artifact.

- The association cannot readily be explained as an effect of confounding.

- There is no evidence that the "effect" precedes the "cause."

There are a number of additional criteria that, taken together, may strengthen or weaken the case for a causal association, although they cannot provide absolute proof that the causal hypothesis is true or false. The following list (based in part on Susser, 1986), states what evidence may be regarded as supporting or weakening the case for a causal association. "Indeterminate" findings that neither strengthen nor weaken the case—such as the *absence* of a dose–response relationship—are not specified.

- *Probability.* Statistical significance supports the case for a causal association. Absence of statistical significance weakens it, but only if the test is powerful (large numbers).

- *Strength of the association.* A strong association supports the case.

- *Dose–response relationship.* If there is a monotonic positive association between the amount, intensity, or duration of exposure to the

301

"cause" and the quantity or severity of the "effect," this supports the case.

- *Time–response relationship.* If the incidence of the "effect" rises to a peak some time after exposure to the "cause" and then decreases, this supports the case.

- *Predictive performance.* If information about the "cause" is predictive of the occurrence of the "effect," this supports the case; if it is not, it weakens it.

- *Specificity.* If the "effect" is related to only one "cause" or constellation of causes, this may be regarded as supporting the case. Specificity of the "effect" (i.e., the "cause" has only one "effect") contributes little to the appraisal.

- *Consistency* (in different populations, circumstances, and studies). If the same association is found repeatedly, this strongly supports the case. If results are inconsistent, and the variation cannot be attributed to modifying factors or differences in study methods, this weakens the case.

- *Coherence* with current theory and knowledge supports the case. Incompatibility with known facts weakens it.

EXERCISE E10

Question E10–1

Table E10–1 shows the association between beer-drinking and rectal cancer in men, according to a case-control study in the United States (Kabat et al., 1986). The odds ratios are based on a multiple logistic regression analysis in which suspected confounders were controlled. Are the results consistent with a causal explanation?

Table E10–1. Association Between Beer-Drinking and Rectal Cancer

Beer Consumption	Odds Ratio	95% Confidence Interval
Never	1.0	—
Occasional	1.4	0.8–2.6
1–7 oz/day	1.4	0.7–2.6
8–31 oz/day	1.6	0.8–3.1
≥32 oz/day	2.7	1.3–5.7

Table E10–2. Evaluation of Studies of Beer Drinking and Rectal Cancer Risk

Criteria	Fit*	Comments
Strength	+	The relative risks, where elevated, are small or borderline.
Specificity	+	Two correlation [group-based] studies have found significant positive correlations between beer and a number of cancers other than the rectum and colon.
Consistency	+	Five of 10 case-control or prospective studies showed no association. Several correlation [group-based] studies showed . . . an association, but one did not.
Dose–response	+	None of the published studies, except the present one, provides evidence of a dose–response relationship.
Temporal sequence	++	Three published prospective studies showed a positive association . . . ; one found no association. . .
Biological rationale	+	Ethanol by itself has not been shown to be a carcinogen. Furthermore, no epidemiological studies have reported an association of wine or whiskey with rectal cancer. . .

*Fit is defined as how well the existing evidence fulfills each of the criteria. +++ = good, ++ = fair, + = poor,
Source: Kabat et al. (1986) (table abbreviated).

Question E10–2

The authors of the paper on beer and rectal cancer provided the review of epidemiological studies shown in Table E10–2. On the basis of this evidence, does beer drinking (in your judgment) increase the risk of rectal cancer?

Unit
E11

EVIDENCE FOR A CAUSAL RELATIONSHIP (CONTINUED)

In answer to *Question E10–1*, the results shown in Table E10–1 are consistent with a causal relationship between beer drinking and rectal cancer. There is evidence of a dose–response relationship: the association is strongest in men who drink most beer. As the confidence intervals show, only in this group is the association statistically significant.

Their review of the available epidemiological evidence on beer and rectal cancer (*Question E10–2*) led Kabat et al. (1986) to the conclusion that

it is clear that the existing studies, at best, provide weak support for a causal association . . . Two explanations can be proposed to explain the conflicting results. . . The first is that some component of beer itself is a weak initiator or promoter of rectal cancer. The alternative explanation is that the association . . . is indirect [i.e., due to confounding] and that beer consumption is associated with an as yet unknown factor, possibly dietary in nature, that is itself a rectal carcinogen . . . we are inclined to favour the second explanation.

You may or may not agree with this appraisal. The interpretation of the criteria of causality is a matter of judgment, and judges may disagree.

THE IMPACT OF A CAUSAL FACTOR

We now leave causes, and pass on to consider their *effects*. Our last topic is the measurement of *impact* on morbidity. Once we have decided that a factor is causal, there are several ways of expressing the magnitude of its influence on the occurrence of a disease in a given population or population group.

For example, we can say how much disease a given factor causes, expressed as a number of cases (the *attributable number*) or as an incidence or prevalence rate; if an incidence rate is used, this is the *attributable risk* or *excess risk.* Alternatively, we can say what *proportion* of the total incidence or prevalence can be attributed to this cause. This is the *attributable* or *etiologic fraction;* it may refer to the impact on the total population (the *population attributable fraction*) or only to the impact on people exposed to the causal factor—that is, the *attributable fraction* (*exposed*).

If the factor is a protective one (not a risk factor), we can speak of the amount of potential disease it *prevents*—that is, the *prevented fraction* in a total population or in people exposed to the factor. We can also speak of the *preventable fraction*—the proportion of the observed incidence that *could* be prevented by removal of a given risk factor or exposure to a given protective factor.

The exercises will use simple calculations only. Depending on what data are available, the calculation of measures of impact—and especially of their confidence intervals—may be more complicated (Note E11).

EXERCISE E11

Watch out for at least one "trick question" in this exercise.

Question E11–1

There is much evidence that prolonged standing is a cause of varicose veins. An association between standing and varicose veins is shown in Table E11–1, which is based on a population study (Abramson et al., 1981).

Using these data, what proportion of the varicose veins in men who work standing can you attribute to their standing? This is the attributable fraction (exposed). To calculate it, assume that if these men had not worked standing, their prevalence of varicose veins would have been 7.7% instead of 12.3%.

Table E11–1. Prevalence of Varicose Veins in Male Workers Aged 20–64 in Jerusalem, by Work Posture

Work Posture	Prevalence Rate %
Standing*	12.3
Other	7.7
Total	8.3

*For at least half the working time.

Question E11–2

What proportion of the varicose veins in this total male working population can be attributed to standing? This is the population attributable fraction. (Assume that if men had not worked standing, the rate would have been 7.7% instead of 8.3%.)

Question E11–3

Table E11–2 presents fictional data from a similar study in Epiville. (This is Epiville's swan song; farewell, Epiville.) Note that the exposure-specific rates of varicose veins are identical to those in Jerusalem.

Using the data in this table, calculate the attributable fraction (exposed) and the population-attributable fraction. Compare your answers with the figures for Jerusalem. How is the difference explained?

Question E11–4

In Table D7, we saw that the annual incidence of CHD was 5.9 per 1,000 in Paris policemen with varicose veins, and 2.9 per 1,000 in those without varicose veins. What proportion of the incidence of CHD in policemen with varicose veins can be attributed to their varicose veins?

Question E11–5

In Table D8, we saw that the annual mortality rate was 4.0% in cigarette-smoking men aged 65–74, and 2.4% in men who had never (or only occasionally) smoked. What proportion of the mortality in the smokers can be attributed to their smoking? (This is the attributable fraction in the exposed.) Do you have any reservations about your answer?

Question E11–6

Suppose that in Question E11–5 you were not told the rates, but only the relative risk in cigarette smokers, which was 1.67. Could you have calculated the attributable fraction in the exposed?

Table E11–2. Prevalence of Varicose Veins in Male Workers Aged 20–64 in Epiville, by Work Posture

Work Posture	Prevalence Rate %
Standing	12.3
Other	7.7
Total	9.7

Question E11–7

For what purposes may attributable fractions be used?

NOTE

E11. Basic measures of impact are explained in all epidemiology text-books. For statistical procedures, see Kahn and Sempos (1989, chap. 4) or Kleinbaum et al. (1982, chap. 9). There is considerable confusion about nomenclature, and you may encounter the same terms used differently.

Unit
E12

THE ATTRIBUTABLE FRACTION

A cause–effect relationship has been established between standing and varicose veins. The difference between the rates of varicose veins in men who stand when at work and those who do not can therefore be used as a measure of the impact of standing. We answer *Question E11–1* by assuming that the men who stood would have had a prevalence rate of 7.7% if they had not stood, instead of 12.3%. The difference, 4.6%, can be attributed to their standing. (If this were a difference between incidence rates, it could be called the attributable risk.) Expressed as a proportion of the total prevalence in men who stand at work, this is 4.6/12.3, or 37%. In other words, 37% of the prevalence of varicose veins among workers who stand can be attributed to their standing. This is the attributable or etiological fraction (exposed).

Similarly, the prevalence of varicose veins in the men as a whole would have been 7.7% if no one had stood when at work, instead of 8.3%. The population attributable fraction (*Question 11-2*) is therefore $(8.3 - 7.7)/8.3$, or 7%.

In Epiville (*Question 11–3*) the attributable fraction (exposed) is again 37%, but the population attributable fraction is now $(9.7 - 7.7)/9.7$, or 21%, which is considerably higher than in Jerusalem, despite the identical exposure-specific rates. The reason, of course, is that in Epiville more men worked standing. Clearly, a population attributable fraction depends not only on the exposure-specific rates, but on the prevalence of the causal factor in the population. It cannot be applied to populations other than the one in which it was calculated.

The attributable fraction is meaningful only if the factor is a causal one or can be regarded as a proxy for a closely correlated, causal, factor. *Question 11–4* therefore cannot be answered. (This is the trick question.)

In *Question 11–5* the proportion of the smokers' mortality attributable to their smoking is $(4.0 - 2.4)/4.0$, or 40%. The main reservation (and this applies to standing and varicose veins also) is that the difference

308

may be partly attributable to confounding factors. *This possibility should be kept in mind whenever attributable fractions are used* (although somehow it often remains unvoiced when they are used to convince decision-makers of the urgency of a problem).

The attributable fraction (exposed) can easily be calculated from the relative risk (RR). It is $(RR - 1)/RR$. In *Question 11–6*, it is $0.67/1.67$, or 40%.

The population attributable fraction can be calculated from the relative risk, provided that the relative risk was derived from a study of representative samples, and additional information is available (Note E12). If the risk is low, the odds ratio can replace the relative risk in these calculations.

In answer to *Question 11–7*, attributable fractions are of use mainly to those concerned with practical aspects of health care. The attributable fraction is based on the absolute difference between rates, and it measures the magnitude of the problem produced by a specific risk factor. The attributable fractions in the population and the exposed are easily understood measures, useful as a basis for determining priorities and for communicating epidemiological findings to nonepidemiologists.

EXERCISE E12

This exercise deals with prevented and preventable fractions.

Question E12–1

A follow-up study in a community in Jerusalem showed that the mortality attributable to hypertension was 23%. This was the population attributable fraction, based on a comparison of ten-year mortality in adults who had raised and normal blood pressures at the outset of the study (Goldbourt and Kark, 1982). Can we infer that this is also the preventable fraction in the population—that is, the proportion of deaths that would be prevented by appropriate intervention with respect to hypertension?

Question E12–2

So far we have considered *risk* factors. This question and the following ones deal with the impact of *protective* factors. Table E12 presents the results of a trial of a whooping cough vaccine performed in England in the 1940s, when this vaccine was still new. Children were randomly allocated to the "vaccinated" and "unvaccinated" groups, and were followed up for two to three years (Hill, 1962).

What proportion of the incidence was prevented, in children who

Table E12. Incidence of Whooping
Cough per 100 Child-Years

Group	Incidence Rate
Vaccinated	1.74
Unvaccinated	8.07

were vaccinated? This is the prevented fraction in the exposed (i.e., in those exposed to this protective factor).

Question E12–3

Fictional data: In England as a whole, the incidence of whooping cough at that time was 6 per 100 child-years. The use of the vaccine throughout the country was patchy, and the number of children who were vaccinated was unknown. Assume that the data in Table E12 refer to representative samples of the vaccinated and unvaccinated children in England. Using these figures, what was the impact of vaccination on incidence in the total child population? That is, what proportion of the potential incidence of whooping cough was prevented by vaccination? (This is the prevented fraction in the population.)

Question E12–4

Using the same figures, what proportion of the actual incidence of whooping cough in the child population would be prevented if all children were vaccinated? (This is the preventable fraction in the population.)

Question E12–5

What was the preventable fraction in unvaccinated children?

Question E12–6

As we have previously seen (Table E5–4), a randomized trial of treatment for mild hypertension in the elderly showed that the mortality rate per 1,000 person-years was 34 in the treated group and 47 in the control (placebo) group. On the basis of these figures, how efficacious was the treatment in preventing cardiovascular deaths? The P value was .037. Do you think your measure of efficacy has a wide or narrow confidence interval?

Question E12–7

For what purposes may prevented fractions be used?

Question E12–8

For what purposes may preventable fractions be used?

NOTE

E12.   The population attributable fraction can be estimated from the relative risk (RR) if we know the proportion (F) of the population exposed to the risk factor. The formula is $F(\text{RR} - 1)/[F(\text{RR} - 1) + 1]$. An alternative formula is $F'(\text{RR} - 1)/\text{RR}$, where F' is the proportion of *cases* who were exposed to the factor. If the risk is low, the odds ratio (OR) can replace RR in these formulae.

Unit
E13

PREVENTED AND PREVENTABLE
FRACTIONS

The attributable fraction is a ceiling estimate of the preventable fraction. To predict what fraction of the mortality can be prevented by controlling hypertension (*Question E12–1*), we also need to know how effectively hypertension can be controlled, and the influence of blood pressure reduction on mortality. We should also consider possible confounding effects: associated risk factors may partly account for the magnitude of the attributable fraction. We might conclude that the preventable fraction is appreciably less than the attributable fraction.

To estimate the prevented fraction in children exposed to vaccination (*Question E12–2*), we can assume that their incidence rate would have been 8.07% instead of 1.74%, if they had not been vaccinated. The difference (6.33%) can be attributed to the preventive effect of vaccination. The prevented fraction is therefore 6.33/8.07—that is, 78% of what the incidence would have been, had they not been vaccinated. This may be termed the *efficacy* of the vaccine, or the "percentage reduction." (Does it matter whether person-time or cumulative incidence rates are used in studies of vaccine efficacy? See Note E13–1.)

The incidence rate in the total child population (*Question E12–3*) would (hypothetically) have been 8.07 per 100 child-years (Table E12) if no children had been vaccinated. The actual incidence was 6%. The difference (2.07%) can be attributed to the preventive effect of vaccination. The prevented fraction in this population is therefore 2.07/8.07 = 26%.

If all children were vaccinated (*Question E12–4*), the expected incidence would be 1.74% (Table E12). In fact, it was 6%. The difference (4.26%) tells us what part of the actual incidence would have been prevented. Expressed as a proportion, the preventable fraction in the population is 4.26/6, or 71%.

The preventable fraction in unvaccinated children (*Question E12–5*) is

6.33/8.07, or 78%. This is of course the same as the prevented fraction in vaccinated children (Question E12–2).

In answer to *Question E12–6*, the prevented fraction in the exposed (treated) sample is a measure of the efficacy of treatment. It is (47 − 34)/47, or 28%. This can also be derived from the relative risk (RR): it is (1 − RR). The relative risk is 34/47 = 0.72, and 1 − 0.72 = 0.28. The "high" *P* value of .037 suggests a wide confidence interval, because the lower confidence limit cannot be far from zero; the 95% interval of the prevented fraction was in fact 1–46%.

In answer to *Question E12–7*, the prevented fraction in people exposed to a preventive procedure is, as we have seen, a measure of efficacy. It is an index commonly used when procedures are tested and compared, both for primary preventive procedures like vaccination and for therapeutic procedures that aim to prevent complications. The prevented fraction in the population measures the effectiveness of a preventive program. (What is the difference between "efficacy" and "effectiveness"? See Note E13–2.)

Preventable fractions (*Question E12–8*) provide both a guide and a stimulus to action. The preventable fraction in people exposed to a risk factor can be applied to individuals as well as to groups, to dramatize the likely effect of change or intervention: "If you stop smoking you will reduce your risk of so-and-so by such-and-such per cent." The preventable fraction in the population is of value to decision-makers who are planning health services, as it provides an estimate of the impact that intervention is likely to have on the public's health.

NOTES

E13–1.   Vaccines are commonly used for diseases with a high incidence. Person-time and cumulative incidence rates may therefore be dissimilar, and give different estimates of vaccine efficacy. Cumulative incidence rates are more appropriate if vaccination is believed to render a proportion of people completely immune (Smith et al., 1984).

E13–2.   "*Efficacy*" and "*effectiveness*" are often used synonymously, but are sometimes distinguished from each other. "Efficacy" often refers to the benefits when a procedure is applied as it "should" be, with full compliance by all concerned (as in a clinical trial subjected to "on randomized treatment" analysis); and "effectiveness," to the benefits at the population level, or among people to whom the procedure or service is offered. According to this usage, a program for the control of hypertension in a community would use drugs known to be efficacious; the program might or might not be effective.

Unit

E14

TEST YOURSELF (E)

- Explain the difference between

  experiments and surveys (E1).
  descriptive and analytic surveys (E1).
  cross-sectional, case-control, and cohort studies (E1).
  a retrospective and a prospective approach (E2).
  retrolective and prolective studies (Note E2).
  an attributable risk and an attributable fraction (E11).
  population attributable risk and attributable risk (exposed) (E11).
  efficacy and effectiveness (Note 13–2).

- Say whether a direct measure of risk can be provided by

  a cross-sectional study (E2).
  a case-control study (E3).

- State some of the possible biases of

  a cross-sectional study (E2).
  a case-control study (E3).
  a cohort study (E4).

- Explain what is meant by

  a group-based study (E1).
  a quasi-experiment (E1, E7).
  a nested case-control study (E3).
  randomization (E6).
  post-stratification (E6).
  a time series (E7).
  a historical prospective study (E8).
  meta-analysis (Note E9–2).
  time–response relationship (E10).

- Calculate

  an attributable fraction (exposed) from rates and from a relative risk (E12).
  a population attributable fraction (E12).
  a prevented fraction (exposed) from rates and from a relative risk (E13).

- State the main drawbacks of group-based studies (E5).

- Say to whom the following can be applied:

  the results of a clinical trial (E6).
  a population attributable fraction (E12).

- Explain the advantages of

  "blind" studies (E6).
  "intention-to-treat" analysis (E6).

- Explain how to use a case-control study to evaluate care (E7).

- Provide a list of

  ways of handling confounding (E9).
  criteria for the appraisal of causality (E10).

- State the uses of

  attributable fractions (E12).
  the prevented fraction (exposed) (E13).
  the preventable fraction (exposed) (E13).
  the preventable fraction (population) (E13).
  the prevented fraction (population) (E13).

- State the conditions for using the following to estimate the relative risk in a target population:

  an odds ratio from a case-control study (E3).
  a relative risk from a cohort study (E4).

Meta-Analysis: Putting It All Together

"That's the most important piece of evidence we've heard yet," said the King, rubbing his hands; "so now let the jury—"

"If any of them can explain it," said Alice, "I'll give him sixpence. I don't believe there's an atom of meaning in it."

"If there's no meaning in it," said the King, "that saves a world of trouble, you know, as we needn't try to find any."

(Carroll, 1865)

Unit
F1

INTRODUCTION

Meta-analysis refers to the critical review and integration of the findings of separate studies (Note F1). Its specific feature is the use of quantitative methods rather than reliance on judgment alone. This feature distinguishes it from most traditional literature reviews. The rapidly increasing volume of research, often with discrepant findings, has led to an increase in the need for and performance of meta-analyses.

This section has two main aims: to help you to adopt reasonable precautions when reviewing the results of a set of studies, by applying the basic principles that underlie good meta-analytic studies, and to help you to appraise published reports of meta-analyses and decide whether to use their results.

Some researchers prefer to speak of "overviews" of research rather than "meta-analysis."

EXERCISE F1

Question F1−1

Meta-analysis is commonly used to integrate the results of different trials of a specific treatment or other intervention (curative or preventive). Can you think of other kinds of study that might be subjected to meta-analysis?

Question F1−2

Table F1 displays the results of 23 randomized controlled trials of long-term treatment with beta-blockers after myocardial infarction (Yusuf et al., 1985). The rate ratios comparing the occurrence of deaths in the treatment and control groups show considerable variation, ranging from 0.56 (i.e., a death rate lower by 44% in the treatment group) to 1.54 (a

Table F1. Results of 23 Randomized Controlled Trials of the Long-Term Use of Beta-Blockers After Myocardial Infarction; Comparison of Deaths in Subjects Allocated to Treatment and Control Groups

Trial	Treatment Group No.	Treatment Group Deaths	Control Group No.	Control Group Deaths	Comparison of Fatality Rates (%) Ratio*	Comparison of Fatality Rates (%) Difference**	P
1	11	1	11	1	1.00	0.0	NS†
2	38	3	39	3	1.03	0.2	NS
3	59	4	52	6	0.59	−4.8	NS
4	69	5	93	11	0.61	−4.6	NS
5	114	7	116	14	0.51	−5.9	NS
6	154	25	147	31	0.77	−4.9	NS
7	151	8	154	6	1.36	1.4	NS
8	174	6	134	3	1.54	1.2	NS
9	251	28	122	12	1.13	1.3	NS
10	207	33	213	38	0.89	−1.9	NS
11	209	32	218	40	0.83	−3.0	NS
12	263	45	266	47	0.97	−0.6	NS
13	278	25	282	37	0.68	−4.1	NS
14	291	9	293	16	0.57	−2.4	NS
15	355	28	365	27	1.07	0.5	NS
16	391	27	364	43	0.58	−4.9	.02
17	632	60	471	48	0.93	−7.0	NS
18	680	22	674	39	0.56	−2.6	.02
19	873	64	583	52	0.82	−1.6	NS
20	858	57	883	45	1.30	1.5	NS
21	945	98	939	152	0.64	−5.8	.0002
22	1,533	102	1,520	127	0.80	−1.7	NS
23	1,916	138	1,921	188	0.77	−2.6	.004
Total	10,452	827	9,860	986	0.79	−2.1	.0000002

*Ratio of rate in treatment group to rate in control group.
**Rate in treatment group minus rate in control group.
†NS = not significant ($P \geq .05$).

death rate higher by 54% in the treatment group). What reasons can you suggest for this variation?

Question F1−3

When reviewing the results of a set of studies of the same topic, would you expect to find more differences between the results of randomized controlled trials, case-control studies, or cohort studies?

Question F1−4

What advantages might there be in drawing conclusions from a series of studies, rather than a single study?

NOTE

F1.   Quantitative methods of combining the results of studies were first
      described in the early 1930s. Interest grew in the 1970s, stimulated
      by the work of Glass (who coined the term "meta-analysis") and
      his colleagues (Glass et al., 1981). Meta-analyses in the health field
      began to appear in the 1970s, and started to flourish in the
      mid-1980s, largely because of the enthusiasm of Peto and his col-
      leagues at Oxford. For a compendious review of principles and
      methods, see Yusuf et al. (1987). Also, see Abramson (1990/91)
      ["pros and cons"], Boden (1992) ["has a tool become a weapon?"],
      T. C. Chalmers (1991) ["problems induced by meta-analysis"], Fel-
      son (1992) ["bias in meta-analytic reearch"], Goodman (1991)
      ["have you ever meta-analysis you didn't like?"], Jenicek (1989)
      ["where we are and where we want to go"], Naylor (1988) ["two
      cheers for meta-analysis"], Spitzer (1991) ["unanswered questions
      about aggregating data"], and Thompson and Pocock (1991) ["can
      meta-analyses be trusted?"]. Methods are described in detail by
      Petitti (1994); statistical methods are described by Hedges and
      Olkin (1985) and (for meta-analyses of nonexperimental studies) by
      Greenland (1987b).

Unit
F2

THE SCOPE OF META-ANALYSIS

In answer to *Question F1–1*, meta-analysis may in principle be applied to quantitative studies of any sort, including clinical trials and other experiments, quasi-experiments, and observational studies (e.g., cohort and case-control studies). Most meta-analyses deal with studies that aim to clarify causal associations; but meta-analysis may also be applied to studies of associations that are not necessarily causal (e.g., studies of risk markers) and to descriptive surveys (e.g., of the magnitude of a health problem). Meta-analysis may be applied to studies of screening or other diagnostic methods for use in individual or community health care (e.g., of their validity and reliability) or to studies of feasibility and cost, factors affecting the feasibility of interventions, and other topics.

Differences between the findings of separate studies (*Question F1–2*) may be due to chance, to differences in the design, execution or circumstances of the studies, or to differences between the people studied. This applies to both experimental and nonexperimental studies. Possible differences between controlled clinical trials include:

1. Differences in the criteria for inclusion in or exclusion from the trial, including differences in diagnostic criteria.
2. Differences in the baseline status of subjects, even if selection criteria are identical.
3. Differences in the manner of allocation to treatment and control groups (randomization or other methods).
4. Differences in the treatment under test, including differences in dosage and timing.
5. Differences in the management of controls (no treatment? placebos? other treatments?).
6. Differences in general management, including the diagnosis and treatment of other conditions, supportive care, responses to complications, etc.

7. Differences in outcome measures (e.g., due to differences in criteria).
8. Differences in follow-up times.
9. Variations in analysis—for example, the use of "intention to treat" or "on randomized treatment" analysis (see *Question E5–7*).
10. Differences in the quality of the study's design or execution—for example, in the precautions taken to avoid bias (e.g., the use of blind methods), in the criteria for withdrawing a subject from the allocated group or from the trial, in the efforts made to trace lost subjects, and in attention to the accuracy of measurements.

The trials listed in Table F1 used different drugs, doses, and exclusion criteria, and they differed in the time at which treatment was started and the duration of treatment and follow-up, which ranged from six weeks to four years.

In answer to *Question F1–3*, randomized control trials and cohort studies are less likely to yield divergent results than case-control studies. The use of randomized controls minimizes the likelihood of confounding, since the only differences in the initial status of the groups compared are those that occur by chance. Divergent results are more likely in nonexperimental studies (or nonrandomized trials or quasi-experiments), where it may be difficult to prevent or adequately control for differences between the groups compared. The possible biases in case-control studies—especially those resulting from an inappropriate selection of controls and from recall bias, exposure suspicion bias, and other forms of information bias (Unit E3)—are in general more difficult to avoid or control than the biases in cohort studies, especially if the cohort studies compare subgroups of the same population.

Possible advantages in drawing conclusions from a series of studies rather than a single study (*Question F1–4*) include the following:

1. If the studies have similar results, this consistency will reinforce the validity of whatever inferences are drawn.
2. Individual studies may be too small to yield statistical significance, especially if the effect is a weak one, but this may be overcome if the results of several studies are combined. As an example, increased infection rates (generally sepsis or pneumonia) were reported in seven randomized control trials of total parenteral (i.e., intravenous) nutrition in cancer patients undergoing chemotherapy, but in no trial was the effect statistically significant; but the combined results showed that the hazard was appreciable: there was a highly significant ($P < .0001$) fourfold increase in the odds in favor of developing infection (Klein et al., 1986).
3. If the findings are similar, combining them will provide better estimates of the effect of an intervention or the strength of other associa-

tions studied. Larger numbers will result in narrower confidence intervals.

4. Consideration of a series of studies may reveal that a result observed in an isolated study is an artifact or chance finding.
5. If there are differences between the findings, inquiry into the reasons for these differences may lead to new knowledge or the formulation of new hypotheses.
6. It may be possible to compare the effects of various interventions (applied in different studies).
7. It may be possible to compare various effects (examined in different studies) of an intervention.

EXERCISE F2

Question F2–1

This question deals with techniques of combining the results of separate studies. Suppose that we wish to use the findings shown in Table F1 as a basis for an overall conclusion about the value of the treatment tested in these trials, and that this is a reasonable thing to do. (In a later unit we consider the precautions that should be taken before results are combined.) What do you think of the following summary statements? What are the main advantages or disadvantages of the techniques used?

1. Altogether there were 827 deaths among the 10,452 subjects in the treatment groups (fatality rate, 7.9%) and 986 among the 9,860 controls (fatality rate, 10.0%). The pooled data thus show a rate ratio of 0.79 and a rate difference of -2.1%. A simple chi-square test shows that the difference between the pooled treatment and control groups is highly significant ($P = .0000002$). Before saying what you think of this method of analysis, look at the fictional data in Table F2.
2. Of the 23 trials, 16 showed a favorable effect (rate ratio less than 1

Table F2. Results of Two Randomized Controlled Trials of the Effectiveness of Fresh Water in the Prevention of Deaths Among Shipwreck Victims: Fictional Data

Trial	Treatment Group			Control Group			Rate Ratio
	No.	Deaths	Rate	No.	Deaths	Rate	
A	50	10	20%	80	32	40%	0.5
B	450	45	10%	80	16	20%	0.5
Total	500	55	11%	160	48	30%	0.37

and rate difference less than zero) and 7 did not. This difference points to the value of the treatment.

3. Of the 23 trials, 16 showed a favorable effect and 7 did not. A chi-square goodness-of-fit test shows no significant difference ($P = .06$) between this distribution (16 and 7) and the 50:50 distribution that might be expected by chance. (If you do not know what a goodness-of-fit test is, see Note 2–1.) The effect of the treatment is thus not statistically significant. Can we conclude that the treatment does not reduce the risk of dying?

4. Significance was tested by computing an overall P value from the 23 separate P values (for simplicity, most of these are not specified in the table). Several methods are available for this purpose (see Note F2–2). The overall P value was .0000005, showing that the difference in fatality between the treatment and control groups is highly significant.

5. Significance was tested by the Mantel–Haenszel chi-square test, which controls for effects connected with a stratifying variable (see Unit D13). The 23 trials were treated as separate strata; the data used were the numbers who died and survived in the treatment and control groups in each trial. The P value was .0000002.

6. The mean value of the rate ratio, computed by summing the 23 rate ratios and dividing by 23, was 0.87. This suggests that treatment prevented 13% of deaths.

7. The mean difference between rates, computed by summing the 23 differences and dividing by 23, was −2.3 per 100. On average the fatality rate was thus lower in the treatment group.

8. Using the Mantel–Haenszel procedure for stratified data (see Unit D13) the point estimate of the common rate ratio was 0.79, with a 99% confidence interval of 0.70 to 0.89. This procedure treats each trial as a separate stratum, as in the Mantel–Haenszel chi-square test, and the findings in the strata are combined, giving an appropriate weight to each stratum (greater weight is given to findings that have narrower confidence intervals). These results indicate that in general, allocation to a treatment group reduces the chance of dying by about 21%, and this reduction can be estimated with 99% confidence to lie between 11% and 30%. (Is 21% the prevented or preventable fraction? See Note F2–3.)

9. By the Mantel–Haenszel procedure, the point estimate of the common difference between the fatality rates in treatment and control groups was −2.1 per 100, with a 99% confidence interval of −1.1 to −3.1 per 100. When might the rate difference be preferable to the rate ratio as a measure of the effect of treatment?

10. The Mantel–Haenszel odds ratio expressing the difference in fatality between the treatment and control groups was 0.77, with a 99% confidence interval of 0.68 to 0.88. Which is preferable—the rate

ratio or the odds ratio? In a similar meta-analysis based on studies of mixed types (trials, cohort studies, and case-control studies) which would be a preferable measure—the rate ratio or the odds ratio?

Question F2–2

What importance may effect modification have in this meta-analysis? May confounding have any relevance?

Question F2–3

Data on nonfatal recurrences of myocardial infarction were available for 19 of the 23 trials listed in Table F1. The Mantel–Haenszel rate ratio, based on these 19 trials, was 0.75 (99% confidence interval, 0.65 to 0.87). The corresponding rate ratio for fatality was 0.79 (99% confidence interval, 0.70 to 0.89). Can it be concluded that treatment prevented nonfatal recurrences about as well as it prevented deaths? Or do you want other information before deciding?

NOTES

F2–1. Goodness-of-fit tests assess the agreement between an observed distribution and a specified expected distribution. A significant result means that the null hypothesis (of a good fit) can be rejected. The closer the agreement with the expected distribution (i.e., the better the fit), the higher the P value. See Siegel and Castellan (1988) pp. 45–55.

F2–2. Various methods of combining P values from independent tests of essentially the same hypothesis are described by DeMets (1987), Hedges and Olkin (1985, chap. 3), and Wolf (1986). Some use the P values, others use the corresponding normal deviates (Z values). In the present instance, the Z values were used (Stouffer et al., 1949), after weighting them by the square root of the sample size (the total number of subjects), a method that may give results close to those of the Mantel–Haenszel and similar tests (Canner, 1987); but there is no agreement on whether weighting should be used or what weights are best. These methods are not always valid; the main condition is that the P values must be one-tailed (Unit D4), and must test the same direction of effect (two-tailed P values should first be halved; if the observed effect in a specific test is opposite to that of the study hypothesis, the halved value should be subtracted from 1); in the present instance the combined one-tailed P was computed and then doubled to yield a two-tailed P.

F2–3. Both! On the assumption that the difference in fatality is attributable to treatment, 21% is the prevented fraction among those exposed to treatment, whose fatality rate is 79% of what it would have been had they not been exposed to treatment. It is also the preventable fraction among those not exposed to treatment, whose deaths would be reduced by 21% if they were exposed to treatment. (See Unit E12.)

U n i t
F3

MEASURES USED IN META-ANALYSIS

In *Question F2–1* the aim is to bring together the results of 23 trials, on the assumption that it is legitimate to do this. Statement (1) is based on simple pooling of the 23 sets of basic data; the numbers are lumped together, as if only one large study had been done, and differences in study design and execution are ignored. This is inadvisable. Not only may the results of large studies overwhelm the results of small ones, but the overall results may be distorted, as clearly shown in Table F2, where the two trials differ in the relative sizes of their treatment and control groups. It is preferable to use techniques that treat each trial as a separate stratum, by comparing each treatment group with its own control group, and then bringing together the stratified findings. This is essentially what is done in statements (2) to (10).

Statements (2) and (3) are based on what has been called "vote counting" (how many in favor? how many against?). Its main drawback is that equal weight is given to each study, however small, so that the conclusions may be misleading. The significance test used in statement (3) has an extremely low power, since it is based on only 23 trials. A significant result might be meaningful, but is hard to achieve (the test has a low power); in this instance it would be attained ($P < .05$) only if at least 17 of the 23 trials showed favorable effects. "Not significant" means only that chance processes might easily account for the observed results, and not that they do; the verdict is "not proven," not "disproved."

Combining the P values, as in statement (4), is an appropriate method, although not often used. Its advantages are that it can be applied to P values based on different kinds of significance tests, and that it is feasible even if only the P values are available, without the basic data on which they were based. It is used much less often than the Mantel–Haenszel test utilized in statement (5) or similar tests for stratified data. Both methods are appropriate, and the difference between the P values—.0000005 versus .0000002—is of course negligible. But significance tests alone are of course of limited value, since they tell us nothing about the strength of the association or its confidence interval.

Calculating an average rate ratio in the way described in statement (6) is not permissible. Imagine two trials: Trial A has fatality rates of 4% and 16% in its treatment and control groups (ratio = 0.25), and trial B has the reverse findings—fatality rates of 16% and 4% respectively (ratio = 4). The mean treated/control group rate ratio is (0.25 + 4) / 2, or 2.125; that is, on average the fatality rate is over twice as high in the treatment group. (Verdict: Shun the treatment like the plague). Now leave the findings unchanged, but instead of the treated/control group rate ratio, use the controls/treated rate ratio; in trial A this is 4, and in trial B it is 0.25. The mean rate ratio is again 2.125, but this time the fatality rate is over twice as high in the control group. (Verdict: Welcome the treatment with open arms). The method is obviously faulty; rate ratios (like percentages) cannot be averaged unless they are based on the same denominators.

On the other hand, it is permissible to take an average of rate differences, as in statement (7). But simple averaging gives every trial the same weight, so that small studies have an unduly large effect on the average.

The Mantel–Haenszel procedure, used in statements (8), (9), and (10), brings together the results of the various studies so as to estimate a common rate ratio, rate difference, or odds ratio. This is one of several techniques available for this purpose (see Note F3–1). Each study is treated as a separate stratum (which, in a meta-analysis of trials, means that the treatment group in each trial is compared only with the control group in the same trial), and the findings in the strata are combined, giving an appropriate weight to each stratum. The assumption is that there is in fact a uniform effect, each study providing a different estimate of this effect (this is called the *fixed-effect model*); the results are valid if this is a reasonable assumption. Alternative methods are available for use in meta-analyses where this assumption is questionable; they will be dealt with in Unit F8.

The rate difference (statement 9) might be used in preference to (or as well as) the rate ratio if we wanted to estimate the absolute number of deaths that the treatment might prevent (see Unit A3).

Both the rate ratio and the odds ratio (statement 10) are satisfactory measures (see Unit B11), but the rate ratio is easier to understand and explain. Case-control studies do not provide direct measures of relative risk, and a meta-analysis including case-control studies would necessarily use the odds ratio.

Effect modification may of course be important in any meta-analysis of studies of an association (*Question F2–2*). In a meta-analysis of clinical trials, the distinctive features of each trial may modify the association between treatment and outcome observed in the trial, resulting in differences between the results of the trials. The uniform measure estimated by the Mantel–Haenszel or similar procedures may not be very meaningful if modifying effects are marked. In such instances, the factors that affect the association may be of more interest than estimation of an imaginary uniform measure. If we are interested only in knowing whether there is a significant association (the null hypothesis being that there is no effect in any of the studies), effect modification has no importance.

Confounding may be of relevance in two contexts. First, the results of the individual studies may be distorted by confounding. This is relatively unlikely in a meta-analysis of randomized controlled trials; but even in such trials, differences between cases and controls (e.g., in the severity of the disease or in other prognostic factors), possibly caused by randomization errors, may distort the results. Second, there may be distortion (as shown in Table F2) when the results are combined, as a consequence of imbalances between the sizes of the treatment and control groups. The Mantel–Haenszel and similar procedures guard against this latter kind of confounding.

Because of the differences between trials, the results of a meta-analysis obviously depend on which trials it covers. The exclusion of four trials from the meta-analysis of nonfatal recurrences (*Question F2–3*) may influence the findings, and this possibility should be explored. Do the missing trials differ in any obvious way from the others? If so, a comparison of the rate ratio with the corresponding rate ratio for fatality, based on all 23 trials, may be misleading. The simplest approach is to perform a meta-analysis of fatality in the 19 trials covered by the meta-analysis of recurrences, and then compare the results. The rate ratio for fatality in these 19 trials is in fact 0.79 (95% confidence interval, 0.70 to 0.80), confirming that treatment prevented nonfatal recurrences about as well as it prevented deaths.

The measures of association used in Unit F2 are obviously not the only ones available, and they are not always appropriate. Use is often made of what is called the *effect size*. This is generally defined as the difference between the mean values in the two groups compared, divided by the standard deviation in the control group; a result of two means that the magnitude of the difference is two standard deviations. The effect sizes in the various trials may then be averaged, for use as an overall measure. The mean effect size can be made more meaningful by looking it up in a table of the normal distribution and translating it to a statement that the average member of one group has a higher value (or a lower value, depending on how the difference was calculated) than a specific proportion of the members of the other group (see Note F3–2). The mean effect size is used in the next three questions. Assume that the necessary precautions were taken before the results were combined.

EXERCISE F3

Question F3–1

Eleven controlled trials of the psychological treatment of asthma all showed a favorable effect. The trials used various outcome measures; these included lung function (the peak expiratory flow), the number of asthma attacks, the amount of medication required, the number of emergency room visits, and so on. The average effect size was 0.86 (Glass et al., 1981); according to a table of the normal distribution, this result indicates that the average patient in a treatment group had a better outcome than did 81% of controls. The mean effect size was significantly greater than zero. What advantages of using the effect size does this example illustrate? Can you think of any disadvantages?

Question F3–2

The results of a meta-analysis of controlled trials of patient education for people with chronic medical problems are summarized in Table F3–1. The outcomes that were measured were compliance with medical advice, physiological progress toward therapeutic goals, and long-term health outcomes. The trials did not use the same outcome measures. Therapeutic progress, for example, was appraised in only 13 trials, and it was measured by changes in blood pressure, body weight, or other characteristics; the long-term outcome was measured in terms of return to work, hospitalization, and so on. The mean effect sizes pointed to a much greater effect on compliance than on therapeutic progress, and a relatively small long-term effect. What advantage of using mean effect sizes is illustrated by this example? What obvious possible source of bias do you see in this study, and how could it be explored?

Table F3–1. Meta-Analysis of 27 Controlled Trials
of Patient Education

Outcome	No. of Studies	Mean Effect Size
Compliance	18	0.67**
Therapeutic progress	13	0.13**
Long-term outcome	5	0.06*

*Significantly greater than zero ($P < .05$).
**Significantly greater than zero ($P < .01$).
From Mazzucca (1983).

Question F3–3

In both the above meta-analyses, there were often two or more outcome measures in the same trial, and these were included when the effect sizes were averaged. In the meta-analysis of patient education, for example, the result in the five trials with data on the long-term outcome is the average of 11 estimates of effect size (1–4 per trial). How may the inclusion of a variable number of outcome measures per trial affect the findings?

Question F3–4

This question deals with a meta-analysis of descriptive surveys. Information on various symptoms was collected in two surveys in California. The samples comprised all adults residing in two small neighborhoods, which had no nearby hazardous waste disposal sites; the populations had very different demographic characteristics. The questions were almost identical, and were administered by interviewers. Table F3–2 shows the prevalence of selected symptoms in women in each survey and in the pooled data. The authors of the meta-analysis suggest that the pooled results might be used as reference (control) rates in studies of communities exposed to suspected environmental hazards. What do you think of this? What precautions would you suggest?

Table F3–2. Prevalence Rates (%) of Four Symptoms
in Women in Two Surveys in California

Symptom	Survey 1 (n = 234)	Survey 2 (n = 170)	Pooled Data (n = 404)
Skin irritation	15.0	11.2	13.4
Eye irritation	30.0	25.3	28.0
Sleep disturbance	15.8	17.2	16.5
Fatigue	15.9	18.9	17.4

From Lipscomb et al. (1992); figures modified slightly.

Question F3–5

In the same meta-analysis, associations between the symptoms and other variables were examined by pooling the data of the two surveys and then performing multiple logistic regression analyses. The variables in the logistic regression model included age, sex, race, education, smoking status, and "study" (i.e., whether the person was included in survey 1 or survey 2). As an example of the findings, Caucasians reported more fatigue than Asians (odds ratio, 2.7), Hispanics (odds ratio,

1.5), or other race groups (odds ratio, 2.3); the difference from Asians was statistically significant. Would it have been better to examine the associations between symptoms and other variables by using the Mantel–Haenszel procedure, treating each survey as a separate stratum? Or are there advantages to the use of multiple logistic regression?

Question F3–6

Enough of statistics for now; quantitative methods are the key feature of meta-analysis, but are not its main problem. This question serves as an introduction to basic principles and predicaments.

The following meta-analysis, dealing with the effect of treating hypertension on coronary mortality, was skimpily described in three sentences in the middle of a narrative review in 1976:

Most trials have shown little or no effect on the incidence of coronary complications. The combined results of a number of studies [9 references] indicate that the risk of coronary mortality among treated hypertensives is about 0.7 times that among the untreated cases; this is a weighted average [using the Mantel–Haenszel procedure] of the relative risks in these trials. Since [this does] not differ significantly from unity ($P = .18$) an effect . . . must be regarded as "not proven," although it cannot be ruled out. (Abramson and Hopp 1976).

What additional information would you like, in order to be convinced that the result is not an artifact attributable to flawed methods? Do not go into detail, but try to list the most important questions.

NOTES

F3–1. See Note D13–1 for references to the Mantel–Haenszel, precision-based, and maximum-likelihood methods. In these and other commonly used procedures for estimating a common measure of association, larger numbers increase the weight assigned to a stratum. Unless numbers are small, the procedures generally provide fairly similar results; for numerical examples, see Kahn and Sempos (1989, chap. 9). One technique frequently used in meta-analyses, the "O minus E" method (Peto, 1987b) is particularly simple; but it may give misleading results if the association is strong and the groups compared are very different in size (Greenland and Salvan, 1990).

F3–2. Since the effect size is expressed in terms of standard deviations (this is what is sometimes called a "Z score"), it can be made more meaningful by referring to a table showing the area in the tail of the normal distribution. Suppose the mean effect size in a meta-analysis of trials is 0.86. The value shown for $Z = 0.86$ in Table A1 of Armitage and Berry (1987) is 0.1949, indicating that the average patient in a treatment group has a better result than 80.51% of controls. If no table is handy, this percentage can be fairly accurately calculated by the formula $49.32 + 45.23es - 10.56es^2$, where es is an effect size between 0.1 and 2; for an effect size of 0.86, the calculated result is 80.41. This way of expressing the results is of course valid only if the variable has a normal or near-normal distribution.

Unit
F4

MEASURES USED IN META-ANALYSIS
(CONTINUED)

Each of the effect sizes used in a meta-analysis is based on a comparison of groups (e.g., treatment and control groups) in the same study. The effect sizes can be weighted before averaging, giving more weight to larger studies (Hedges and Olkin, 1985), although in this instance (*Question F3–1*) the same weight was given to every study.

A special advantage illustrated in *Question F3–1* arises from the fact that the effect size is "unitless"—that is, it is expressed in terms of standard deviations (of whatever variable is measured) rather than in terms of number of attacks, number of visits, and so on. This permits the calculation of average effect sizes based on various dependent variables, in meta-analyses where the latter can be regarded as indicators of a general effect.

This may be misleading, however, if the effect sizes are different for different dependent variables. Moreover, a measure based on standard deviations has little meaning in terms of health implications, and a change of 0.86 standard deviations in one variable may not have the same importance as a change of 0.86 standard deviations in another. This problem remains if the effect measures are interpreted in terms of the normal distribution (as explained in Note F3–2): The statement that the average member of a treatment group has a better result than 84% of controls may have a different health relevance for one variable than for another. Unless logic or necessity dictates otherwise, it may be preferable to conduct a separate meta-analysis for each dependent variable.

Even if effect sizes based on a single outcome variable (such as peak expiratory flow) are used, their magnitude depends on the standard deviations in the studies, which may vary because of population differences or for other reasons. Effect sizes should therefore be used with circumspection; some experts deprecate their use (Greenland, 1987).

As illustrated in *Question F3–2*, the unitlessness of effect sizes also permits comparisons of different kinds of outcome. Here too there may be a problem of interpretation, as there is no simple way of comparing the importance (in terms of health relevance) of one standard deviation of different outcome measures.

Also, a comparison of mean effect sizes based on different sets of trials may be misleading. The differences in mean effect sizes shown in Table F3–1 may be partly or wholly due to differences (e.g., in the mode of education or in the nature of the medical problem) between the trials included in the three sets. This problem may be approached by comparing the descriptions of the trials in the three sets, and/or by comparing mean effect sizes (for each pair of outcomes) based on the same trials, if there is enough overlap to permit this.

If different trials contribute different numbers of outcome measures to the calculation of a mean effect size (*Question F3–3*), trials with more outcome measures may have an undue influence on the mean. If they differ from other trials, this may produce a bias. In the study of patient education, trials of behavioral (rather than didactic) educational methods tended to have more "compliance" than "therapeutic progress" or "long-term outcome" measures per study. As a result, over two-thirds of the effect sizes in the "compliance" set were based on behavioral methods, as compared with half of the effect sizes in the other two sets—a difference that may have contributed to the contrast seen in Table F3–1.

When prevalence findings are combined by simple pooling (*Question F3–4*), the weight given to each study is determined by the size of the sample studied; the "pooled" prevalence rate is therefore to some extent arbitrary, since it reflects the relative sizes of the study samples. A more important consideration—and this applies to any meta-analysis of descriptive studies of characteristics whose frequency varies—is that generalizations to other populations may be of uncertain validity, whatever technique of combination is used. Unless the studies were performed in samples that represent a total population, generalizations to a total population may be debatable. The authors of this meta-analysis advise caution in applying the pooled results to populations that differ demographically from the populations studied. They also warn that the results should be compared only if the questions are identical and are administered by interviewers; in a third survey, which used self-administered questionnaires asking the same questions, symptom rates were two- to fivefold higher.

In answer to *Question F3–5*, there is no compelling reason to prefer the Mantel–Haenszel procedure to multiple logistic regression in this analysis. Both methods can control for confounding, and the inclusion of "study" as an independent variable in the logistic regression model serves the same purpose as handling the studies as separate strata in the Mantel–Haenszel procedure. The two methods generally yield very similar odds ratios; if these differ, the Mantel–Haenszel value is probably preferable because it does not depend on the validity of the logistic model (Kahn and Sempos, 1989). In a meta-analysis of randomized controlled trials, where it is to be hoped that most confounders are taken care of by the randomization, the Mantel–Haenszel procedure has the advantage that it can be used even without a computer. But this procedure is awkward in studies where there are many uncontrolled potential confounders, so that elaborate substratification (e.g., by study, age, sex, race, and education, etc.) is required. It is also awkward if the independent variable has more than two categories, since a separate analysis is required for each comparison (Caucasians vs. Asians, Caucasians vs. Hispanics, etc.). Multiple logistic regression also has the advantages that it permits the simultaneous study of several independent variables and the exploration of interactions (effect modification), and provides a risk-predicting equation (see Unit D–15).

Linear regression methods may also be used in meta-analyses, sometimes using "meta-regression" techniques based on weighting of the study results (see Note F4).

BASIC INFORMATION

In reply to *Question F3–6*, every meta-analysis should include the answers to at least the following basic questions:

1. How were the studies found? There is a possibility of bias if the meta-analysis does not include all relevant studies.
2. How were studies selected for inclusion? (What were the inclusion and/or exclusion criteria?)
3. What are the distinctive features of the studies, with respect to their design, execution, study populations, and other characteristics, and are these features sufficiently similar to justify combining the studies' results?
4. How well were the studies designed and executed?
5. What are the results of the studies, and are the results consistent enough to justify combining them?

EXERCISE F4

How to find studies, and how to select studies for the meta-analysis— these are the topics of this exercise and the next.

Question F4–1

A meta-analysis obviously requires a systematic search of the literature, using (for example) *Index Medicus*, *Current Contents*, or a computerized data-base. To test the validity of computer methods, randomized controlled trials in liver disease during a 17-year period were first sought manually in 34 selected journals, and then a MEDLARS computer search was conducted (Poynard and Conn, 1985). Can you guess what proportion of the trials identified in the journals were found by the computer search? Can you suggest any other ways of finding published studies? What method would you recommend?

Question F4–2

Do you think that the omission of unpublished studies may bias the results of a meta-analysis? If so, what would you expect the direction of the bias to be?

Question F4–3

Should unpublished studies be sought and included? If not, why not?

Question F4–4

How can the results of unpublished studies be sought?

Question F4–5

Can you suggest a way of assessing how important the omission of unidentified unpublished studies may be, with respect to a specific meta-analysis? This is a difficult question. Clue: See statement (4) in *Question F2–1*.

NOTE

F4.   "Meta-regression," in which each study's result is "precision-weighted" by multiplying it by the reciprocal of its variance, is described by Greenland (1987b).

Unit
F5

FINDING THE STUDIES

In the test described in *Question F4–1*; the manual search of the 34 journals revealed 208 randomized controlled trials; only 51% of these were found by the MEDLARS search. The manual search found 244 trials in all, including 36 mentioned in reference lists but published elsewhere; the MEDLARS search of 3,686 journals led to the identification of 154 (63%) of the 244, and missed 90 (37%); it found an additional 35 trials published elsewhere. Clearly, reliance should not be placed on any single method of searching the literature, and use of a combination of methods is recommended. In the meta-analysis of trials of beta blockers (Table F1), a systematic literature search for published studies (including those listed in conference abstracts) was supplemented by an informal search for studies known to the investigators and their colleagues, and perusal of reference lists in the reports found. The meta-analysis of trials of patient education (Table F3–1) used a MEDLARS search plus two annotated bibliographies on the subject.

There is much evidence for publication bias in the health field. In general (*Question F4–2*) it is the negative or inconclusive studies that are rejected or remain "tucked away in file drawers." In Oxford, for example, a survey of 487 clinical research projects approved in 1984–87 showed that the odds in favor of publication by 1990 were over twice as high if the results were statistically significant (Easterbrook et al., 1991). Omission of unpublished studies from a meta-analysis may thus be expected to bias the results by making overall effects stronger and exaggerating their statistical significance. Bias in the opposite direction has also been occasionally reported, with smaller effects found in published studies; studies that contradict conventional wisdom may be less likely to appear in print, even if they show strong effects, unless they are especially newsworthy. In principle, unpublished studies should be included if possible, to avoid bias in any direction (*Question F4–3*), although some investigators oppose this on the grounds that unreported studies are likely to be of poor quality; surprisingly, however, follow-up studies of medical researches have shown no independent relationship between the quality of research design and the likelihood of publication (Chalmers et al., 1990, Easterbrook et al., 1991).

Unpublished studies may be sought in several ways (*Question F4–4*). In the beta-blocker meta-analysis, the investigators interrogated colleagues. Other methods include the scanning of conference proceedings and lists of dissertations, and contacts with funding organizations. Emphasis has recently been placed on registers of clinical trials; in one instance, where there was a relatively complete register for comparison, a MEDLINE search revealed only 28 of 96 known trials (Dickersin et al., 1985). If unpublished studies are identified, it becomes necessary to ask the investigators for information on their methods and results.

An easy way of handling possible bias due to the omission of unidentified studies (*Question F4–5*) is to take the "worst-case" view that these are all "null studies" (that show no association whatever between the variables studied), and calculate how many such studies (the "fail-safe *N*") would be needed to change the observed overall *P* value to a nonsignificant level or reduce the observed overall effect to a trivial value (Note F5). In the beta-blocker meta-analysis (Table F1), the number of null studies required to push the observed overall *P* value (.0000005) up to .05 turns out to be 108. Since is it is very unlikely that there are 108 unreported null randomized controlled trials of beta-blockers, the possibility that the finding is attributable to this source of bias can be disregarded. By contrast, the fail-safe *N* was only 2 in a meta-analysis of trials of total parenteral nutrition in cancer patients undergoing surgery, which showed a significant reduction in operative mortality (Klein et al., 1986).

EXERCISE F5

Question F5–1

A MEDLARS search, together with screening of *Current Contents*, review articles and reference lists, revealed 12 controlled trials showing the effect of vitamin A supplements on child mortality. Four of the trials were conducted in hospitals, and dealt with children with measles. Eight were community-based trials in which children living in different villages, districts, or households were assigned to treatment or control groups (Fawzi et al., 1993). Can all 12 trials be included in a meta-analysis?

Question F5–2

A meta-analysis of studies of age trends in the prevalence of senile dementia was limited to studies conducted since 1980 (Ritchie et al.,

1992). It was also restricted to studies of moderate and severe (not mild) dementia. Can you suggest reasons for these limitations?

Question F5–3

Can you suggest why old studies might be excluded from a meta-analysis of clinical trials?

Question F5–4

The selection of studies for a meta-analysis obviously influences the results; a biased selection may lead to biased results. Assuming that an appropriate search has been conducted, can you suggest what precautions should then be taken to make the selection of studies as objective as possible?

Question F5–5

It is plainly advisable that findings that are to be combined in a meta-analysis should be independent of each other. If two papers report the same study (one of them perhaps including additional cases and controls), it is obviously wrong to include both in the meta-analysis. But what should be done if one paper reports the results of a short-term follow-up and a later paper describes a long-term follow-up of the same subjects; should both papers be included? What should be done if the short-term and long-term results are reported in the same publication; should both sets of findings be included?

Question F5–6

Controlled trials of work-site smoking cessation programs were identified by searches of MEDLINE and 11 other literature data bases, an index of theses and dissertations, and reports of meetings of two associations, and by contacts with other investigators (Fisher et al., 1990). Twenty trials were found; Since some programs were conducted in 2–4 different treatment groups (e.g., in different companies), 34 experimental–control comparisons were available. The outcome variable was the long-term quit rate—that is, the proportion (of smokers who were exposed to the program) who quit smoking, as measured 12 months later. The 34 effect sizes were calculated and averaged, after weighting them by a method that gives more weight to larger samples. A weak mean effect size of 0.21 (95% confidence interval, 0.16 to 0.26) was found, indicating that (by the method described in Note F3–2) the average smoker who was exposed to a program had a better result (i.e., was more likely to quit) than about 56–60% of smokers who were not $P <$ .01). How may the inclusion of all 34 comparisons affect the mean effect size? What solutions can you suggest?

Question F5-7

A MEDLINE search was performed for controlled clinical studies of acupuncture for chronic pain, supplemented by screening of *Excerpta Medica*, the *Journal of Traditional Chinese Medicine*, and bulletins from a documentation service for alternative medicine, as well as correspondence with and visits to colleagues. The search revealed 71 reports that met the following criteria: (1) Needles were used; studies in which only surface electrodes or laser acupuncture were used were excluded; (2) the word "chronic" was mentioned in the title or abstract, or the duration of pain was stated to be at least six months; (3) a reference (control) group was used, which was exposed to another treatment or sham treatment (placebo). Some reports were excluded because they turned out not to deal with chronic pain or because they replicated descriptions of the same studies or patients, and one because it was totally uninterpretable. This left 51 studies for analysis. Can you suggest why the above three criteria were used?

Question F5-8

The 51 trials of acupuncture were of uneven quality, as shown in Table F5; only six were randomized and double-blind. Should some of the studies be excluded from the meta-analysis? What arguments might be

Table F5. Methods Used in 51 Controlled Trials of Acupuncture

	Blind?		
Randomized?	*Patients*	*Evaluator*	*Number of Trials*
Yes	Yes	Yes	6
Yes	?*	Yes	3
Yes	No	Yes	7
Yes	Yes	No	1
Yes	?	?	3
Yes	?	No	1
Yes	No	?	2
Yes	No	No	11
?	?	?	1
?	No	Yes	1
?	No	No	4
No	Yes	Yes	1
No	?	?	1
No	No	Yes	2
No	No	No	7

*? = maybe; the study report is unclear.
From Ter Riet et al. (1990).

offered in favor of including studies that are not of the best quality in a meta-analysis?

NOTE

F5.   Formulae for the fail-safe N (if the meta-analysis yields a significant effect) are provided by Rosenthal (1979), Orwin (1983), Klein et al. (1986), and Wolf (1986). More elaborate statistical approaches are considered by Iyengar and Greenhouse (1988) and discussants of their paper.

Unit
F6

SELECTING STUDIES

The inclusion or exclusion of a study should be determined, in the first instance, by the objective of the meta-analysis. If the question asked is a general one, broad selection criteria may be used; if it is a more specific one—for example, what is the effect of a particular drug on a particular outcome with respect to a particular disease in a particular kind of patient?—stricter criteria must be used.

The answer to *Question F5–1* thus depends on what we want to learn from the meta-analysis. If the question of interest is the value of vitamin A in the treatment of children with measles, the first four trials should be selected. If interest lies in the prophylactic administration of vitamin A supplements to children living in the community, the eight community-based trials should be selected. If both these questions are of interest, both sets of trials can be included in the meta-analysis, but they should be analyzed separately; this might also permit comparison of its value in the two situations. And if the question asked is a general one—can vitamin A supplements reduce child mortality? (without reference to any specific situation)—all 12 trials can legitimately be included in a single analysis. But if the effects of vitamin A in the two situations are very different, the overall effect in the 12 trials will of course depend on the relative numbers of trials in the two sets (4 and 8), and may not be a very meaningful quantitative measure.

Appropriate rules may be applied for the inclusion or exclusion of studies, in order to reduce excessive differences that may make it difficult to integrate findings in a meaningful way. If it is known or suspected that there have been changes over time, for example, a time limitation may be built in. Plausible reasons for the exclusion of pre-1980 studies from a meta-analysis of senile dementia (*Question F5–2*) might include known changes in the epidemiology of this condition or in diagnostic methods. The actual reason was the development of the *DSM-III* and other standardized sets of diagnostic criteria in and after 1980. Widely varying definitions were used in earlier years, when reported prevalence rates in the elderly ranged from 1.3% to 15.8%, whereas the range was from 2.0% to 7.8% in the main studies of moderate and severe senile dementia conducted after 1980.

Studies of mild senile dementia were excluded from the meta-analysis because of the questionable reliability of diagnoses; reported rates range from 2.6% to 52.7%.

The exclusion of old studies might be advisable in a meta-analysis of clinical trials (*Question F5–3*) if there have been changes in medical or nursing care that may influence the outcome, changes in diagnostic methods, or changes in the natural history of the condition under study.

In answer to *Question F5–4*, precautions for ensuring an objective selection of studies center around the formulation and application of inclusion and/or exclusion criteria. These should be explicitly stated, should be as clear and specific as possible, and (if feasible) should be applied "blind": Decisions concerning the inclusion of specific studies should not be influenced by knowledge of their results.

Short-term and long-term outcomes (or any different outcomes) in the same subjects (*Question F5–5*) can be included in a meta-analysis— whether they appear in the same or different reports—provided that each outcome is analyzed separately. If some studies or individuals contribute more outcome measures than others to the estimation of an overall effect, they may have an undue influence on the overall effect (as illustrated in *Question F3–3*).

Question F5–6 presents another example of overrepresentation of some trials in a meta-analysis. Since the trials differed in educational methods and other respects, the mean effect size may well be biased. Also, it may have a spurious degree of precision (i.e., an unduly narrow confidence interval) because it is based on more results although these include clusters of results that are similar because they come from the same trial. These problems could be avoided by using only one effect size for each trial. This might be the average effect size for the experimental–control comparisons in the trial, or a single one of the effect sizes in the trial, randomly or systematically selected. These methods obviously entail the loss of specific information. The investigators found that the mean effect size was 0.27 (95% confidence interval, 0.22 to 0.33) if it was based on the average results in the 20 trials, and it was 0.26 (95% confidence interval, 0.20 to 0.32) if it was based on a single result per trial (the result that the author of the study regarded as the strongest). They decided, as a calculated risk, to use all 34 measures in subsequent analyses aimed at investigating modifying factors affecting the success of the programs, so as not to waste data.

Criteria for the inclusion of studies should reflect the objectives of the meta-analysis. The reason for the first two criteria used in the overview of acupuncture studies (*Question F5–7*) is obviously the investigators' interest in the effectiveness of needle acupuncture (and not laser acupuncture) in chronic pain (and not in other conditions). The third criterion (the use of a control group) relates to study quality, and represents an effort to restrict the meta-analysis to studies with a potential for giving an adequate answer to the research question.

Opinions differ as to whether studies of a poor quality should be excluded from a meta-analysis (*Question F5-8*). Some experts suggest that acceptable standards should always be set in advance, in the form of criteria for inclusion, and studies that do not meet them should not be accepted. The extreme view is that in a meta-analysis of clinical trials "it is important to restrict inclusion to randomized trials, ideally with intention-to-treat analysis, complete follow-up information, and objective or blinded outcome assessment" (Thompson and Pocock, 1991). Some suggest that the best of the available studies should be used (Slavin, 1986, 1987). Others advise the inclusion of all studies except those that are really bad: "[I]f it is clear that a certain study is fundamentally flawed, say with obvious numerical errors, I find it hard to argue for its inclusion. I do not believe that wrong information is better than no information" (Light, 1987).

The main arguments for including studies that are not of the best quality are that increasing the number of studies permits the examination of the topic in more circumstances, and that it boosts numbers. If an effect truly exists in all circumstances, this consistency may be demonstrated more convincingly if more studies are included. On the other hand, if the effect is not consistent, the inclusion of more studies may make it easier to detect this inconsistency and explore its sources. Other things being equal, larger numbers will increase the power of statistical tests and make confidence intervals narrower.

In some instances the appraisal of study quality is the main purpose or main contribution of the meta-analysis, and all studies must of course then be included. An overview of papers on the effectiveness of health education programs in developing countries, for example, revealed that only 3 of 67 studies met four simple criteria, and it led to specific recommendations for improvements in health education research (Loevinsohn, 1990). A meta-analysis of studies of lumbar spine fusion revealed widely variable results and numerous flaws in study design, leading to the conclusion that the indications for this surgical procedure were not scientifically established, and that randomized controlled trials were required (Turner et al., 1993).

The advantages of including more studies in an analysis must of course be balanced against the obvious disadvantages of including questionable results. If poor studies are included, the differences in quality should be taken into account; it may be possible to control bias in the analysis, or make allowances for it. Often there are no really good studies, and the choice is between making the best use of what there is, or not doing a meta-analysis at all.

There is thus no "correct" answer to the question: Should studies that are not of the best quality be included in a meta-analysis? The best answer is probably a qualified yes: They should be included, but only on condition that due regard is paid to the possible problems.

One way of taking account of differences in study quality is to pay separate attention to studies that are of higher and lower quality. This is what was done by the authors of the acupuncture meta-analysis, who scored the trials by giving points for randomization, blinding, and other features, and found that even the better studies (which were mediocre) gave contradictory results. They concluded that "the efficacy of acupuncture in the treatment of chronic pain remains doubtful," and called for research of a higher quality. Their summary table shows that only 2 of the 17 trials that used randomization and blind methods gave "positive" results (i.e., better results for acupuncture, according to the investigators' own statements), as compared with 22 of the 34 other trials ($P < .0001$).

EXERCISE F6

Question F6-1

The importance of appraising the scientific quality of the individual studies is clear. This may be done as part of the selection procedure or after the studies have been selected for inclusion, or even after the analysis. Can you suggest what precautions might be taken to make the appraisal of quality as objective as possible?

Question F6-2

A meta-analysis of 375 controlled evaluations of psychotherapy, using various outcome measures, revealed a mean effect size of 0.68, indicating that the average patient receiving treatment had a better outcome than 75% of controls (Smith and Glass, 1977). A critic called this study an "exercise in mega-silliness," and fulminated against "the abandonment of critical judgments of any kind. A mass of reports—good, bad, and indifferent—are fed into the computer in the hope that people will cease caring about the quality of the material on which the conclusions are based. . . . The notion that one can distill scientific knowledge from a compilation of studies mostly of poor design, relying on subjective, unvalidated, and certainly unreliable clinical judgments, and dissimilar with respect to nearly all the vital parameters, dies hard. . . . 'Garbage in—garbage out' is a well-known axiom of computer specialists; it applies here with equal force" (Eysenck, 1978). Assuming that the studies were uneven in their quality, can you suggest any additional analyses that might counter this criticism?

Question F6–3

Guess whether the following statements are true or false:

1. In the meta-analysis of trials of work-site smoking cessation programs (*Question F5–6*) the effect was largest in trials in which reported smoking habits were not verified by biochemical tests.
2. In an overview of studies of anticoagulants for acute myocardial infarction (Gifford and Feinstein, 1990) the benefit of anticoagulant therapy (in comparison with no therapy) was more often observed in studies that failed to meet defined quality standards.
3. In a meta-analysis comparing coronary artery bypass surgery with nonsurgical intervention (Wortman and Yeaton, 1983), the results were better in nonrandomized than in randomized trials.
4. A meta-analysis of the effect of physical activity in preventing coronary heart disease (Berlin and Colditz, 1990) showed a larger preventive effect in methodologically stronger studies than in less well designed ones.
5. In a meta-analysis of trials of the treatment of mild hypertension, in which trials using different treatments were compared (Andrews et al., 1982), the effect was largest in the trials of higher quality.
6. In a meta-analysis of cohort studies of the relationship between mammary dysplasia (dense areas seen in a mammogram) and subsequent breast cancer (Goodwin and Boyd, 1988), the association was strongest in the studies of higher quality.
7. In a meta-analysis of randomized controlled trials of antibiotic prophylaxis in biliary tract surgery (Meijer et al., 1990), the effect was unrelated to study quality.

Question F6–4

In which (if any) of the following situations might it be worthwhile to contact the investigators and ask for further information:

1. The study report does not describe the methods clearly (as in the acupuncture meta-analysis, Table F5).
2. The study is reported in an abstract, with incomplete information on methods and results.
3. In a meta-analysis of trials, some of the reports use "while-on-randomized-treatment" analysis only, and provide no information on what happened to subjects after they abandoned the allocated regimen.

4. In a meta-analysis of trials of intravenous beta-blockers in acute myo-cardial infarction, it is found that three studies report significant re-ductions in cardiac arrest, with prevented fractions of 61–79%, but many other trials provide no information on this outcome.

Question F6–5

Suppose that a meta-analysis of epidemiological studies of the asso-ciation between calcium intake and fractures includes a case–control study (Kreiger et al., 1992) in which postmenopausal women with hip and wrist fractures were compared with a group of controls. The report of this study provides separate findings for hip and wrist fractures, and for each kind of fracture there are five measures of the association with calcium intake: (1) the crude difference in mean daily calcium intake; (2) an odds ratio (adjusted by multiple logistic regression for age, obesity, and other variables) comparing women with a low and moderate dietary calcium intake; (3) a similar odds ratio comparing women with a low and high dietary calcium intake; (4) an odds ratio (adjusted for the above factors and dietary calcium intake) expressing the association with long-term calcium supplements; and (5) a similar odds ratio expressing the association with recent calcium supplements. When an overall measure is calculated in the meta-analysis, would the inclusion of more than one of these ten measures carry any disadvantages? Would restriction of the meta-analysis to only one of the measures carry any disadvantages?

Question F6–6

What solutions can you suggest to the problem of multiple measures, illustrated in the previous question?

Unit
F7

THE QUALITY OF THE STUDIES

Appraising the scientific quality of a study is not easy. Judgements of the same study may differ, and there is no "gold standard" for comparison. The best approach is to ask questions about the presence of a number of features generally regarded as important determinants of the internal or external validity of studies. The studies can then be classified and ranked according to their quality (e.g., randomized controlled trials with blinding, randomized controlled trials without blinding; nonrandomized controlled trials; uncontrolled trials). If points are allotted to the various features, a quality score can be assigned to each study.

To make the appraisal as objective as possible (*Question F6–1*), the questions should be explicitly stated, and they should be phrased as clearly and specifically as possible. If a quality score is used, the method of scaling should be explicitly specified (see Note F7–1). Since expertise both in research methods and in the study topic may be needed to answer some of the questions (e.g., is the statistical analysis appropriate?), it may be advisable to have each study appraised by two reviewers, who can compare their verdicts and reach a consensus. One recommendation is that material that might bias the reviewers (e.g., the names and affiliations of the researchers) should first be blotted out, and the methods appraised without knowledge of the study results; the appraisal can then be completed by looking at the results section (T. C. Chalmers, 1991); these precautions are often not feasible.

When there are differences in the quality of the studies, as in *Question F6–2*, the possible approaches are:

- To discard studies of poor quality before combining the results.

- To compare the combined results in all studies with the results when poor-quality studies are excluded; this is a form of "sensitivity analysis" (a term used for examinations of the extent to which the results of an analysis are affected by changes in methods or assumptions).

- To compare the results of studies that differ in quality; the relationship between quality and the result can be shown graphically, especially if quality scores are used.

- To give each study a weight determined by its quality, before combining results, so that better studies have a larger impact on the overall result (Note F7–2).

- If regression analysis is employed, to use a measure of study quality as an independent variable in the model, and to control statistically for the effect of differences in quality (Note F7–2).

- If few or no studies reach an acceptable standard, to abandon the meta-analysis and issue a call for better research.

In their reply to the criticism of their meta-analysis of controlled trials of psychotherapy, the authors said that in their analysis, "good, bad, and indifferent" studies showed almost the same results; "such features as use of randomization versus matching and double versus single versus no-blinding had virtually no correlation with study findings." Also, their findings were confirmed by multiple regression analyses using a model that included a score measuring the subjectivity of each outcome measure (Glass and Smith, 1978). A careful reanalysis, restricted to trials that used randomization and whose control groups received placebo or no treatment, yielded almost the same findings as the overall analysis: The mean effect size was 0.78, suggesting that the average patient receiving treatment had a better outcome than 78% of untreated controls (Landman and Dawes, 1982).

All the statements in *Question F6–3* are true. The influence of methodological shortcomings may not be easy to guess. In comparison with better studies, studies of a poorer quality can show an enhanced, reduced, or similar effect.

Often, of course, studies with methodological weaknesses (and there are those who put all nonexperimental studies in this category) are the only ones available. For example, a meta-analysis of studies of bone marrow transplantation in acute nonlymphocytic leukemia was based only on nonrandomized controlled trials and uncontrolled follow-up studies, because no randomized controlled trials had yet been done; after adjustment for a number of biases, the analysis showed a consistent advantage over chemotherapy in long-term disease-free survival (Begg et al., 1989).

Requests to investigators for further information about their methods or results may often add to the value of a meta-analysis, and might be worthwhile in all the situations listed in *Question F6–4*. They are least likely to be successful if they demand further action by the investigators, as they probably do in situation 3. In a meta-analysis in which unreported means and correlation coefficients were required, "letters were sent to 10 authors, but the necessary information was provided by 1 of those 10" (Gray et al., 1991). Collecting complete data on all subjects is "often . . . the most difficult and time-consuming aspect of doing overviews and can take 3 to 4 years!" (Yusuf, 1987a). Additional data on unreported outcomes, obtained by correspondence, reduced the summary prevented fraction for cardiac arrest in situation 4 from over 60% to 15% (Yusuf, 1987a). (Can you suggest why the unpublished data changed the overall result? See Note F7–3.) In a meta-analysis of randomized controlled trials comparing two forms of chemotherapy for advanced cancer of the ovary, it was found that the difference was larger (and significant) when the analysis was based on published reports than when it used full data on all randomized patients, including those excluded from published analyses and those studied in unpublished trials; the full data showed a nonsignificant difference (Stewart and Parmar, 1993).

EXTRACTING THE FINDINGS

Question F6–5 exemplifies a common situation: A single study offers more than one measure of effect, and a decision must be made as to what should be used when an overall measure is calculated in the meta-analysis. This is a difficult problem. If more than one measure is included, extra weight is given to that study. Moreover, the different measures in a single study cannot be completely independent of each other; this dependence is particularly obvious in the study under consideration, where both fracture groups are compared with the same set of controls, whose calcium intake will influence each one of the measures. If only one measure is included, the specific choice may affect the overall result; in this study, fractures of the wrist were associated with a low intake of calcium, but fractures of the femur were not.

This dilemma occurs most often in observational studies. Not only may there be alternative dependent and independent variables and a choice between crude and adjusted measures, as in the present instance, but there may also be a choice between different adjusted or specific measures (controlling for different sets of potential confounders, or using different methods of adjustment), and there may be comparisons with different control groups. A choice may also be required in trials, since the same trial may provide two or more outcome measures, as we saw in the meta-analyses of asthma treatment and patient education (*Question F3–3*), smoking cessation programs (*Question 5–6*), and beta-blockers (*Question F2–3*).

There is no simple universal way of handling the problem of multiple measures (*Question F6–6*), and it must be considered anew in each meta-analysis. To reduce possible bias, explicit rules or guidelines should be formulated (preferably in advance), and (unless these are very simple) two or more reviewers should independently extract the findings and later resolve their disagreements by discussion. Preference should of course be given to measures that control for confounding. Sometimes an average of the measures is used, or a randomly or systematically selected one—for example, "the largest estimate, the smallest estimate, or, in order to be fair, the estimate closest to the average of the individual ones" (Fleiss and Gross, 1991). Analyses may be conducted using different choices, and the results compared. It is sometimes decided to take a calculated risk and use more than one measure from the same study; this was done in the study of work-site smoking cessation programs (*Question F5–6*) in order to have more data for the examination of modifying factors.

APPLES AND ORANGES

Most writings on meta-analysis are packed with fruity metaphors (Note F7–4). A recurrent theme is the disadvantage of "mixing apples and oranges"—that is, combining the results of studies that are so different that "it may be uncertain to which fruit or to what specific combination of fruits, the results apply." "By mixing apples and oranges and an occasional lemon, one may end up with an artificial product." "Interpreting a weighted average of different odds ratios can be like describing an 'average fruit'." If different dependent variables are used, "a good meta-analysis capitalizes on this by coding apples as apples and oranges as oranges." If important differences between studies are overlooked, "the problem of 'apples' and 'oranges' . . . may render the entire exercise—dare one say it?—fruitless."

A meta-analysis can, of course, include both apples and oranges if what is wanted is general information about fruit. But even then, "the trials used . . . are not likely to be a random sample of all the trials that might conceivably have been done to provide information about 'fruit'; that is, the proportion of 'apples' and 'oranges' may be wrong." There will accordingly remain some uncertainty about the accuracy of the picture provided by "the 'fruit salad' created in our meta-analysis."

Also, "a miscellany of fruit is not necessarily a disadvantage. . . . Comparisons of apples and oranges may . . . provide useful additional information."

With respect to study quality: "Rotten apples in the basket may invalidate the results. . . . Some apples are healthy, some are slightly spoiled, some have a moderate degree of decay, and some are really rotten. Due account should be taken of the quality of whatever studies are included in the analysis."

And finally, publication bias: "Only the big apples may get to the market."

Studies are usually selected in the expectation that their results can be combined, and narrowly defined inclusion criteria may be used for this purpose. But the results may still turn out to be so dissimilar that it does not make sense to combine them as if they were all expressions of a single overall result. It is therefore essential to appraise the consistency of the results. Heterogeneous findings should be combined only with reservations, or by using statistical methods that are specifically designed for this situation.

The next exercise deals with the appraisal of combinability. Both a statistical test for heterogeneity (Note F7–5) and visual inspection of the results (preferably after plotting them graphically) should be performed before combined results are used.

EXERCISE F7

Question F7–1

In 1991 a meta-analysis was performed of epidemiological studies of the association between passive smoking in the home and lung cancer (in nonsmokers) in the United States (Fleiss and Gross, 1991). Different methods were employed in the nine studies that were identified. For example, one study was a cohort study and the others were case-control studies. Some of the case-control studies used hospital patients as controls, others used healthy people living at home. In only two studies were the interviewers explicitly "blinded" as to whether the subject was a case or control. The proportion of proxy informants about smoking habits ranged from zero (in a study confined to living cases) to nearly 70%. Definitions of "nonsmoker" and exposure to smoking varied: In one study the subjects who reported occasional smoking were classified as nonsmokers, and in another the comparison was not between subjects exposed and not exposed to smoking, but between those exposed for more or less than four hours a day. Can the odds ratios provided by these nine studies be combined?

Question F7–2

A recent meta-analysis of epidemiological studies showed a weak but statistically significant association between cigarette smoking and leukemia (Brownson et al., 1993). In cohort studies the summary rate ratio was 1.3 (95% confidence interval, 1.3 to 1.4). In case-control studies the summary odds ratio was 1.1 (95% confidence interval, 1.0 to 1.2). Can you suggest why cohort studies provided a higher estimate of the increased risk associated with smoking? Can the cohort and case-control studies be combined in a single analysis?

Question F7–3

Statistical tests for the heterogeneity of findings have a low power; that is, they may fail to show heterogeneity when actually it exists, unless the number of studies is very large. How, therefore, would you interpret a P value of .001? .04? .09? .15? .8?

Question F7–4

In the meta-analysis of 23 trials of beta-blockers (Table F1), the Mantel–Haenszel summary rate ratio was 0.79, indicating that "on average" (controlling for the differences between the trials) the beta-blockers prevented 21% of deaths. A heterogeneity test yielded a P value of .38, indicating that the differences between the trial results could easily be accounted for by chance variation. Now suppose that the heterogeneity test had yielded a P value of .001 instead of .38, so that the differences could not be regarded as fortuitous. How would this modify the interpretation of the summary rate ratio?

Question F7–5

In the same meta-analysis the overall P value, based on the results of one-tailed significance tests in each study (see Note F2–2), was .0000005, indicating that the effect on fatality could safely be regarded as nonfortuitous. The Mantel–Haenszel test gave a similar P value, .0000002. Would the interpretation of these results be different if the heterogeneity test had yielded a P value of .001 instead of .38?

Question F7–6

The results of 14 randomized controlled trials of hypertension treatment, showing the effect on the occurrence of strokes, are summarized in Table F7. The reduction in strokes was highly significant; by the Mantel–Haenszel test, $P = 2.82E-13$ (what does this number mean? See Note F7–6). The rate ratios are shown graphically in Fig. F7(A), together with their 95% confidence intervals. They are plotted on a logarithmic scale (why? And what scale would you use for plotting rate differences? odds ratios? effect sizes? See Note F7–7). For convenience the results are arranged in decreasing sequence. Can you tell which of the 14 values were statistically significant (i.e., significantly different from 1)? Do you think the results are acceptably consistent? Would you expect a test to show significant heterogeneity?

Question F7–7

Figure F7(B) shows the same results, but here the sequence is determined by the size of the study sample (treatment and control groups combined). The smallest trial (on the left) had 87 subjects, and the largest (on the right) had 17,354 subjects. What do you observe, with respect to (1) the point estimates of the rate ratios, and (2) the confidence intervals? Can you suggest an explanation?

Question F7–8

The rate differences listed in Table F7 are charted in Fig. F7(C) [not in the same sequence as in Fig. F7(A)]. What is your impression of the con-

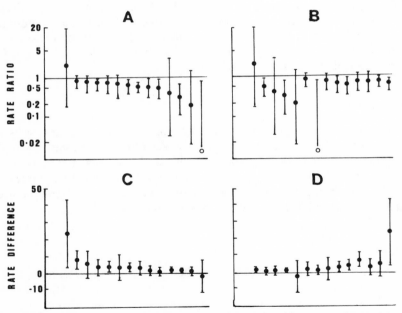

Figure F7. Comparisons of stroke rates in 14 trials of hypertension treatment: rate ratios (ratio of rate in treatment group to rate in control group) and rate differences (rate in control group minus rate in treatment group), with 95% confidence intervals. The rate ratio marked "0" is zero; only its upper confidence limit is shown. (A) Rate ratios. (B) Rate ratios, arranged in sequence of sample sizes (smallest on left). (C) Rate differences. (D) Rate differences, arranged in sequence of stroke rates in control group (lowest on left).

Table F7. Results of 14 Randomized Controlled Trials of Antihypertensive Drugs; Comparison of Stroke Rates in Subjects Allocated to Treatment and Control Groups

Trial	Strokes Per 100		Ratio (a/b)	Difference (b − a)
	Treatment Group (a)	Control Group (b)		
1	1.51	2.24	0.67	0.73
2	0	1.32	0	1.32
3	0.76	1.29	0.59	0.53
4	0.69	1.26	0.55	0.57
5	2.69	10.31	0.26	7.62
6	0.52	3.06	0.17	2.54
7	2.39	3.59	0.67	1.20
8	18.46	23.74	0.78	5.29
9	1.47	4.76	0.31	3.29
10	4.44	2.38	1.87	−2.06
11	20.41	43.75	0.47	23.34
12	3.37	6.43	0.52	3.06
13	7.69	11.32	0.68	3.63
14	4.77	8.39	0.57	3.61
Pooled*			0.61	0.72

*Using precision weighting (i.e., each value was weighted by the reciprocal of its variance). The smaller the variance, the greater the weight.
Based on Collins et al. (1990).

sistency of the values? Would you expect a test to show significant heterogeneity? When two different measures of an effect are used, it is possible for one to exhibit heterogeneity and the other not?

Question F7–9

In a meta-analysis of controlled trials it is generally advisable to see whether the outcomes in the control groups are similar. Why? Table F7 shows marked heterogeneity of the stroke rates in the control groups. What are the most likely explanations for this variation?

Question F7–10

In Fig. F7(D) the trials are arranged in the sequence of the stroke rates in their control groups (with the lowest rate on the left), and rate differences are plotted. The graph shows a clear association (correlation coefficient = .91). Can this explain the heterogeneity of rate differences? There was no such association between the rate ratios and the stroke rates in the control groups (correlation coefficient = .08).

NOTES

F7–1.   Methods for assigning quality scores to trials are described by (inter alia) Chalmers et al. (1981), Klein et al. (1986), Liberati et al. (1986), Zelen (1983), and Detsky et al. (1992). The simplest method (I. Chalmers, 1981; T. C. Chalmers, 1991) examines three aspects: method of treatment assignment (full marks for true randomization), control of selection bias after treatment assignment (full marks if both intention-to-treat and on-randomized-treatment analyses were done), and blinding of participants and investigators (full marks if subjects, care-givers, and investigators assessing outcomes were all kept unaware of the treatment assignment). Criteria for case-control studies are listed by Feinstein (1985) and Lichtenstein et al. (1987). Quality scores are arbitrary, in the sense that they depend on the items included and the weight given to each; but different systems tend to rank studies in the same order (Detsky et al., 1992). It may be necessary to add criteria based on the specific requirements for the particular topic studied.

F7–2.   A formula for weighting by quality when results are combined are provided by Fleiss and Gross (1991). The use of quality scores as weights in multiple logistic regression analysis is described by Detsky et al. (1992). These methods are not yet widely accepted.

F7–3.   Although different outcomes may be measured in a trial, investigators may tend to report only those that show statistically significant findings; other results may be merely reported as "not significant," or omitted. One way of handling this "reporting bias" is to assume that unreported results were statistically null and give them effect sizes of 0 (Felson, 1992).

F7–4.   The quotations come from Abramson (1990–91), Furbery and Morgan (1987), Goodman (1991), Naylor (1988), and Wolf (1986).

F7–5.   For references describing the heterogeneity tests usually used, see Note D13–1. Heterogeneity tests for effect sizes are described by Hedges and Olkin (1985) and Wolf (1986), and testing of heterogeneity in a multiple logistic regression analysis by Detsky et al. (1992).

F7–6.   2.82E–13 is expressed in scientific notation. It means 2.82×10^{-13}; to convert the number to ordinary (fixed point) notation, multiply 2.82 by 10^{-13} (−13 is the exponent of 10). In other words, move the decimal point 13 spaces to the left, which gives

0.00000000000282. If there is no minus, move the decimal point to the right; 2.82E4 is 28200.

F7–7. Rate ratios and odds ratios are measures of relative difference, and a logarithmic scale is therefore appropriate (see Unit A4). Absolute differences, such as rate differences and effect sizes, should be plotted on an ordinary scale.

Unit
F8

APPRAISING COMBINABILITY

Opinions differ as to whether nonexperimental studies in which non-randomly selected groups are compared should be combined (*Question F7–1*). At one extreme is the view that these studies have so many possible biases that they should never be submitted to a meta-analysis; at the other is a permissive approach that accepts all studies that conform to the objectives and inclusion criteria of the meta-analysis (i.e., those that are relevant and have sufficiently similar features, according to the rules laid down for the meta-analysis), provided that their results are reasonably consistent. The results of the studies of passive smoking were fairly similar, and the summary odds ratio was 1.12 (95% confidence interval, 0.95 to 1.30)—a finding that did not convincingly support a relationship to lung cancer in the United States. The odds ratio of 1.17 for the cohort study was similar to the summary odds ratio of 1.07 for the case-control studies.

Question F7–1 serves to highlight the importance of knowing (and, in a published meta-analysis, of reporting) the methods and possible biases of the studies included in a meta-analysis. This knowledge may help to explain any heterogeneity of the results, and may influence the inferences from the findings of the meta-analysis. Sometimes, possible biases can be reduced before the findings are combined. In a trial, this generally involves collecting additional information—for example, about the outcome in subjects who did not continue the regimen to which they had been randomized. In an observational study, it may involve statistical procedures to control for differences in sociodemographic or other characteristics between the groups compared or to compensate for misclassification of subjects with regard to the independent or dependent variable (see Note F8–1).

The authors of the meta-analysis of smoking and leukemia (*Question F7–2*) could not explain the difference between the results of the cohort and case-control studies. They suggested that it might be due to the biases commonly found in case-control studies, such as those arising from the manner of selection of controls. The use of different measures—the rate ratio for the cohort studies and the odds ratio for the case- control studies—is a red herring. It cannot explain the difference, since simple algebra (see Note F8–2) shows that an odds ratio would, in this instance, exceed a rate ratio based on the same data. If a summary odds ratio had been estimated from the cohort studies, it would have been more than 1.3. Before combining the cohort and case-control studies in a single analysis (using odds ratios throughout), the heterogeneity of the odds ratios in the combined studies should be assessed. It is probably advisable not to combine the results of the cohort and case-control studies; if this is done, it should be done with reservations, since the overall result will depend on how many studies there are of each type.

The results of different studies are never identical. The issue is not whether differences exist, but whether they can reasonably be ignored. If a statistical test for heterogeneity yields a low *P* value (*Question F7–3*), the differences between study results should not be ignored. But these tests have a low power, and there is no clearly defined critical level; .05 may be regarded as too low a critical level. As an arbitrary rule of thumb, *P* values below .1 can usually be taken to mean that the differences should not be ignored; and if the number of studies is small, even higher *P* values than this should not be regarded as safe. However few the studies may be, a value exceeding .5 can usually be taken as convincing support for homogeneity; in the meta-analysis of passive smoking studies (*Question F7–1*) the *P* value was .71. Unless the *P* value is very high, possible heterogeneity should also be assessed by visual inspection.

In answer to *Question F7–4*, a heterogeneity test result of $P = .001$ would mean that the study results should be regarded as heterogeneous. The assumption that there is a single underlying true effect—a "fixed effect"—that can be estimated from the results in the separate studies, then becomes untenable. We have an "apples and oranges" situation, with different true effects, and the Mantel–Haenszel summary measure can be regarded only as a convenient weighted average of the measures, but not as an estimate of a single fixed effect. An average of discrepant results may be misleading (remember the statistician with his head in a freezer and his feet in an oven, who felt comfortable on the average).

Even if the results were heterogeneous (*Question F7–5*), overall tests showing a significant effect on fatality would mean that we can confidently reject the null hypothesis that there is no effect in any trial. In the presence of heterogeneity it would be wrong, however, to use the Mantel–Haenszel test result as an indication of the significance of a common measure of association.

Charting the results, as in Fig. F7(A), often makes the appraisal of homogeneity or heterogeneity relatively easy. The values need not be arranged in sequence, as they are here. The confidence intervals show how precise each estimate is; but they may be confusing, since the studies with the largest and therefore most eye-catching confidence intervals are the most imprecise ones. The confidence intervals also show which results are statistically significant: If 1 is not included in the 95% confidence interval, P can be taken to be under .05. (In answer to *Question F7–6*, the 4th, 7th, 8th, 9th, 10th, 12th, and 14th values are significant). The impression provided by a diagram is of course subjective, and judgments may differ. But it is clear that most of the values are similar, with only one divergent result on the left and a few on the right. Also, the aberrant results have especially wide confidence intervals, and all the confidence intervals overlap. It is probably safe to decide that the results are consistent enough to warrant use of the overall measure. This combinability was confirmed by the test for the heterogeneity of the rate ratios, which yielded a P value of .73.

Figure F7(B) is an example of a "funnel display," in which results are plotted against a measure of precision (this is generally sample size or the reciprocal of the variance). The idea is that if all studies are in fact estimating a similar value, the spread of results should become narrow as precision increases, forming a funnel-like shape. This (in answer to *Question F7–7*) is what is seen here. The point estimates in the left half of the diagram vary, whereas those on the right almost form a straight line. The confidence intervals based on small samples are broad, whereas those associated with larger samples are narrow. With a little imagination the picture resembles a funnel, and this suggests that random variation is the main explanation for the inconsistencies among the values.

Close inspection of Fig. F7(C), which displays the rate differences in the same 14 studies (*Question F7–8*), suggests more heterogeneity than Fig 7(A), with special reference to the two left-hand values, which are "outliers." The first confidence interval has no overlap with the 9th, 10th, 11th, 12th, or 13th confidence interval, and the second confidence interval has no overlap with the 10th, 11th, 12th, or 13th confidence interval. It would not be surprising if a test showed significant heterogeneity. The test result was, in fact, $P = .006$, indicating that the pooled value should not be used as an overall measure of effect.

As this example shows, one measure of an effect may manifest heterogeneity whereas another does not. The odds ratios in this meta-analysis, like the rate ratios, were not significantly heterogeneous ($P = .50$). We can therefore express the effect of antihypertensive treatment in terms of a single rate ratio or odds ratio, but not in terms of the absolute reduction in the rate of stroke occurrence. (Does this matter? See Note F8–3). An extreme discrepancy of this kind is unusual. For the meta-analysis of 23 trials of beta blockers shown in Table F1, for example, the heterogeneity test results were $P = .40$, .38, and .14 for rate ratios, odds ratios, and rate differences, respectively.

EXPLAINING HETEROGENEITY

Once it has been decided that there is more heterogeneity than can easily be attributed to chance, that it is too marked to be ignored, and that it cannot be avoided by switching to a different measure of effect, the next step is to consider and examine possible explanations. Differences should be brought to the surface and examined, rather than drowning them in a statistical pool.

Obvious possible explanations are that the methods or circumstances of the studies were very different, or that the people studied were very different. One simple way of exploring this possibility, in studies in which treatment groups, cases, or groups exposed to a supposed risk or protective factor are compared with control groups, is a comparison of the findings in the various control groups. The most likely explanation for the wide variation in stroke rates in control groups seen in Table F7 (*Question F7–9*) is that the follow-up periods differed; there may also have been differences (especially in age) between the samples studied, or differences in definitions or in methods of ascertainment. Careful reading of the study reports would probably clarify the main reasons.

The heterogeneity of stroke rates in the control groups, together with the association between these rates and the rate differences, can easily account for the observed heterogeneity of rate differences (*Question F7–10*). The two "outliers" with respect to rate differences (trials 5 and 11 in Table F7) were among those with high stroke rates in their control groups. If antihypertensive treatment reduces the stroke rate to about 0.61 of the rate in the control group (as the pooled value in Table F7 suggests), the absolute rate differences can be similar only if the rates in the control groups are similar.

If the heterogeneity in this instance is accounted for by differences in the follow-up period, it may be regarded as an artifact, as also in meta-analyses where it can be attributed to methodological flaws (such as insufficiently objective methods of measurement) in some or all studies. If heterogeneity of this sort cannot be sidestepped (e.g., as in this study, by the use of odds or rate ratios rather than rate differences) or somehow controlled in the analysis, it may preclude any conclusions, or lead to qualified conclusions.

On the other hand, heterogeneity may be an expression of interesting effect modification. Comparisons of the results of different studies may be used for testing or developing hypotheses concerning factors that affect the association under study, so that heterogeneity becomes an asset rather than a liability. The strategy of meta-analysis is to "combine results if you can, compare them if you can't." Instead of the fixed-effect model (which assumes that the association under investigation is equally strong in every study, apart from random variation), use may then be made of a *fixed-effects* [plural] model, which assumes that there are different fixed effects in different sets of studies, or a regression model, which assumes that the effect is altered by a specific amount by each variable included in the model. (What is the assumption if the dependent variable in the regression model is the logarithm of the rate ratio or odds ratio? See Note F8–4.)

If there is unexplained heterogeneity, it is difficult to draw useful conclusions, since there are unknown biases or unknown modifying factors. In such circumstances a *random-effects model* is sometimes used to summarize the findings. This model is based on the assumption that the true effects in the different studies differ, and are randomly positioned about some central value. Allowance is made for the variation between studies as well as within studies. Some experts query the usefulness of the random-effects approach (see Note F8–5), on the grounds that its assumptions are difficult to justify. The random-effects model is sometimes used even when there is little heterogeneity; its results are then very similar to those provided by the Mantel–Haenszel procedure and other methods that use the fixed-effect model.

EXERCISE F8

Question F8–1

A meta-analysis of eight community-based controlled trials of vitamin A supplementation (previously referred to in *Question F5–1*) showed a beneficial effect on mortality in children aged 6 to 72 months. The Mantel–Haenszel summary odds ratio was 0.72 (95% confidence interval, 0.66 to 0.79). However, the results, which are listed in Table F8–1,

Table F8–1. Results of Eight Controlled Trials of Vitamin A Supplementation; Odds Ratios Showing Effect on Mortality in Children Aged 6 to 72 Months

		Odds Ratio	
Trial	Location	Point Estimate	95% Confidence Interval
1	Sarlahi, Nepal	0.70	0.57–0.87
2	Northern Sudan	1.04	0.81–1.34
3	Tamil Nadu, India	0.45	0.31–0.67
4	Aceh, Indonesia	0.73	0.56–0.95
5	Hyderabad, India	1.00	0.64–1.55
6	Jumla, Nepal	0.73	0.58–0.93
7	Java, Indonesia	0.69	0.57–0.84
8	Bombay, India	0.20	0.09–0.45

showed significant heterogeneity ($P = .0004$). [Do the results look heterogeneous? This may be easier to answer if you chart them, using the format of Fig. F7(A); use a logarithmic scale, or plot the logarithms of the odds ratios and their confidence limits on an ordinary scale. When you have answered, see Note F8–6.] Suggest at least three possible reasons for the heterogeneity.

Question F8–2

The results of a sensitivity analysis, exploring the possibility that the heterogeneity was related to the quality of the studies, are listed in Table F8–2; combined results were recomputed after omitting first the worst study, then the two of lowest quality, then the three worst, etc. The criteria of study quality suggested by Chalmers et al. (1981) were used. The numbers used in Table F8–1 indicate the ranking of the trials according to their quality; trial 1 was the best and trial 8 the worst. What light do the new results throw on the reasons for heterogeneity?

Table F8–2. Combined Results of Eight Controlled Trials of Vitamin A Supplementation; Summary Odds Ratios for Mortality in Children Aged 6 to 72 Months: Sensitivity Analysis

Studies Pooled	Heterogeneity Test (P)	Summary Odds Ratio (With 95% C.I.)
All eight	.0004	0.72 (0.66–0.79)
All but the poorest study	.01	0.74 (0.67–0.81)
All but the two poorest studies	.006	0.76 (0.68–0.84)
All but the three poorest studies	.005	0.76 (0.67–0.86)
All but the four poorest studies	.004	0.75 (0.66–0.85)
All but the five poorest studies	.001	0.75 (0.65–0.87)
All but the six poorest studies	.020	0.82 (0.70–0.97)

Question F8–3

Vitamin A was administered in small frequent doses in trials 3 and 7, and in large doses once or every 4–6 months in other trials. The summary odds ratio was lower (i.e., the apparent protective effect was larger) in the former two trials (odds ratio, 0.58; 95% confidence interval, 0.37 to 0.92) than in the latter trials (odds ratio, 0.81; 95% confidence interval, 0.68 to 0.97). What, in general terms, are the possible explanations for this difference? Would it be helpful if we knew that the difference was statistically significant? Why is it worth knowing that the two sets of trials yielded different summary odds ratios?

Question F8–4

If we wish to make this meta-analysis the basis for a policy decision concerning the use of vitamin A supplementation to reduce child mortality in developing countries, should we use the Mantel–Haenszel odds ratio, which is based on the fixed-effect model, or an odds ratio (the DerSimonian–Laird odds ratio) that is based on the random-effects model? The respective 95% confidence intervals are 0.66 to 0.79 (Mantel–Haenszel) and 0.58 to 0.85 (DerSimonian-Laird). Or should we use neither? Can a certainty of 95% be ascribed to a 95% confidence interval?

Question F8–5

In another kind of sensitivity analysis, which is recommended if there are few studies, the impact of each study is examined by seeing how its removal influences the overall findings. As an example, a meta-analysis of six randomized controlled trials of the effectiveness of aspirin in preventing death after a myocardial infarction provided a Mantel–Haenszel odds ratio of 0.90 (95% confidence interval, 0.80 to 1.02), with a heterogeneity P of .076. The DerSimonian–Laird odds ratio (using the random-effects model) was 0.84 (95% confidence interval, 0.70 to 1.02). Table F8–3 shows the findings of each trial and the summary results after exclusion of each trial in turn. What conclusion can be reached about the value of aspirin in reducing the risk of death after myocardial infarction? There was no obvious reason for the discrepant result of trial F; should this trial be excluded?

Table F8–3. Results of Six Randomized Controlled Trials of the Effect of Aspirin in Preventing Deaths (From Any Cause) Within Two Years After Myocardial Infarction*: Sensitivity Analysis

				Combined Results, Excluding Specified Study	
Study	Aspirin: Deaths /Total	Placebo: Deaths /Total	Odds Ratio**	Heterogeneity Test (P)	Odds Ratio** (Mantel–Haenzel)
A	49/615	67/624	0.72 (0.48–1.08)	.075	0.93 (0.81–1.06)
B	44/758	64/771	0.68 (0.45–1.03)	.099	0.93 (0.82–1.06)
C	102/832	126/850	0.80 (0.60–1.07)	.058	0.93 (0.81–1.07)
D	32/317	38/309	0.80 (0.57–1.36)	.045	0.91 (0.80–1.03)
E	85/810	52/406	0.80 (0.54–1.17)	.050	0.92 (0.80–1.05)
F	246/2267	219/2257	1.13 (0.96–1.34)	.960	0.76 (0.65–0.90)

*A meta-analysis cited by Bailey (1987) and Fleiss and Gross (1991).
**95% confidence intervals shown in parentheses.

Question F8-6

A subsequent meta-analysis (Fleiss and Gross, 1991) was able to include a large new randomized controlled trial of the effect of aspirin, in which the odds ratio was 0.89. The Mantel–Haenszel odds ratio for the seven trials was 0.90 (95% confidence interval, 0.84 to 0.96), and the DerSimonian–Laird odds ratio was 0.88 (95% confidence interval, 0.77 to 0.99). The heterogeneity P was .126. Do you want to change your conclusion about the value of aspirin in reducing the risk of death after myocardial infarction?

NOTES

F8–1. Greenland (1982) describes methods of manipulating the results of epidemiological studies to adjust for confounding, selection bias, and misclassification. Spitzer (1991) provides a list of "unanswered questions" about the combinability of nonexperimental studies, including those raised in *Question F7–1* and others (e.g., "Should control groups assembled by matching be combined with independent samples of . . . populations?"), and expresses the view that until they are answered the widespread application of meta-analysis to these studies is not warranted, except as methodological research.

F8–2. Call the risk in smokers $P1$ and the risk in nonsmokers $P2$ (both $P1$ and $P2$ are between zero and 1). The relative risk is $P1/P2$. As we saw in Unit B11, odds $= P/(1 - P)$. Therefore, the odds ratio is $P1/(1 - P1)$ divided by $P2/(1 - P2)$. This is the same as $P1/P2$ (the relative risk) multiplied by $(1 - P2)/(1 \times P1)$. Since in this instance $P2$ is less than $P1$, $(1 - P2)$ must exceed $(1 - P1)$, and $(1 - P2) / (1 - P1)$ must thus be more than 1. Hence the odds ratio must be larger than the relative risk. In the beta-blocker example (statements 8 and 10 in *Question F2–1*) the odds ratio was lower than the rate ratio, because $P1$ was less than $P2$.

F8–3. A general rule of thumb for preferring the absolute difference or a relative difference (like a rate ratio) was suggested in Unit A3.

F8–4. In a regression equation with the format

$$\text{log rate ratio} = a + b_1x_1 + \ldots + b_ix_i,$$

each regression coefficient b_i tells us the mean increase in the log rate ratio associated with a rise of one unit in the value of independent variable x_i (see Units D11 and D13). Increasing the log rate ratio by b_i is equivalent to multiplying the rate ratio by b_i.

The assumption is that each independent variable included in the model has a specific multiplicative effect on the rate ratio. This principle is illustrated in a meta-analysis of studies of senile dementia (Ritchie et al., 1992), in which simple regression analysis, using the log of the prevalence as the dependent variable, showed that prevalence increases exponentially with age, with a doubling of the rate for each 6-year increase in age.

F8–5. The *random-effects* model assumes that the studies are representative of a hypothetical universe of studies with a specific statistical distribution of effects, and it estimates the findings in this hypothetical universe. Allowance is made for the variation between as well as within studies, so that the summary measure has a wider confidence interval than that provided by the fixed-effects model, and its statistical significance is lower (Berlin et al., 1989); the results are similar, however, if heterogeneity is slight. The random-effects model gives more weight to small studies than the fixed-effect model. Methods are described (inter alia) by DerSimonian and Laird (1986), Whitehead and Whitehead (1991), and Fleiss and Gross (1991). Proponents of the random-effects model suggest that it is more appropriate than the fixed-effect model if the intention is (as usually it is) to make generalizations that go beyond the studies actually included (Berlin et al., 1989, Fleiss and Gross, 1991): "The fixed effects model leads to valid inferences about the particular studies that have been assembled. The random-effects model leads to inferences about all studies in the hypothetic *population* of studies" (Berlin et al., 1989). Other experts query the usefulness of the random-effects approach, on the grounds that it is based on assumptions that are difficult to justify (Hedges, 1987; Thompson and Pocock, 1991; Jones, 1992). Pocock and Hughes (1990) conclude that "neither the fixed effect nor the random effects model can be trusted to give a wholly informative summary of the data when heterogeneity is present."

F8–6. The point estimate of the odds ratio for study 8 is much lower than the other point estimates, and the 95% confidence interval for this study shows no overlap with any other confidence interval, except that for study 3. Also, there is no overlap between the confidence intervals for study 2 (which has the highest point estimate) and study 3.

Unit
F9

EXPLAINING HETEROGENEITY
(CONTINUED)

Some of the most obvious possible reasons for the heterogeneity of the effects of vitamin A in preventing child mortality (*Question F8–1*) are differences between the populations studied (especially with respect to their nutritional and morbidity status), the use of different dosages, different durations of intervention, and differences in the quality of the trials.

When studies of poor quality were omitted from the analysis, the heterogeneity remained statistically significant. This indicates that the observed heterogeneity was not attributable, or at least not attributable solely to the poor quality of some studies (*Question F8–2*).

The difference observed between the findings of studies using different dosage schedules (*Question F8–3*) may reflect the modifying effect of the dosage schedule (which may have various mechanisms), but it may also be due to an artifact, a chance occurrence, or confounding. We have previously (in Unit F3) considered two possible manifestations of confounding in a meta-analysis: distortion of the results of individual studies and (as a consequence of imbalances between the sizes of the groups compared) distortion of the combined results. Here we are concerned with a third possibility: that studies with different dosage schedules may differ in other respects too—such as the nutritional status of children in the communities studied—and the different results may be due to these other differences rather than, or in addition to, the differences in dosage.

The difference between the findings in the two groups of studies obviously explains part of the overall inconsistency of findings, whatever the reason for the difference—even if it is a chance occurrence.

The meaning of a significance test depends on whether the association tested (in this instance, the association with dosage schedules) was postulated as a study hypothesis before inspection of the findings (a priori). If so, the result can be taken at its face value. But if the test is done only because a difference was noticed when the findings were examined (a posteriori), a significant result may be misleading. Chance differences occur in every set of data, and any difference observed when the data are searched for interesting findings (a process of "data dredging" or "panning for gold") may be a chance one. The same data cannot then be validly used for a conventional test of significance, and hence "we are unable to separate the phantom effects from real ones" (Furberg and Morgan, 1987). As an illustration of the "statistically significant" chance associations that may be brought to light by data dredging, in a randomized controlled trial of the treatment of acute myocardial infarction with intravenous atenolol, with over 16,000 subjects, the percentage reduction in the odds of death was 48% among subjects born under Scorpio ($P < .04$), and only 12% (not significant) among subjects born under other astrological birth signs (Collins et al., 1987). The problem of spurious significance did not arise in the instance described in *Question F8–3*, since the significance test yielded a P value of .21.

The difference between the findings in the two groups of studies obviously explains part of the overall inconsistency of findings, whatever the reason for the difference—even if it is a chance occurrence. The value of knowing that the difference exists depends on whether the hypothesis was derived from the data. If the hypothesis was formulated in advance (and if we decide that the difference is probably not due to chance, flawed methods, or confounding), the finding has obvious practical implications. If not, detection of the difference—even if the role of chance or other factors cannot be excluded—is still of value, since it permits the generation of a hypothesis for subsequent testing. This is an example of how a comparison of apples and oranges can raise new questions—which may be one of the main fruits of a meta-analysis.

In an "apples and oranges" situation, the Mantel–Haenszel odds ratio or any other summary measure based on the fixed-effect model can be used only as a weighted average of the results of the studies included in the meta-analysis, but not as an estimate of the effect that might be expected elsewhere (*Question F8–4*). A summary measure based on the random-effects model (see Note F8–3) is often regarded as a more appropriate basis for generalizations that go beyond the studies included, and for policy decisions. If nothing else, it provides a wider confidence interval, which seems to express the variety of the findings better. Some experts would not use this summary measure either, because of reservations about the basic assumptions of the model, and might merely utilize the variety of observed results, together with the fact that the effect was statistically significant, as rough guides for a policy decision.

Since the studies included in a meta-analysis do not constitute a random sample of all the situations in which the findings of the meta-analysis might be applied (although the random-effects model makes this assumption), the confidence intervals of summary measures cannot be taken too literally. It is prudent to regard them as underestimates of the range of variation in the real world, and to attach less than 95% certainty to a 95% confidence interval (Fleiss and Gross, 1991). One recommendation is that 99% confidence intervals should be used in meta-analyses (Peto, 1987b). In the vitamin A meta-analysis the 99% confidence intervals for the odds ratio were .64 to .82 (Mantel–Haenszel) and .54 to .90 (random-effects model). The latter figures may be translated into a preventable fraction of 10–46%.

In the meta-analysis of trials of aspirin after myocardial infarction (*Question F8–5*), the sensitivity analysis shows that the results were heterogeneous only if trial F was included. This was the only trial that did not show a reduction in the risk of death, and it was so large that it had a very appreciable impact on the summary odds ratio. If trial F is included, the effect on fatality is not statistically significant; whereas if it is excluded the preventive effect is larger (odds ratio = 0.76) and significant. Trial F was actually reported some years after the other five; previously, the summary odds ratio had been significant; with the addition of trial F to the meta-analysis, the effect became nonsignificant. If the discrepant result is obviously due to flawed methods, trial F can legitimately be excluded; but we have no evidence that this is so. The findings are therefore inconclusive. Maybe aspirin is helpful; maybe it is not.

The addition of a new trial (*Question F8–6*) changes the picture. The combined results now indicate that aspirin has a modest but statistically significant effect. But the basic heterogeneity remains; the heterogeneity P is now .126, a value which, in a comparison of only seven results, is not high enough to provide assurance that the differences can be ignored. The overall result may still be so fragile that another new trial might alter it. The authors' conclusion was expressed very cautiously:

Aspirin seems to be a modestly effective agent . . . with a percentage reduction in the odds for dying relative to placebo equal to approximately 10%. The limits of uncertainty about this value are unsure, with the conservative random effects approach yielding a much wider confidence interval than the anticonservative fixed effects approach. . . . It would be prudent always to attach greater uncertainty than provided by traditional confidence intervals to the results of a meta-analysis of studies conducted to date. (Fleiss and Gross, 1991)

The kind of sensitivity analysis shown in Table F8–3 may be advisable in all meta-analyses of small numbers of studies, to appraise the influence of each study. At the very least, the analysis should be repeated with the largest study excluded to assess the influence of that study (Andersen and Harrington, 1992). It may be unwise to draw a conclusion that hinges on a single study.

EXERCISE F9

Question F9–1

In the meta-analysis of controlled trials of work-site smoking cessation programs referred to in *Question F5–5*, the mean effect size was significantly higher in the six comparisons conducted at work sites with under 250 employees than in the 28 conducted at larger work sites. What is the value (if any) of this finding? (Ignore the possible bias caused by the overrepresentation of trials that embraced more than one comparison, as explained in Question F5–5.)

Question F9–2

A meta-analysis of eight randomized controlled trials of intravenous streptokinase for acute myocardial infarction showed a summary risk ratio for fatality of 0.80, with significant heterogeneity. It was afterwards shown that the risk ratio was different in trials with different eligibility rules (Zelen, 1983). In the two trials that excluded patients whose symptoms had lasted for more than 72 hours, the risk ratio was 1.29. In the three trials where the maximum duration of symptoms was 24 hours, the risk ratio was 0.80. And in the three trials where the maximum duration of symptoms was 12 hours, the risk ratio was 0.69. These differences were significant ($P = .01$). What is the value (if any) of these findings?

Question F9–3

Do older men have less testosterone (male sex hormone) in their blood? A meta-analysis of 88 studies (Gray et al., 1991) displayed heterogeneous findings, with age–testosterone correlations ranging from $-.68$ (a moderate decrease with age) to $+.68$ (a moderate increase). Weighted regression analyses (see Note F4) showed that the direction and degree of change with age varied significantly with the health status of the subjects and the time of day at which blood was taken. For example, in studies that included ill men there was no decline with age, whereas in studies of healthy subjects there was a decline with age. How can the significance of modifying effects be tested in a regression analysis? How can possible confounders be controlled in a regression analysis? What is the value (if any) of the findings of this meta-analysis? Do not try to explain the findings.

Question F9–4

Let us return to the meta-analysis of 23 beta blocker trials, with which we started (Table F1). There seemed to be no reason not to combine the

Table F9–1. Results of 23 Randomized Controlled Trials of the Effect
on Fatality of Long-Term Use of Beta-Blockers After Myocardial Infarction;
Comparison of Trials of Beta Blockers With and Without Intrinsic
Sympathomimetic Activity (ISA)

Type of Beta Blocker	No. of Trials	Heterogeneity Test (P)	Summary Rate Ratio* (With 95% C.I.)
Without ISA	12*	0.70	0.72 (0.64–0.81)
With ISA	11+	0.60	0.91 (0.81–1.02)
Total	23	0.38	0.79 (0.73–0.87)

*The summary rate ratios are precision-based.
**Trials 1, 3, 6, 9, 13–16, 18, 19, 21, and 23 in Table F1.
+Trials 2, 4, 5, 7, 8, 10, 11, 12, 17, 20, and 22 in Table F1.

results; the heterogeneity P was 0.38. However, the results of trials
using different kinds of beta blocker were compared, in order to see
whether different beta blockers differed in their preventive value. This
revealed no differences related to the drug's cardioselectivity or its
membrane-stabilizing difference, but there was a difference related to
intrinsic sympathomimetic activity (ISA). As shown in Table F9–1, the
effect on mortality was larger in the 12 trials that used beta blockers
without ISA than in the other 11 trials, where the effect was weak and
not statistically significant. The two summary odds ratios were significantly different from each other ($P <= .01$). The authors conclude that
"it appears that [beta blockers with appreciable ISA] may confer less
benefit," but say this "remains uncertain, for the distinction between
these two categories of agent was a data-derived hypothesis" (Yusuf et
al., 1985). Were they right to draw attention to the difference? Was it
right to soft-pedal it?"

Question F9–5

A meta-analysis of 19 randomized controlled trials of measures to reduce
plasma cholesterol (Holme, 1993) showed a significant reduction of coronary heart disease incidence, with a summary odds ratio of 0.91 (95%
confidence interval, 0.87 to 0.96). The results were very heterogeneous
($P = .027$). So were the trials: Some used drugs, some used dietary or
other measures; several trials were multifactorial ones that tried to control other risk factors also; some were concerned with preventing first
episodes (primary prevention), others with recurrences (secondary prevention). A weighted regression analysis was performed, with the log
odds ratio for coronary heart disease incidence as the dependent variable (see Note F8–4) and the mean percentage decrease in cholesterol in
the study as the independent variable. This led to the conclusion that on
average the incidence rate decreased by 2.5% (95% confidence interval,

2.0% to 3.0%) for each 1% reduction in cholesterol. The heterogeneity P rose to .14 when differences in cholesterol response were controlled in the analysis. This study suggests that the inconsistent effects on incidence are largely explained by differences in plasma cholesterol reduction. In the context of this meta-analysis, is plasma cholesterol reduction a modifying factor, a confounding factor, or what?

Question F9–6

In the meta-analysis of eight community-based trials of the value of vitamin A supplements in preventing child mortality, the modifying effect of age was examined not by comparing different trials or subsets of trials, but by comparing different subsets of individuals. The results are summarized in Table F9–2. Why do you think that different sets of studies are used for different age groups? Does this matter? Why do you think study 8 does not appear at all?

Table F9–2. Effects of Vitamin A Supplementation on Child Mortality in Controlled Community-Based Trials, by Age

Age (Months)	Studies Pooled*	Summary Odds Ratio** (With 95% C.I.)
0–11	1,2,3,4,6,7	0.76 (0.84–0.91)
12–23	1,2,4,6	0.90 (0.70–1.15)
24–35	1,2,4,6	0.89 (0.57–1.39)
36–47	1,2,4,6	0.94 (0.49–1.79)
48–59	1,2,4,6	0.80 (0.38–1.70)
≥60	2,4	0.55 (0.11–2.77)

*Numbered as in Table F8–1.
**DerSimonian–Laird method (random effects model).

Question F9–7

Suppose that we wish to see whether smoking habits modify the effect of the long-term use of beta blockers after myocardial infarction, by comparing the results in individuals with different smoking habits who were included in the trials listed in Table F1. What difficulties might we encounter?

Unit
F10

EFFECT MODIFICATION

The investigation of effect modifiers—factors that influence the outcomes of trials or the associations examined in nonexperimental studies—can be an important feature and sometimes the main contribution of a meta-analysis. It is usually done by comparing the results of different studies, either to test previously formulated hypotheses or to explain inconsistent findings. What is learned may have important theoretical and practical implications.

In the meta-analysis of smoking cessation programs (*Question F9–1*), the significantly greater success observed at small work sites is not necessarily attributable to the size of the work force or factors related to the size of the work force, such as (maybe) the degree of social interaction, integration, or support. It might be due to other (confounding) influences. But if confounders unrelated to the operation of the program (e.g., age and sex differences) can be excluded, careful examinations of how the programs at small and large work sites operated may point to ways of enhancing effectiveness.

An obvious possible explanation for the findings described in *Question F9–2* is that streptokinase is more effective if it is given early, and might even be harmful if given very late. The association may be attributable to other differences between the groups of trials, and the significance test may be misleading because the hypothesis was not formulated in advance. But the ostensible explanation may have practical importance, and can be tested in subsequent trials. In this meta-analysis it was not possible to compare the results in individuals with different duration of symptoms, because these data were not available (Stampfer et al., 1982).

Modifying effects can be studied not only by comparing mean effect sizes (as in *Question F9–1*), summary odds ratios (as in *Question F8–3*) or risk ratios (as in *Question F9–2*), or other measures of effect, but also by using regression analysis. In such an analysis the significance of a modifying effect can be tested in two ways (*Question F9–3*). First, if regression coefficients are calculated separately for different samples (e.g., for studies of healthy men and those including ill men), using the simple regression equation $y = a + bx$ (see Unit D11), where (in this instance) $y =$ testosterone level, $x =$ age, and b is the slope of the regression line, the difference between the b coefficients is an expression of a modifying effect (in this instance, of health status on the testosterone–age association), and its significance can be tested. Second, if multiple linear regression is used (Unit D16), the suspected modifier can be included in the model, together with a term that expresses its interaction with age. The significance of the latter term is the significance of the modifying effect. In this meta-analysis, a multiple regression analysis showed that the interactions between age and health status and between age and time of day were both significant ($P = .02$ and $.01$, respectively); that is, both health status and time of day modified the age–testosterone relationship. Suspected confounders can be controlled by adding them to the regression model.

The demonstration of factors that modify the age trend of testosterone in the blood may be a stimulus to research to explain these influences. It also has practical implications with respect to the performance of testosterone assays, the appraisal of their findings, and the way in which the results of future studies should be reported.

The comparison of two subgroups of beta blocker trials—those using beta blockers with and without ISA (*Question F9–4*)—raises the same problems as those considered in the comparison of vitamin A trials with different dosage schedules (in *Question F8–3*). There may be confounding because of other differences between the studies, and statistical testing may be misleading because the hypothesis was derived from the data and not formulated in advance.

One of the authors of the beta-blocker meta-analysis gave the following answer to *Question F9–4* some years after the report was published:

This difference was conventionally significant at the 0.01 level. At the time this seemed rather impressive—and it did not take long to think up a biological 'explanation' for it—but it is interesting that all the data that has turned up since has tended to contradict this finding. . . . More recently we have seen results of two more trials. . . . These two extra trials demolish that statistically significant interaction. In retrospect, we were wrong to give it as much credence as we did. It was right to observe it and report it; but it was wrong to believe it. (Peto, 1987a)

"You should look for subgroups, you should report what you find, and half the time you shouldn't believe it" (Peto, 1987b).

In the meta-analysis of trials of cholesterol-lowering measures (*Question F9–5*), heterogeneity with respect to one outcome (reduction of coronary heart disease incidence) is explained, or partly explained, by heterogeneity with respect to another outcome (plasma cholesterol reduction). Since the reduction in plasma cholesterol is presumably a link in the chain of causation between the cholesterol-lowering measures and the reduced incidence, it is an intermediate cause (see Unit A14) rather than a modifier or confounder.

When modifying effects are investigated by comparing the findings in various subsets of individuals, as in *Question F9–6*, it frequently happens that findings for specific subsets are not available from all studies. In this meta-analysis, studies 3 and 7 were apparently confined to children less than one year old, and studies 1 and 6 were apparently restricted to children less than five years old. Comparisons based on the data shown in Table F9–2 might therefore be misleading. In the table published in the study report, the odds ratio for the 0- to 11-month group is based only on studies 1, 2, 4, and 6; it is 0.70 (95% confidence interval, 0.58 to 0.92), so that the larger protective effect in young infants remains apparent. The published table does not include the ≥ 60-month age group. Study 8 apparently provided no age-specific information.

Comparisons of subsets of individuals—for example, those with different smoking habits (*Question F9–7*)—present numerous difficulties. As in the previous example, some studies may not provide the required information at all, and others (e.g., a study restricted to nonsmokers) may not supply it for all categories. If information is available, categories and definitions may differ in different studies. The information on different sets of individuals may thus be based on different sets of studies, raising possibilities of bias; exploration of this bias may require additional information at an individual level, which may not be available. Moreover, the shrinkage of sample sizes due to the fact that separate categories of individuals are analyzed, and their further shrinkage due to incomplete information, may produce summary measures with very wide confidence intervals.

One suggestion made to overcome some of these difficulties is that, where possible, meta-analyses should be based not on study reports but on the collection and analysis of full data on all the individuals studied (Note F10); this is seldom possible.

EXERCISE F10

Question F10–1

A meta-analysis (cited in *Question F7–2*) showed a statistically significant association between cigarette smoking and leukemia; the summary risk ratio based on seven cohort studies was 1.3. Can it be concluded that smoking is a cause of leukemia; and if not, why not? What additional information from the meta-analysis might strengthen the case?

Question F10–2

Assuming that smoking is a cause of leukemia, what extra information is required in order to estimate how many cases of leukemia are caused by smoking each year in a given population?

Question F10–3

A clinician finds an up-to-date meta-analysis that shows that a particular treatment is effective in the treatment of a particular disease. The reported effect is statistically significant, and it is stronger, to a clinically meaningful degree, than the effect of the usual current treatment. Suppose that there is no difference from the usual treatment in safety, side effects, cost, convenience of use, or acceptability to patients. What should the clinician look for in the report of the meta-analysis before deciding to apply the treatment to his or her own patients?

Question F10–4

In what ways can a meta-analysis help future research? If a meta-analysis of clinical trials clearly shows that a treatment is effective, does this mean that additional trials of the treatment are superfluous?

Question F10–5

Several studies have assembled samples of meta-analyses, reviewed their methods, and examined their quality. An overview of these meta-meta-analyses (such an overview might be called a meta-meta-meta-analysis) would show that the evaluations were based partly on how well the meta-analyses were done and partly on how fully they were reported. Both these aspects are dealt with in this question, which is the last question in this book ("O frabjous day! Callooh! Callay! He chortled in his joy"; Carroll, 1872).

1. What information should the report of a meta-analysis provide, in order to permit the reader to make an appraisal of quality?
2. Suggest a set of questions that you could ask about a meta-analysis in order to appraise its quality.

NOTE

F10.   Stewart and Parmar (1993) compare what they call MAP (meta-analysis of individual patient data) with MAL (meta-analysis of the literature). Using information collected by a group of investigators conducting cancer trials, they show that these two methods can provide different estimates of the effectiveness of a treatment, and they point out that MAP provides a less biased means of comparing results in different groups of patients.

Unit
F11

USING THE RESULTS

Although the meta-analysis of cohort studies (Question F10–1) showed an association between smoking and leukemia, this alone is not convincing evidence for a cause–effect relationship. The overall association is statistically significant, and the "cause" apparently precedes the "effect," but we do not know whether other criteria for the appraisal of causality (see Unit E10) are met. The observed association is not strong, and a weak association, especially one found in nonexperimental studies, can easily be caused by flawed methods or confounding.

The following additional information might be helpful: (1) How were the studies done? Can the association be readily explained as an artifact caused by flawed methods? (2) Were the smokers and nonsmokers in each study similar in age, social class, ethnic or racial group, alcohol consumption, occupation, and other characteristics? And if not, were adequate measures taken to control for possible confounding? (3) Were the results of the studies consistent? What was the finding of each study, and were the findings tested for heterogeneity? Evidence of consistency and (if this is lacking) evidence of modifying effects are probably the main potential contributions of meta-analyses to etiological research. (4) Was there a dose–response relationship?

This meta-analysis did not include a systematic assessment of study quality. All the studies matched or controlled for at least age and sex, but no information is provided on the comparability of smokers and nonsmokers with respect to ethnic group or other characteristics; the authors say that "since the causes of leukemia are largely unknown . . . analyses cannot completely control for potential confounding." The findings of the studies were not very similar; two studies had risk ratios below one and confidence intervals that did not overlap with the confidence intervals of most other studies; a heterogeneity test was apparently not performed. An association with the number of cigarettes smoked per day was found in most but not all of the studies. The summary rate ratio was 1.4 (95% confidence interval, 1.3 to 1.6) for smokers of 1 to 19 cigarettes a day and 1.6 (95% confidence interval, 1.5 to 1.8) for smokers of ≥20 cigarettes a day; the report does not say how many studies supplied the data required for these comparisons of sub-sets of individuals. In the light of the evidence you now have, would you conclude that smoking is a cause of leukemia? (See Note F11.)

If it is assumed that smoking is a cause of leukemia, the population attributable fraction (*Question F10–2*) can be estimated from the risk ratio and the rate of smoking in the population (see Note E12 for the formula). If the number of new cases of leukemia per year in the population is also known, this fraction can be translated into an absolute number. The finding of this meta-analysis led to an estimate that about one in seven adult leukemia cases in the United States, or about 3,600 new cases per year, may be caused by smoking.

For a clinician who is deciding whether to adopt the findings of a meta-analysis of clinical trials (*Question F10–3*), the first prerequisite is confidence in the scientific quality of the meta-analysis and of the trials on which it is based. This requires careful reading of the report to see whether anything about the way the trials were found, selected, or analyzed gives rise to doubts about the validity of the results, and to see whether the quality of the trials was appraised and found satisfactory.

Next, the clinician should see whether the results of the trials were consistent: What were the findings, and were they tested for hetero-geneity? If they were consistent, and the trials encompassed a varied collection of patients, the treatment can probably be considered for any patient. However, if the meta-analysis includes a summary measure of effect based on a subset of trials or individuals (e.g., trials conducted in a specific age group, or patients of a specific age group) that seems partic-ularly relevant to a specific patient, the clinician may prefer to use this. Opinions on this issue differ. On the one hand, "when treating Ms Jones, the clinician may want to focus on the single trial or subset of trials conducted in patients most like Ms Jones" (Goodman, 1991), since the summary measure of effect may be "only a rough answer to a rough question about the average effectiveness . . . for a broad class of pa-tients" (Simon, 1991). On the other hand, as samples get smaller, the random error gets bigger, and use of the broad picture may therefore be preferable, even if this provides an apparently less specific indication of the results to be expected in a particular patient. One expert says: "Knowing the pitfalls, or the variations and the errors that there are— the random noises—even if in a particular subset the treatment did not seem to be particularly beneficial, and I've got a patient who belongs to that subset, but on average the benefit was 25%, I would say I would use the average figure rather than what I saw in that particular subset" (Yusuf, 1987b). "An overview allows a look at the forest through the trees" (Furberg and Morgan, 1987).

If there is appreciable heterogeneity of the findings in the various trials, the overall finding may have little relevance to a particular patient even if the random-effects model is used. The physician should then comb the report of the meta-analysis for descriptions of the kinds of patient included in each trial and the conditions in which each trial was administered, to see whether any trials are particularly relevant to his or her specific patient, and should rather use the results of these trials. If the meta-analysis provides a summary measure of effect based on a particularly appropriate subset of trials or individuals, this too may be preferred to the overall measure.

Whichever summary measure is used, its confidence interval should be sought and used as a guide to the decision on use of the treatment and to the prognosis if the treatment is used. There is, however, "invariably a leap of faith between formal statistical inference . . . and extrapolation to the true population of future patients." This uncertainty can be recognized by using broad confidence intervals if these are available: 99% rather than 95% intervals, and/or intervals based on the random-effects model rather than the fixed-effect model.

The bottom line in the answer to this question, as in the answer to the question (F10–1) on the meta-analysis of nonexperimental studies, is that the results of meta-analyses should be regarded at least as critically and applied with at least as much caution, as would the results of any individual study.

A meta-analysis can help future research (Question F10–4) in at least three ways. First, however inconclusive its results may be, it may draw attention to flaws in the design, conduct, or reporting of previous studies and thereby stimulate improved methods and reporting in future studies; "in order to do meta-analyses with a high degreee of certainty tomorrow, one must do meta-analyses with a certain degree of uncertainty today!" (O'Rourke and Detsky, 1992). Second, it may resolve uncertainties and consolidate present knowledge, thus providing a firm basis for new research. And third, it can identify unexplained inconsistencies and unanswered questions, leading to the formulation of hypotheses for subsequent testing.

It is tempting to say that if a meta-analysis clearly shows that a treatment is effective, further trials of the treatment are unnecessary. Repeated (cumulative) meta-analyses of trials of many treatments for myocardial infarction have in fact shown that once a significant effect has been detected, the main consequence of adding new trials is narrowing of the confidence interval. For example, the summary odds ratio expressing the effect of intravenous streptokinase on mortality in myocardial infarction, based on eight trials involving 2,432 patients between 1959 and 1972, was 0.74 (95% confidence interval, 0.59 to 0.92). In 1988, 25 trials and 34,542 experimental patients later, the summary odds ratio was almost the same, but the confidence interval was much narrower (Lau et al., 1992).

But there may be surprises. We had an example in *Questions F8–5 and F8–6*: The addition of a sixth trial made a significant and consistent effect nonsignificant, and the addition of a seventh trial made it significant again; similarly, a meta-analysis of small trials of phenobarbital for intracranial hemorrhage in premature infants showed a positive effect, but a larger subsequent trial showed a detrimental effect (T. C. Chalmers, 1991). Also, new trials may permit a better look at the effects of specific modes of treatment in specific kinds of patient. For example, a meta-analysis of trials of calcium antagonists in myocardial infarction "did not indicate any overall beneficial effect" (Held et al., 1989), but later meta-analyses showed a significant and marked benefit for patients with infarction of the non–Q-wave type who received calcium antagonists that reduce the heart rate (Yusuf et al., 1991; Boden, 1992). It is probably safe to conclude that if a meta-analysis based on many trials and several thousand subjects clearly shows a consistent and statistically significant effect, further trials are generally needed only if there is interest in questions (e.g. about modifying factors) that have not been adequately answered, or if there is reason to suspect that the effect may be modified by time-related or other differences.

EVALUATING A META-ANALYSIS

An appraisal of the quality of a meta-analysis may require the following information (*Question F10–5a*). This may be regarded as a checklist of items that should be considered for inclusion in the report of any meta-analysis.

I. *Objectives*
   A. What were the objectives of the meta-analysis? Were the questions asked general or specific ones?

II. *Identification and selection of studies*
   A. How were the studies found? Were unpublished papers sought? And if so, how were their findings obtained?
   B. How were the studies selected? What inclusion and exclusion criteria were used? What precautions were taken to avoid bias?
   C. What studies were excluded, and why?
   D. What is the fail-safe N?

III. *Information about the studies*
   A. What studies were included?
   B. How well were they designed and executed? What criteria were used for appraising their quality? What precautions were taken to avoid bias in the appraisal? If data were incomplete, what efforts were made to fill the gaps?

    C. How did the characteristics of the studies differ? For example, what differences were there in study design, the source, selection, and characteristics of subjects, inclusion and exclusion criteria, diagnostic criteria, definitions of variables, the manner of allocation to groups, follow-up times, and (for trials) details of management of treatment and control groups, outcome criteria, and the use of "intention to treat" or "on randomized treatment" analysis.

    D. What were the results of the studies? If groups were compared in the studies, what were the results in each group?

IV. *Methods of analysis*
    A. How was heterogeneity tested?
    B. How were differences in study quality taken into account in the analysis?
    C. Were the results of studies adjusted to control suspected bias?
    D. What method was used for combining results? Was a fixed-effect, fixed-effects, or random-effects model used?
    E. Was sensitivity analysis used?
    F. Were subsets of trials or individuals compared? If so, was this done to test a priori or data-derived hypotheses? How were possible confounding factors taken into account in the comparison?

V. *Results*
    What was the result of the heterogeneity test?
    What are the confidence intervals of the combined findings?

The questions that might be asked about a meta-analysis in order to appraise its quality (*Question F10–5b*) include the following. This may be regarded as a checklist of precautions to be taken in conducting a meta-analysis.

I. *Identification and selection of studies*
    A. Was the search for relevant studies conducted in a satisfactory way, so as to find as many of the wanted studies as possible, and without bias in the search?
    B. Is the fail-safe N small?
    C. Were studies selected in an objective manner, using explicit inclusion and exclusion criteria, and with precautions to avoid bias (e.g., through knowledge of the study results)?
    D. Are the selection criteria concordant with the objectives of the meta-analysis?

II. *Quality of the studies*
    A. Was the quality of the studies appraised?

B. Was the appraisal made in an acceptably objective manner, using explicit criteria, and with precautions to avoid bias?
C. Was appropriate attention given to the quality of the studies in the analysis?

III. *Extraction of results*
A. Were precautions taken to avoid bias in the extraction of results (especially those of observational epidemiological studies)?

IV. *Combining of results*
A. Was the combining of results justifiable, in terms of:
  1. The relevance of the studies to the study objectives
  2. Differences in design, the source, selection, and characteristics of subjects, inclusion and exclusion criteria, diagnostic criteria and definitions, the manner of allocation to groups, follow-up times, the management of treatment and control groups, outcome criteria, and the use of "intention to treat" or "on randomized treatment" analysis
  3. The consistency of the results?
B. Were appropriate statistical methods used to pool the findings?
C. Was attention given to the possibility that the combined result might be unduly affected by one large study?
D. Is the measure of effect an appropriate one, in the light of the study objectives?

V. *Comparisons of results*
A. If the findings were heterogeneous, were possible explanations explored?
B. If subgroups of trials or individuals were compared, was appropriate attention paid to possible confounding and to the pitfalls of tests of data-derived hypotheses?

VI. *Analysis*
A. Was sensitivity analysis used to see how the results were affected by decisions about the inclusion of studies or the extraction of findings or by other choices of methods?
B. Was appropriate attention paid, in the analysis or in interpreting the findings, to possible biases in the results of individual studies?

VII. *Interpretation of findings*
A. Were the results interpreted correctly, and are the conclusions and practical implications presented with appropriate reservations?

As an example of the application of questions of this sort, the findings of a meta-meta-analysis of meta-analyses of randomized controlled trials published in English between 1966 and 1986 were summarized as follows: "We found indications of a written protocol in very few. Attempts to include all relevant trials seemed optimal in a minority and in none was the determination of suitability for inclusion made in a blinded manner (i.e., without knowledge of source or results of the trial). Interrater disagreement rates in the selection of papers and in the extraction of data were almost never reported. Statistical methods of combining the data were considered adequate in most, but only a few carried out sensitivity analyses by employing more than one method, or considered the problem of heterogeneity of results. . . . Publication bias was rarely considered. . . . Quality of the original trials was considered in few of the meta-analyses" (Chalmers et al., 1987b; Sacks, et al., 1987).

It is difficult to determine how these shortcomings affect validity, since a "gold standard" is hard to find. One suggestion is that the findings should be compared with those of subsequent large randomized trials, since "assessing the predictive power of meta-analyses is as close as we are likely to come to a 'gold standard'" (I. Chalmers, 1991). But there is no reason to assume that the result of a large trial is more valid than meta-analyses of small ones; "in fact, one might argue that the results of combining multiple small trials are more applicable to the practice of medicine in which the encountered patients are rarely homogeneous." (T. C. Chalmers, 1991). Results may also be compared with those of other published meta-analyses addressing the same topic. Such comparisons usually show differences in degree rather than in the direction of the effect, with greater differences in authors' interpretations concerning clinical implications than in the statistical findings. Using the majority finding of meta-analyses of the same topic as a gold standard (or, if there were less than three, the finding of the other meta-analysis), disagreements in statistical findings were more frequent if crude pooling was used than if a Mantel–Haenzel measure or the mean effect size was used, and they were more frequent in meta-analyses of published trials than in those that included unpublished trials as well. "Hopefully," say the authors, "disagreements will disappear as meta-analyses methodology becomes more rigorous" (Chalmers et al., 1987a).

The last self-test follows.

NOTE

F11.   In an editorial commenting on this meta-analysis, Severson and Linet (1993) say, "On balance, the evidence suggests a causal relationship between cigarette smoking and leukemia, but many questions remain." This is a matter of judgment, and you are entitled to disagree with this verdict.

Unit
F12

TEST YOURSELF (F)

- Explain what is meant by

  meta-analysis (F1).
  a goodness-of-fit test (Note F2–1).
  a heterogeneity test (F8).
  a mean effect size (F3).
  unitlessness (F4).
  the fail-safe N (F5).
  sensitivity analysis (F7).
  a funnel display (F8).
  data dredging (f9).
  an a priori hypothesis (F9).
  an a posteriori hypothesis (F9).

- State arguments for and against the inclusion of unpublished studies in a meta-analysis (F5).

- Provide a list of

  possible explanations for differences between the results of clinical trials of the same topic (F2).
  possible benefits of drawing conclusions from a series of studies (F2).
  possible reasons for excluding old studies from a meta-analysis (F6).
  possible reasons for including poor studies in a meta-analysis (F6).
  possible procedures if the studies vary in quality (F7).
  possible procedures if a study to be included in a meta-analysis offers more than one measure (F7).
  possible reasons for differences between the results of different sets of studies (F9)

- Explain (in general terms)

  how to minimize bias when deciding whether to include a study in a
    meta-analysis (F6).
  how to minimize bias when appraising the quality of a study (F7).
  how the combinability of studies can be appraised (F8).

- State the disadvantages (if any) of

  simply pooling study results, as if only one large study had been
    done (F3).
  combining study results by "vote counting" (F3).
  combining P values from separate studies (F3).
  calculating an average of rate ratios (F3).
  using effect sizes (F4).
  data dredging (9).
  comparing subsets of individuals in a meta-analysis (F10).
  using the findings of a specific trial or set of trials rather than the
    overall findings of a meta-analysis of trials (F11).
  using the overall findings of a meta-analysis of trials rather than the
    findings of a specific trial or set of trials (F11).

- Explain (in general terms)

  how the results of separate significance tests can be combined (Note
    F2–2).
  how the confidence interval of a summary measure should be in-
    terpreted (F9, F11).
  how a modifying effect can be investigated in regression analysis
    (F10).
  how a confounding effect can be controlled in regression analysis
    (F10).

- Explain the following models:

  a fixed-effect model (F3).
  a fixed-effects model (F8).
  a random-effects model (F8 and Note F8–5).
  a regression model (F8).
  a regression model with the logarithm of the rate ratio as the depen-
    dent variable (F8).

- Explain

  how to interpret a goodness-of-fit test with a low P value (Note
    F2–1).
  how to interpret a heterogeneity test with a low P value (F8).

the advantages (if any) of the Mantel–Haenszel procedure over multiple logistic regression analysis (F4).

the advantages (if any) of multiple logistic regression analysis over
the Mantel–Haenszel procedure (F4).

why the results in the control groups of different studies should be
compared (F8).

what should be done if the results of a meta-analysis would be
appreciably modified by the exclusion of one study (F9).

how a meta-analysis can throw light on causation (F11).

what should be looked for in the report of a meta-analysis of trials
before a decision is made to apply the treatment to a specific
patient (F11).

why a meta-analysis that clearly shows the effectiveness of a treatment does not necessarily rule out the need for new trials of the
treatment (F11).

• Give a list of

information that the report of a meta-analysis should provide in
order to permit the reader to appraise the quality of the meta-
analysis (F11).

questions that could be asked about a meta-analysis in order to
appraise its quality (F11).

"Would you tell me, please, which way I ought to go
from here?"

"That depends a good deal on where you want to get
to," said the Cat.

"I don't much care where—" said Alice.

"Then it doesn't matter which way you go," said the
Cat.

(*Carroll, 1865*)

REFERENCES

Polonius: What do you read, my lord?
Hamlet: Words, words, words.

(Shakespeare 1603)

Abramson JH. *Survey methods in community medicine: Epidemiological studies, programme evaluation, clinical trials,* 4th edn. Edinburgh: Churchill Livingstone, 1990.

Abramson JH. Meta-analysis: a review of pros and cons. *Public Health Reviews* 18: 1–47, 1990/91.

Abramson JH, Hopp C. The control of cardiovascular risk factors in the elderly. *Preventive Medicine* 5: 32–47, 1976.

Abramson JH, Hopp C, Epstein LM. The epidemiology of varicose veins: a survey in western Jerusalem. *Journal of Epidemiology and Community Health* 35: 213–217, 1981.

Abramson JH, Kark SL, Palti H. The epidemiological basis for community-oriented primary care. In: *Epidemiologie et médecine communautaire* (Lellouche J, ed). Paris: INSERM, 1983, pp. 231–263.

Abramson JH, Sacks MI, Cahana E. Death certificate data as an indication of the presence of certain common diseases at death. *Journal of Chronic Diseases* 24: 417–431, 1971.

Amery A, Birkenhager W, Brixko P, Bulpitt C, Clement D, Deruyttere M, de Schaepdryver A, Dollery C, Fagard R, Forette F, Forte J, Hamdy R, Henry JF, Joossens JV, Leonetti G, Lund- Johansen P, O'Malley K, Petrie J, Strasser T, Tuomilehto J, Williams B. Mortality and morbidity results from the European Working Party in High Blood Pressure in the Elderly trial. *Lancet* 1: 1349–1354, 1985.

Andersen JW, Harrington D. Meta-analyses need new publication standards. *Journal of Clinical Oncology* 10: 878–880, 1992.

Anderson S, Auquier WW, Hauck WW, Oakes D, Vandaele W, Weisberg HI. *Statistical methods for comparative studies.* New York: Wiley, 1980.

Andrews G, MacMahon SW, Austin A, Byrne DG. Hypertension: comparison of drug and non-drug treatments. *British Medical Journal* 284: 1523–1526, 1982.

Armitage P, Berry G. *Statistical methods in medical research,* 2nd edn. Oxford: Blackwell, 1987.

Bailey KR. Inter-study differences: how should they influence the interpretation and analysis of results? *Statistics in Medicine* 6: 351–358, 1987.

Ban R and Peritz E. Longitudinal study of borderline hypertension. Paper presented at International Symposium on Hypertension Control in the Community, Tel Aviv, Nov. 1982.

Begg CB, Pilote L, McGlave PB. Bone marrow transplantation versus chemotherapy in acute non-lymphocytic leukemia: a meta-analytic review. *European Journal of Cancer and Clinical Oncology* 25: 1519–1523, 1989.

Berlin JA, Colditz GA. A meta-analysis of physical activity in the prevention of coronary heart disease. *American Journal of Epidemiology* 132: 612–628, 1990.

Berlin JA, Laird NM, Sacks HS, Chalmers TC. A comparison of statistical methods for combining event rates from clinical trials. *Statistics in Medicine* 8: 141–151, 1989.

Boden WE. Meta-analysis in clinical trial reporting: has a tool become a weapon? *American Journal of Cardiology* 69: 681–686, 1992.

Boivin J-F, Wacholder S. Conditions for confounding of the risk ratio and of the odds ratio. *American Journal of Epidemiology* 121: 152–158, 1985.

Boyce WJ, Vessey MP. Rising incidence of fracture of the proximal femur. *Lancet* 1: 150–151, 1985.

Breslow NE, Day NE. Statistical methods in cancer research, Vol. 1: *The analysis of case-control studies*. Lyon: International Agency for Research on Cancer, 1980.

Brett M, Barker DJP 1976. The world distribution of gallstones. *International Journal of Epidemiology* 5: 335–341, 1976.

Bross IDJ. Spurious effects from an extraneous variable. *Journal of Chronic Diseases* 19: 637–647, 1966.

Bross IDJ. Pertinency of an extraneous variable. *Journal of Chronic Diseases* 20: 487–495, 1967.

Brownson RC, Novotny TE, Perry MC. Cigarette smoking and adult leukemia: a meta-analysis. *Archives of Internal Medicine* 153: 469–475, 1993.

Brunekreef B, Fischer P, Remijn B, van der Lende R, Schouten J, Quanjer P. Indoor air pollution and its effect on pulmonary function of adult non-smoking women: III. Passive smoking and pulmonary function. *International Journal of Epidemiology* 14: 227–230, 1985.

Buck C. Popper's philosophy for epidemiologists. *International Journal of Epidemiology* 4: 159–168, 1975.

Bulpitt CJ, Beilin LJ, Clifton P, Coles EC, Dollery CT, Gear JSS, Harper GS, Johnson BF, Munro-Faure AD. Risk factors for death in treated hypertensive patients: report from the D.H.S.S. Hypertension Care Computing Project. *Lancet* 2: 134–137, 1979.

Campbell DT. Factors relevant to the validity of experiments in social settings. In: *Program evaluation in the health fields* (Schulberg HC, Sheldon A, Baker F, eds). New York: Behavioral Publications, 1969, pp. 165–185.

Campbell DT, Stanley JC. *Experimental and quasi-experimental designs for research*. Chicago: Rand McNally, 1966.

Canner PL. An overview of six clinical trials of aspirin in coronary heart disease. *Statistics in Medicine* 6: 255–263, 1987.

Carmines EG, Zeller RA. Reliability and validity assessment. Beverley Hills: Sage Publications, 1979, pp. 22–26.

Carroll L. *Alice's adventures in Wonderland*. 1865.

Carroll L. *Through the looking glass (and what Alice found there)*. 1872.

Chalmers I. Can meta-analyses be trusted? *Lancet* 338: 971–972, 1991.

Chalmers I, Adams M, Dickersin K, Hetherington J, Tarnow-Mordi W, Meinert C, Tonascia S, Chalmers TC. A cohort study of summary reports of clinical trials. *JAMA* 263: 1401–1405, 1990.

Chalmers TC. Problems induced by meta-analyses. *Statistics in Medicine* 10: 971–980, 1991.

Chalmers TC, Berrier J, Sacks HS, Levin H, Reitman D, Nagalingam R. Meta-analysis of clinical trials as a scientific discipline. II: Replicate variability and comparison of studies that agree and disagree. *Statistics in Medicine* 6: 733–744, 1987a.

Chalmers TC, Levin H, Sacks HR, Reitman D, Berrier J, Nagalingam R. Meta-analysis of clinical trials as a scientific discipline. I: Control of bias and comparison with large cooperative trials. *Statistics in Medicine* 6: 315–325, 1987b.

Chalmers TC, Smith H, Blackburn B, Silverman B, Schroeder B, Reitman D, Ambroz A. A method for assessing the quality of a randomized clinical trial. *Controlled Clinical Trials* 2: 31–49, 1981.

Clark VA, Aneshensel CS, Frerichs RR, Morgan TM. Analysis of non-response in a prospective study of depression in Los Angeles County. *International Journal of Epidemiology* 12: 193–198, 1983.

Cochran WG. *Planning and analysis of observational studies*. New York: John Wiley, 1983, p. 20.

Cochrane AL, St Leger AS, Moore F. Health service 'input' and mortality 'output' in developed countries. *Journal of Epidemiology and Community Health* 32: 200–205, 1978.

Cole TJ. The influence of height on the decline in ventilatory function. *International Journal of Epidemiology* 3: 145–152, 1974.

Collins R, Gray R, Godwin J, Peto R. Avoidance of large biases and large random errors in the assessment of moderate treatment effects: the need for systematic overviews. *Statistics in Medicine* 6: 245–250, 1987.

Collins R, Peto R, MacMahon S, Herbert P, Fiebach NH, Eberlein KA, Godwin J, Qizilbash N, Taylor JO, Hennekens CH. Blood pressure, stroke, and coronary heart disease: Part 2, short-term reductions in blood pressure: overview of randomized drug trials in their epidemiological context. *Lancet* 335: 827–838, 1990.

Connor E, Mullan F (eds.). Community-oriented primary care: new directions for health service delivery. Washington, D.C.: National Academy Press, 1983.

Cook TD, Campbell DT. *Quasi-experimentation: design and analysis issues for field settings.* Chicago, Illinois: Rand McNally, 1979.

Davies AM. Epidemiological reasoning: comments on 'Popper's philosophy for epidemiologists' by Carol Buck. *International Journal of Epidemiology* 4: 169–170, 1975.

Davies TW, Williams DRR, Whitaker RW. Risk factors for undescended testis. *International Journal of Epidemiology* 4: 169–170, 1975.

DeMets DL. Methods for combining randomized clinical trials: strengths and limitations. *Statistics in Medicine* 6: 341–348, 1987.

Department of Clinical Epidemiology and Biostatistics, McMaster University, Hamilton, Ont. Clinical epidemiology rounds. *Canadian Medical Association Journal* 129: 429–432, 559–564, 705–710, 832–835, 947–954, 1093–1099, 1983.

Depue RH. Maternal and gestational factors affecting the risk of cryptorchidism and inguinal hernia. *International Journal of Epidemiology* 13: 311–318, 1984.

DerSimonian R, Laird N. Meta-analysis in clinical trials. *Controlled Clinical Trials* 7: 177–188, 1986.

Detsky AS, Naylor CD, O'Rourke K, McGeer AJ, L'Abbe KA. Incorporating variations in the quality of individual randomized trials into meta-analysis. *Journal of Clinical Epidemiology* 45: 255–265, 1992.

Dickersin K, Hewitt P, Mutch L, Chalmers I, Chalmers TC. Comparison of MEDLINE searching with a perinatal clinical trials database. *Controlled Clinical Trials* 6: 306–317, 1985.

Ducimitiere P, Richard JL, Pequignot GP, Warnet JM. Varicose veins: a risk factor for atherosclerotic disease in middle-aged men? *International Journal of Epidemiology* 10: 329–335, 1981.

Easterbrook PJ, Berlin JA, Gopalan R, Matthews DR. Publication bias in clinical research. *Lancet* 337: 867–872, 1991.

Ellenberg JH, Nelson KB. Sample selection and the natural history of disease: studies of febrile seizures. *JAMA* 243: 1337–1340, 1980.

Elwood JM, Lee JAH, Walter SD, Mo T, Green AES. Relationship of melanoma and other skin cancer mortality to latitude and ultraviolet radiation in the United States and Canada. *International Journal of Epidemiology* 3: 325–332, 1974.

Epstein LM. Validity of a questionnaire for diagnosis of peptic ulcer in an ethnically heterogeneous population. *Journal of Chronic Diseases* 22: 49–55, 1969.

Evans AS, Wells AV, Ramsay F, Drabkin P, Palmer K. Poliomyelitis, rubella and dengue antibody survey in Barbados. A follow-up study. *International Journal of Epidemiology* 8: 235–241, 1979.

Eysenck HJ. An exercise in mega-silliness. *American Psychologist* 35: 517, 1978.

Fawzi WW, Chalmers TC, Herrera MG, Mosteller F. Vitamin A supplementation and child mortality: a meta-analysis. *JAMA* 269: 898–903, 1993.

Feinstein AR. *Clinical biostatistics.* St. Louis: Mosby, 1977, p. 91.

Feinstein AR. *Clinical epidemiology: the architecture of clinical research.* Philadelphia: W. B. Saunders, 1985.

Felson DT. Bias in meta-analytic research. *Journal of Clinical Epidemiology* 45: 885–892, 1992.

Fisher KJ, Glasgow RE, Terborg JR. Work site smoking cessation: a meta-analysis of long-term quit rates from controlled studies. *Journal of Occupational Medicine* 32: 429–439, 1990.

Fisher L, Patil K. Matching and unrelatedness. *American Journal of Epidemiology* 100: 347–349, 1974.

Fleiss JL. *Statistical methods for rates and proportions.* New York: John Wiley, 2nd edn., 1981.

Fleiss JL. Significance tests have a role in epidemiologic research: reactions to A. M. Walker. *American Journal of Public Health* 76: 559–560, 1986a.

Fleiss JL. Dr Fleiss responds. *American Journal of Public Health* 76: 1033–1034, 1986b.

Fleiss JL. *The design and analysis of clinical experiments.* New York: John Wiley, 1986c.

Fleiss JL, Gross AJ. Meta-analysis in epidemiology, with special reference to studies of the association between exposure to environmental tobacco smoke and lung cancer: a critique. *Journal of Clinical Epidemiology* 44: 127–139, 1991.

Fletcher RH, Fletcher SW, Wagner EH. *Clinical epidemiology—the essentials.* Baltimore: Williams & Wilkins, 1982.

Forman MR, Graubard BI, Hoffman HJ, Beren R, Harley EE, Bennett P. The Pima Infant Feeding Study: breastfeeding and respiratory infections during the first year of life. *International Journal of Epidemiology* 13: 447–453, 1984.

Freedman D, Pusani R, Purves R. *Statistics*. New York: Norton, 1978.

Friedman GD. *Primer of epidemiology*, 2nd edn. New York: McGraw-Hill, 1980.

Furberg CD, Morgan TM. Lessons from overviews of cardiovascular trials. *Statistics in Medicine* 6: 295–303, 1987.

Giagnoni E, Secchi MB, Wu SC, et al. Prognostic value of exercise EKG testing in asymptomatic normotensive individuals. *New England Journal of Medicine* 309: 1085–1089, 1983.

Gifford RH, Feinstein AR. A critique of methodology in studies of anticoagulant therapy for acute myocardial infarction. *New England Journal of Medicine* 280: 351–357, 1969.

Glass GV, McGaw B, Smith ML. Meta-analysis in social research. Beverley Hills: Sage Publications, 1981.

Glass GV, Smith ML. Reply to Eysenck. *American Psychologist* 35: 517–519, 1978.

Godfrey CM, Morgan P. A controlled trial of the theory of acupuncture in musculoskeletal pain. *Journal of Rheumatology* 5: 121–124, 1978.

Gofin J, Kark E, Mainemer N, Kark SL, Abramson JH, Hopp C, Epstein LM. Prevalence of selected health characteristics of women and comparisons with men: a community health survey in Jerusalem. *Israel Journal of Medical Sciences* 17: 145–149, 1981.

Goldbourt U, Kark JD. The epidemiology of coronary heart disease in the ethnically and culturally diverse population of Israel. *Israel Journal of Medical Sciences* 18: 1077–1097, 1982.

Goodman SN. Have you ever meta-analysis you didn't like? *Annals of Internal Medicine* 114: 244–246, 1991.

Goodwin PJ, Boyd NF. Mammographic parenchymal pattern and breast cancer risk: a critical appraisal of the evidence. *American Journal of Epidemiology* 127: 1097–1107, 1988.

Gray A, Berlin JA, McKinlay JB, Longcope C. An examination of research design effects on the association of testosterone and male aging: results of a meta-analysis. *Journal of Clinical Epidemiology* 44: 671–684, 1991.

Grayson DA. Confounding confounding. *American Journal of Epidemiology* 126: 546–553, 1987.

Grayson DA. The author replies. *American Journal of Epidemiology* 129: 1089–1091, 1989.

Green M. Use of predictive value to adjust relative risk estimates biased by misclassification of outcome status. *American Journal of Epidemiology* 117: 98–105, 1983.

Greenland S (ed.). *Evolution of epidemiologic ideas: annotated readings on concepts and methods*. Chestnut Hill, Massachusetts: Epidemiology Resources, Inc., 1987a.

Greenland S. Quantitative methods in the review of epidemiologic literature. *Epidemiologic Reviews* 9: 1–30, 1987b.

Greenland S, Morgenstern H, Poole C, Robins J. Re: "Confounding confounding." *American Journal of Epidemiology* 129: 1086–1089, 1989.

Greenland S, Robins JM. Identifiability, exchangeability, and epidemiological confounding. *International Journal of Epidemiology* 15: 413–419, 1986.

Greenland S, Salvan A. Bias in the one-step method for pooling study results. *Statistics in Medicine* 9: 247–252, 1990.

Gupta PC, Bhonsle RB, Mehta FS, Pindborgh JJ. Mortality experience in relation to tobacco chewing and smoking habits from a 10-year follow-up study in Ernakulam District, Kerala. *International Journal of Epidemiology* 13: 184–187, 1984.

Hammond EC, Selikoff IJ, Seidman H. Asbestos exposure, cigarette smoking and death rates. *Annals of the New York Academy of Sciences* 330: 473–495, 1979.

Hedges LV. Commentary. *Statistics in Medicine* 6: 381–385, 1987.

Hedges LV, Olkin I. *Statistical methods for meta-analysis*. Orlando: Academic Press, 1985.

Held PH, Yusuf F, Furburg CD. Calcium channel blockers in acute myocardial infarction and unstable angina: an overview. *British Medical Journal* 299: 1187–1192, 1989.

Hennekens CH, Buring JE. *Epidemiology in medicine*. Boston: Little, Brown, 1987.

Hill AB. *Statistical methods in clinical and preventive medicine*. Edinburgh: Livingstone, 1962.

Hofman A, Valkenburg HA, Maas J, Groustra FN. The natural history of blood pressure in childhood. *International Journal of Epidemiology* 14: 91–96, 1985.

Holland WW, Detels R, Knox G. *Oxford textbook of public health*, 2nd edn., Vol. 2: *Methods of public health*. Oxford: Oxford University Press, 1991.

Holme I. Relation of coronary heart disease incidence and total mortality to plasma cholesterol reduction in randomised trials: use of meta-analysis. *British Heart Journal* 69 (Suppl.): S42–7, 1993.

Ibrahim MA. *Epidemiology and health policy.* Rockville, Maryland: Aspen, 1985.

Iyengar S, Greenhouse JB. Selection models and the file-drawer problem. *Statistical Science* 3: 109–135, 1988.

Jacobsen M. Against Popperized epidemiology. *International Journal of Epidemiology* 5: 9–11, 1976.

Jenicek M. Meta-analyses in medicine: where we are and where we want to go. *Journal of Clinical Epidemiology* 42: 35–44, 1989.

Jones DR. Meta-analysis of observational epidemiological studies: a review. *Journal of the Royal Society of Medicine* 85: 165–169, 1992.

Kabat GC, Howson CP, Wynder EL. Beer consumption and rectal cancer. *International Journal of Epidemiology* 15: 494–501, 1986.

Kahn HA. The Dorn study of smoking and mortality among U.S. veterans: report on eight and one-half years of observation. In: *Epidemiological approaches to the study of cancer and other chronic diseases* (Haenszel W, ed.), National Cancer Institute Monograph 19, 1966.

Kahn HA, Herman JB, Medalie JH, Neufeld HN, Riss E, Goldbourt U. Factors related to diabetes incidence: a multivariate analysis of two years observation on 10,000 men. The Israel Ischemic Heart Disease Study. *Journal of Chronic Diseases* 23: 617–629, 1971.

Kahn HA, Sempos CT. *Statistical Methods in Epidemiology.* New York: Oxford University Press, 1989.

Kark SL. *Epidemiology and community medicine.* New York: Appleton-Century-Crofts, 1974.

Kark SL. *The practice of community-oriented primary health care.* New York: Appleton-Century-Crofts, 1981.

Kark SL, Abramson JH. Community oriented primary care: meaning and scope. In: *Community-oriented primary care: new directions for health service delivery* (Connor E, Mullan F, eds.). Washington, D.C.: National Academy Press, 1983, pp. 21–59.

Kark SL, Gofin J, Abramson JH, Makler A, Mainemer N, Kark E, Epstein LM, Hopp C. Prevalence of selected health characteristics of men: a community health survey in Jerusalem. *Israel Journal of Medical Sciences* 15: 732–741, 1979.

Kark SL, Kark E. An alternative strategy in community health care: community-oriented primary health care. *Israel Journal of Medical Sciences* 19: 707–713, 1983.

Kelsey JL, Thompson WD, Evans AS. *Methods in observational epidemiology.* New York: Oxford University Press, 1986.

Khaw K-T, Rose G. Population study of blood pressure and associated factors in St Lucia, West Indies. *International Journal of Epidemiology* 11: 372–377, 1982.

Klein S, Simes J, Blackburn GL. Total parenteral nutrition and cancer clinical trials. *Cancer* 58: 1378–1386, 1986.

Kleinbaum DG, Kupper LL, Morgenstern H. *Epidemiologic research: principles and quantitative methods.* Belmont, California: Lifetime Learning Publications, 1982.

Knox EG (ed.) *Epidemiology in health care planning.* Oxford: Oxford University Press, 1979.

Kono S, Ikeda M, Tokudome S, Nishizumi M, Kuratsune M. Alcohol and mortality: a cohort study of male Japanese physicians. *International Journal of Epidemiology* 15: 527–532, 1968.

Kreiger N, Gross A, Hunter G. Dietary factors and fracture in postmenopausal women: a case-control study. *International Journal of Epidemiology* 21: 953–958, 1992.

Landman JT, Dawes RM. Psychotherapy outcome: Smith and Glass' conclusions stand up under scrutiny. *American Psychologist* 37: 504–516, 1982.

Last JM (ed.), with Abramson JH, Greenland S, Thuriaux MC. *A dictionary of epidemiology.* New York: Oxford University Press, 1983.

Last JM, Foege WH. International health. In: *Maxcy-Rosenau Public health and preventive medicine* (Last JM, ed.), 12th edn. Norwalk, Connecticut: Appleton-Century-Crofts, 1986.

Lau J, Antman EM, Jimenez-Silva J, Kupelnick B, Mosteller F, Chalmers TC. Cumulative meta-analyses of therapeutic trials for myocardial infarction. *New England Journal of Medicine* 327: 248–254, 1992.

Lee J. An insight on the use of multiple logistic regression analysis to estimate association between risk factor and disease occurrence. *International Journal of Epidemiology* 15: 22–29, 1986.

Lehtonen A, Luutinen S. Serum lipids of very old people without dementia or with different types of senile dementia. In: *8th Scandinavian Congress of Gerontology: congress proceedings*. Tampere: Societas Gerontologica Fennica, 1986, pp. 489–491.

Lellouch J, Rokotovao R. Estimation of risk as a function of risk factors. *International Journal of Epidemiology* 5: 349–352, 1976.

Lemeshow S, Hosmer DW Jr. A review of goodness of fit statistics for use in the development of logistic regression models. *American Journal of Epidemiology* 115: 92–106, 1982.

Liberati A, Himel HN, Chalmers TC. A quality assessment of randomized clinical trials of primary treatment of breast cancer. *Journal of Clinical Oncology* 4: 942–951, 1986.

Lichtenstein MJ, Mulrow CD, Elwood PC. Guidelines for reading case-control studies. *Journal of Chronic Diseases* 40: 893–903, 1987.

Light RJ. Accumulating evidence from independent studies: what we can win and what we can lose. *Statistics in Medicine* 6: 221–228, 1987.

Lilienfeld AM, Lilienfeld DE. *Foundations of epidemiology*, 2nd edn. New York: Oxford University Press, 1980.

Lindquist C. Risk factors in lip cancer. *American Journal of Epidemiology* 109: 521–530, 1979.

Lipscomb JA, Satin KP, Neutra RR. Reported symptom prevalence rates from comparison populations in community-based environmental studies. *Archives of Environmental Health* 47: 263–269, 1992.

Loevinsohn BP. Health education interventions in developing countries: a methodological review of published articles. *International Journal of Epidemiology* 19: 788–794, 1990.

MacMahon B, Pugh TF, Ipsen J. *Epidemiologic methods*. Boston: Little, Brown, 1960.

Maffei FHA, Magaldi C, Pinho SZ, Lastoria S, Pinho W, Yoshida WB, Rollo HA. Varicose veins and chronic venous insufficiency in Brazil: prevalence among 1755 inhabitants of a country town. *International Journal of Epidemiology* 15: 210–217, 1986.

McMichael AJ, Hetzel BS. An epidemiological study of the mental health of Australian university students. *International Journal of Epidemiology* 3: 125–134, 1974.

Mainland D. *Elementary medical statistics*, 2nd edn. Philadelphia: W. B. Saunders, 1964.

Mantel N. Chi-square tests with one degree of freedom: extensions of the Mantel–Haenszel procedure. *American Statistical Association Journal* 58: 690–700, 1963.

Matthews KA, Jamison JW, Cottington EM. Assessment of type A, anger, and hostility: a review of scales through 1982. In: *Measuring psychosocial variables in epidemiologic studies of cardiovascular disease* (Ostfeld AM, Eaker ED, eds.). NIH publication No. 85–2270, U.S. Department of Health and Social Services, 1985.

Maxwell GF, Prujit JFM, Arntzenius AC. Comparison of the conical cuff and the standard rectangular cuffs. *International Journal of Epidemiology* 14: 468–472, 1985.

Mazzuca SA. Does patient education in chronic disease have therapeutic value? *Journal of Chronic Diseases* 35: 521–529, 1983.

McGee DL. Epidemiologic programs for computers and calculators: a program for logistic regression on the IBM PC. *American Journal of Epidemiology* 124: 702–705, 1986.

Meijer WS, Schmitz PIM, Jeekel J. Meta-analysis of randomized, controlled clinical trials of antibiotic prophylaxis in biliary tract surgery. *British Journal of Surgery* 77: 283–290, 1990.

Miettinen OS. *Theoretical epidemiology: principles of occurrence research in medicine*. New York: John Wiley, 1985.

Miettinen OS, Cook EF. Confounding: essence and detection. *American Journal of Epidemiology* 114: 593–603, 1991.

Morris JN. *Uses of epidemiology*, 3rd edn. Edinburgh: Churchill Livingstone, 1975.

Moss AJ, Parsons VL. *Current estimates from the National Health Interview Survey*. Vital and Health Statistics Series 10, No. 160, 1986.

Mulder PGH, Garretsen HFL. Are epidemiological and sociological surveys a proper instrument for detecting true problem drinkers? (The low sensitivity of an alcohol survey in Rotterdam.) *International Journal of Epidemiology* 12: 442–444, 1983.

National Center for Health Statistics. *Health, United States, 1986*. Washington, D.C.: U.S. Public Health Service. DHHS Publication No. (PHS) 87–1232, 1986.

Naylor CD. Two cheers for meta-analysis: problems and opportunities in aggregating results of clinical trials. *Canadian Medical Association Journal* 138: 891–895, 1988.

Niswander K, Henson G, Elbourne D, Chalmers I, Redman C, MacFarlane A, Tizard P. Adverse outcome of pregnancy and the quality of obstetric care. *Lancet* 2: 827–831, 1984.

Nutting PA (ed.) Community-oriented primary care: from principle to practice. Washington, D.C.: U.S. Department of Health and Human Services. HRSA Publication No. HRS-A-PE 86–1, 1987.

O'Rourke K, Detsky AS. Second thoughts: meta-analysis in medical research: strong encouragement for higher quality in individual research efforts. *Journal of Clinical Epidemiology* 42: 1021–1026, 1989.

Orwin RG. A fail-safe N for effect size. *Journal of Educational Statistics* 8: 157–159, 1983.

Ostfeld AM, Shekelle RB, Klawans H, et al. Epidemiology of stroke in an elderly welfare population. *American Journal of Public Health* 64: 450–458, 1974.

Owen R. Reader bias. *Journal of the American Medical Association* 247: 2533–2534, 1982.

Palti H. Use of control groups in evaluating the effectiveness of community health programs in primary care. *Israel Journal of Medical Sciences* 19: 756–759, 1983.

Palti H, Adler B, Tepper D. An early infant stimulation program in the maternal and child health service—evaluation at 5 years of age—preliminary findings. In: *Stimulation and intervention in infant development* (Tamir D, ed.), London: Freund, 1986, pp. 195–201.

Pearson K. *A grammar of science*. London: Scott, 1892.

Petitti DB. *Meta-analysis, decision analysis, and cost-effectiveness analysis: methods for quantitative synthesis in medicine*. New York: Oxford University Press, 1994.

Peto R. Why do we need systematic overviews of randomized trials? *Statistics in Medicine* 6: 233–240, 1987a.

Peto R. Discussion. *Statistics in Medicine* 6: 241–244, 1987b.

Peto R, Pike MC, Armitage P, Breslow NE, Cox DR, Howard SV, Mantel N, McPherson K, Peto J, Smith PG. Design and analysis of randomized clinical trials requiring prolonged observation of each patient: I. Introduction and design. *British Journal of Cancer* 34: 585–612, 1976.

Peto R, Pike MC, Armitage P, Breslow NE, Cox DR, Howard SV, Mantel N, McPherson K, Peto J, Smith PG. Design and analysis of randomized clinical trials requiring prolonged observation of each patient: II. Analysis and examples. *British Journal of Cancer* 35: 1–39, 1977.

Philipp R, Evans EJ, Hughes AO, Grisdale SK, Enticott RG, Jephcott AE. Health risks of snorkel swimming in untreated water. *International Journal of Epidemiology* 14: 624–627, 1985.

Pocock SJ, Hughes MD. Estimation issues in clinical trials and overviews. *Statistics in Medicine* 9: 657–671, 1990.

Popiela T, Jedrychowski W, Filipek A, Dolzycki E, Kulig J, Olszanecki S. Validity of questionnaire criteria in mass screening for the diagnosis of peptic ulcer. *International Journal of Epidemiology* 5: 251–253, 1976.

Popper KR. *The logic of scientific discovery*. New York: Harper and Row, 1968 (revised edn.).

Poynard T, Conn HO. The retrieval of randomized clinical trials in liver disease from the medical literature: a comparison of MEDLARS and manual methods. *Controlled Clinical Trials* 6: 271–279, 1985.

Ritchie K, Jildea D, Robine J-M. The relationship between age and the prevalence of senile dementia: a meta-analysis of recent data. *International Journal of Epidemiology* 21: 763–769, 1992.

Roberts CJ. *Epidemiology for clinicians*. Tunbridge Wells: Pitman Medical, 1977.

Roberts RS, Spitzer WO, Delmore T, Sackett DL. An empirical demonstration of Berkson's bias. *Journal of Chronic Diseases* 31: 119–128, 1978.

Rona RJ, Chinn S, Florey CduV. Exposure to cigarette smoking and children's growth. *International Journal of Epidemiology* 14: 402–409, 1985.

Rona RJ, Swan AV, Altman DG. Social factors and height of primary schoolchildren in England and Scotland. *Journal of Epidemiology and Community Health* 32: 147–154, 1978.

Roper HP, David TJ. Decline in deaths from choking on food in infancy: an association with change in feeding practice? *Journal of the Royal Society of Medicine* 80: 2–3, 1987.

Rosenthal R. The "file drawer problem" and tolerance for null results. *Psychological Bulletin* 85: 185–193, 1979.

Rothman KJ. *Modern epidemiology*. Boston: Little, Brown, 1986.

Rothman KJ (ed.) *Causal inference*. Chestnut Hill, Massachusetts: Epidemiology Resources, 1988.

Sackett DL. Bias in analytic research. *Journal of Chronic Diseases* 32: 51–63, 1979.

Sackett DL, Haynes RB, Tugwell P. *Clinical epidemiology: a basic science for clinical medicine.* Boston: Little, Brown, 1985.

Sacks HS, Berrier J, Reitman D, Ancona-Berk VA, Chalmers TC. Meta-analyses of randomized controlled trials. *New England Journal of Medicine* 316: 450–455, 1987.

Schlesselman JJ. *Case-control studies: design, conduct, analysis.* New York: Oxford University Press, 1982.

Schull WJ, Cobb S. The intrafamilial transmission of rheumatoid arthritis—III. The lack of support for a genetic hypothesis. *Journal of Chronic Diseases* 22: 217–222, 1969.

Severson RK, Linet MS. Does cigarette smoking lead to the subsequent development of leukemia? *Archives of Internal Medicine* 153: 425–427, 1993.

Shakespeare W. *Hamlet, prince of Denmark.* 1603.

Shapiro S. Evidence on screening for breast cancer from a randomized trial. *Cancer* 39 (Suppl. 6): 2772–2782, 1977.

Shapiro S, Slone D, Rosenberg L, Kaufman DW, Stolley PD, Miettinen OS. Oral-contraceptive use in relation to myocardial infarction. *Lancet* 1: 743–747, 1979.

Shapiro S, Venet W, Strax P, Venet L, Roeser R. Ten- to fourteen-year effect of screening on breast cancer mortality. *Journal of the National Cancer Institute* 69: 349–355, 1982.

Shirlow MJ, Mathers CD. Caffeine consumption and serum cholesterol levels. *International Journal of Epidemiology* 13: 422–427, 1984.

Shirlow MJ, Mathers CD. A study of caffeine consumption and symptoms: indigestion, palpitations, tremor, headache and insomnia. *International Journal of Epidemiology* 14: 239–248, 1985.

Siegel S, Castellan NJ Jr. *Nonparametric statistics for the behavioral sciences,* 2nd edn. New York: McGraw-Hill, 1988.

Simon R. A decade of progress in statistical methodology for clinical trials. *Statistics in Medicine* 10: 1789–1817, 1991.

Slavin RE. Best-evidence synthesis: an alternative approach to traditional and meta-analytic reviews. *Educational Researcher* 15(9): 5–11, 1986.

Slavin RE. Best-evidence synthesis: why less is more. *Educational Researcher* 16(5): 15–16, 1987.

Smith A. Epidemiological reasoning: comments on 'Popper's philosophy for epidemiologists' by Carol Buck. *International Journal of Epidemiology* 4: 171–172, 1975.

Smith ML, Glass GV. Meta-analysis of psychotherapy outcome studies. *American Psychologist* 35: 752–760, 1977.

Smith PG, Rodriguez LC, Fine PEM. Assessment of the protective efficacy of vaccines against common diseases using case-control and cohort studies. *International Journal of Epidemiology* 13: 87–93, 1984.

Sommer A. *Epidemiology and statistics for the ophthalmologist.* New York: Oxford University Press, 1980.

Sosenko JM, Gardner LB. Attribute frequency and misclassification bias. *Journal of Chronic Diseases* 40: 203–207, 1987.

Spitzer WO. Meta-meta-analysis: unanswered questions about aggregating data. *Journal of Clinical Epidemiology* 44: 103–107, 1991.

Sprackling ME, Mitchell JRA, Short AH, Watt G. Blood pressure reduction in the elderly: a randomised controlled trial of methyldopa. *British Medical Journal* 283: 1151–1153, 1981.

Stampfer MJ, Goldhaber SZ, Yusuf S, Peto R, Hennekens CH. Intravenous streptokinase for acute myocardial infarction. *New England Journal of Medicine* 308: 593–594, 1982.

Stark CR, Mantel N. Effects of maternal age and birth order on the risk of mongolism and leukemia. *Journal of the National Cancer Institute* 37: 687–698, 1966.

Stellman SD, Garfinkel L. Artificial sweetener use and one-year weight change among women. *Preventive Medicine* 15: 195–202, 1986.

Stewart AL, Ware JE Jr, Brook R, Davies-Avery A. Conceptualization and measurement of health for adults in the Health Insurance Study, Vol. II: *Physical health in terms of functioning.* Santa Monica, California: Rand Corporation, 1978.

Stewart AW, Jackson RT, Ford MA, Beaglehole R. Underestimation of relative weight by use of self-reported height and weight. *American Journal of Epidemiology* 125: 122–126, 1987.

Stewart LA, Parmar MKB. Meta-analysis of the literature or of individual patient data: is there a difference? *Lancet* 341: 418–422, 1993.

Stouffer SA, Suchman EA, De Vinney LC, Star SA, Williams RM Jr. *The American soldier: adjustment during army life*, Vol. 1. Princeton, New Jersey: Princeton University Press, 1949.

Sukwa TY, Bulsara MK, Wurapa FK. The relationship between morbidity and intensity of *Schistosoma mansoni* infection in a rural Zambian community. *International Journal of Epidemiology* 15: 248–251, 1986.

Susser M. *Causal thinking in the health sciences: concepts and strategies in epidemiology.* New York: Oxford University Press, 1973.

Susser M. The logic of Sir Karl Popper and the practice of epidemiology. *American Journal of Epidemiology* 124: 711–718. 1986.

Ter Riet G, Kleijnen J, Knipschild P. Acupuncture and chronic pain: a criteria-based meta-analysis. *Journal of Clinical Epidemiology* 43: 1191–1199, 1990.

Thompson SG, Pocock SJ. Can meta-analyses be trusted? *Lancet* 338: 1127–1130, 1991.

Tillett HE. Statistical analysis of case-control studies of communicable diseases. *International Journal of Epidemiology* 15: 126–133, 1986.

Tuomilehto J, Morelos S, Yason J, Guzman SV, Geizerova H. Trends in cardiovascular disease mortality in the Philippines. *International Journal of Epidemiology* 13: 168–176, 1984.

Turner JA, Herron L, Deyo RA. Meta-analysis of the results of lumbar spine fusion. *Acta Orthopaedica Scandinavica* 64 (Suppl. 251): 120–122, 1993.

Walker AM. Reporting the results of epidemiologic studies. *American Journal of Public Health* 76: 556–558, 1986.

Weddell JM, McDougall A. Road traffic accidents in Sharjah. *International Journal of Epidemiology* 10: 155–159, 1981.

Weinberg CR. Toward a clearer definition of confounding. *American Journal of Epidemiology* 137: 1–8, 1993.

Whitehead A, Whitehead J. A general parametric approach to the meta-analysis of randomized clinical trials. *Statistics in Medicine* 10: 1665–1677, 1991.

WHO Expert Committee on Diabetes Mellitus. Second report. WHO Technical Report Series No. 646, Geneva: WHO, 1980.

Wolf FM. *Meta-analysis: quantitative methods for research synthesis.* Beverly Hills: Sage Publications, 1986.

Wortman PM, Yeaton WH. Synthesis of results in controlled clinical trials of coronary bypass graft surgery. In: Evaluation Studies Review Annual, Vol. 8. (Light RJ, ed.). Beverly Hills, California: Sage Publications, 1983.

Wright HJ, MacAdam DB. *Clinical thinking and practice: diagnosis and decision in patient care.* Edinburgh: Churchill Livingstone, 1979.

Yusuf S. Discussion. *Statistics in Medicine* 6: 287–294, 1987b.

Yusuf S. Obtaining medically meaningful answers from an overview of randomized clinical trials. *Statistics in Medicine* 6: 281–286, 1987a.

Yusuf S, Held P, Furburg CD. Update of effects of calcium antagonists in myocardial infarction or angina in light of the Second Danish Verapamil Infarction Trial (DAVIT-II) and other recent studies. *American Journal of Cardiology* 67: 1295–1297, 1991.

Yusuf S, Peto R, Lewis J, Collins R, Sleight P. Beta blockade during and after myocardial infarction: an overview of the randomized trials. *Progress in Cardiovascular Diseases* 27: 335–371, 1985.

Yusuf S, Simon R, Ellenberg S. (eds.) Proceedings of "Methodologic Issues in Overviews of Randomized Clinical Trials." *Statistics in Medicine* 6: 217–409, 1987.

Zelen M. Guidelines for publishing papers on cancer clinical trials: responsibilities of editors and authors. *Journal of Clinical Oncology* 1: 164–169, 1983.

Zoloth S, Michaels D, Lacher M, Nagin D, Drucker E. Asbestos disease screening by non-specialists: results of an evaluation. *American Journal of Public Health* 76: 1392–1395, 1986.

INDEX

"Are there many crabs here?" said Alice.
"Crabs, and all sorts of things," said the Sheep:
"plenty of choice, only make up your mind."

(Carroll, 1872)

Misclassification, 158–61, 164–67, 168–69,
  201–2
  differential, 160, 162, 168–69
  nondifferential, 160
Mode, 135
Models
  additive, 241
  chance, 204
  epidemiological, 65–66
  in meta-analysis, 329, 361, 363–64, 368,
    370
  in multiple linear and logistic
    regression, 247
  interaction, 253, 255
  main effect (no-interaction), 252–53, 255
  mathematical, 218
    validity of, 248, 250, 256, 260–61
  multiplicative, 241, 247
Modifier. *See* Effect modification
Monotonic trend, 12
Multicollinearity, 256, 262
Multiple linear regression, 247
Multiple logistic regression, 247, 251–52,
  255–56
  impact of effect modification, 255
Multivariate analysis, 216–17, 219, 246–48.
  See also Multiple linear regression;
  Multiple logistic regression
  in meta-analysis, 336–37, 358, 367–68

Normal, meaning of, 191
Numerator of rate, 28

Occam's razor, 21, 23
Odds, 127
  calculated from probability, 131
  disease and exposure, 127
  pretest and posttest, 188–89, 190–91
Odds ratio, 127, 130–33
  based on multiple logistic regression,
    247, 255
  based on paired data, 238
  disease and exposure, 128–29, 132
O minus E method, 333
Ordinal scale, 173
Overviews of research, 319

P, 202
  combining values of, 326, 328–29
Percentage agreement, 176
Person-time, 101–2
Pie chart, 19, 20
Population at risk, 100
Post-stratification, 288
Posttest probability, 189, 190–91, 227
Power of a test, 208
Precision
  of estimate, 96
  of measurements, 171

Predictive value
  of risk marker, 222–23
  of test results, 184–85, 187
Pretest probability, 99, 188, 190–91
Prevalence, changes in, 89–90
Prevalence rate. *See* Rates, prevalence
Prevalence studies. *See* Cross-sectional
  studies
Preventable and prevented fractions, 305,
  312–13, 327
Prevention, levels of, 78
Probability, calculated from odds, 131
Prolective studies, 276
Proportions, 86, 103
Prospective approach, 43, 273
Prospective studies. *See also* Cohort
  studies
  historical, 298
Protective (preventive) factor, 226

Quality of studies, 346–47, 350–52
  score 358–59
Quasi-experiments, 269, 292–93

Random-effects model, 364, 368, 370
Randomization (random allocation), 285,
  323
Rate difference, 227, 230
Rate ratio, 199, 231–32, 273
Rates, 28, 31–32, 36–37, 64–65, 85–86
  adjusted, 139. *See also* Standardization,
    direct; Standardization, indirect
  appraisal of, 92–93
  calculation of, 85–86, 89, 101–2, 103–4,
    105–6, 126–27
  case fatality, 113
  crude, 36
  cumulative incidence, 101
  false positive and negative, 155–56
  incidence, 28, 100–2, 105–6
    mathematical relations between, 103–4
    uses of, 75, 77, 114–16
  infant mortality, 28
  mortality, 102
  prevalence, 86, 89–91
    uses of, 98–99, 114
  secondary attack, 126
  specific, 36
  standardized, uses of, 146–47. *See also*
    Standardization, direct;
    Standardization, indirect
  survival, 115–16
Ratio scale, 175
Ratios, 42, 86
Reference category, 199, 209
Reference population
  for generalizations, 96, 287
  for standardization, 139, 143, 145, 146
Refinement of variables, 52